Core Topics in Airway Management

Third Edition

Management of the airway is an important and challenging aspect of many clinicians' work and is a source of complications and litigation.

The new edition of this popular book remains a clear, practical and highly-illustrated guide to all necessary aspects of airway management. The book has been updated throughout, to cover all changes to best practice and clinical management, and provides extensive coverage of the key skills and knowledge required to manage airways in a wide variety of patients and clinical settings. The best of the previous editions has been preserved, whilst new chapters on videolaryngoscopy, awake tracheal intubation, lung separation, airway ultrasonography, airway management in an epidemic and many more have been added.

This is an essential text for anyone who manages the airway including trainees and specialists in anaesthesia, emergency medicine, intensive care medicine, prehospital medicine as well as nurses and other healthcare professionals.

Tim Cook is a Consultant in Anaesthesia and Intensive Care Medicine at the Royal United Hospital in Bath, UK, and is also Director of National Audit Projects and College Advisor on Airway at the Royal College of Anaesthetists.

Michael Seltz Kristensen is a Consultant in Anaesthesia and Intensive Care Medicine and Head of Airway Anaesthesia Research and Development at Rigshospitalet, Copenhagen University Hospital in Denmark and is also President of the European Airway Management Society (EAMS).

Core Topics in Airway Management

Third Edition

Edited by

Tim Cook
Royal United Hospitals, Bath, UK

Michael Seltz Kristensen
Rigshospitalet, Copenhagen University Hospital, Copenhagen, Denmark

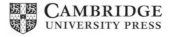

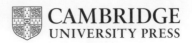

Shaftesbury Road, Cambridge CB2 8EA, United Kingdom

One Liberty Plaza, 20th Floor, New York, NY 10006, USA

477 Williamstown Road, Port Melbourne, VIC 3207, Australia

314–321, 3rd Floor, Plot 3, Splendor Forum, Jasola District Centre, New Delhi – 110025, India

103 Penang Road, #05–06/07, Visioncrest Commercial, Singapore 238467

Cambridge University Press is part of Cambridge University Press & Assessment, a department of the University of Cambridge.

We share the University's mission to contribute to society through the pursuit of education, learning and research at the highest international levels of excellence.

www.cambridge.org
Information on this title: www.cambridge.org/9781108419536

DOI: 10.1017/9781108303477

First published 2005
Second edition 2011
Third edition 2021 (version 3, May 2023)

Printed in the United Kingdom by Bell and Bain Ltd, Glasgow

A catalogue record for this publication is available from the British Library

ISBN 978-1-108-41953-6 Hardback

Cambridge University Press & Assessment has no responsibility for the persistence or accuracy of URLs for external or third-party internet websites referred to in this publication and does not guarantee that any content on such websites is, or will remain, accurate or appropriate.

....

Every effort has been made in preparing this book to provide accurate and upto-date information that is in accord with accepted standards and practice at the time of publication. Although case histories are drawn from actual cases, every effort has been made to disguise the identities of the individuals involved. Nevertheless, the authors, editors and publishers can make no warranties that the information contained herein is totally free from error, not least because clinical standards are constantly changing through research and regulation. The authors, editors and publishers therefore disclaim all liability for direct or consequential damages resulting from the use of material contained in this book. Readers are strongly advised to pay careful attention to information provided by the manufacturer of any drugs or equipment that they plan to use.

Contents

Contributors

Basem Abdelmalak
Professor of Anesthesiology,
Director, Anesthesia for Bronchoscopic Surgery and
Director, Center for Procedural Sedation,
Anesthesiology Institute,
Cleveland Clinic,
Cleveland, Ohio, USA

Hanne Abildstrøm
Senior Consultant,
Department of Anaesthesia,
Centre of Head and Orthopaedics,
Rigshospitalet,
University of Copenhagen,
Copenhagen, Denmark

Imran Ahmad
Consultant Anaesthetist,
Clinical Lead & Airway Lead,
Guy's Hospital,
Guy's & St Thomas' NHS Foundation Trust,
London, UK

Takashi Asai
Department of Anaesthesiology,
Dokkyo Medical University Saitama
Medical Centre,
Koshigaya City, Japan

Michael Aziz
Professor of Anesthesiology & Perioperative
Medicine,
Oregon Health & Science University,
Portland, Oregon, USA

Paul A. Baker
Department of Anaesthesiology,
University of Auckland,
Auckland, New Zealand and
Consultant Anaesthetist,
Starship Children's Hospital,
Auckland, New Zealand

Lauren Berkow
Professor of Anesthesiology,
University of Florida College of Medicine,
Gainesville, Florida, USA

Morten Bøttger
Consultant Anaesthetist,
Department of Anaesthesia,
Center of Head and Orthopaedics,
Rigshospitalet,
University of Copenhagen,
Copenhagen, Denmark

Jay B. Brodsky
Professor,
Department of Anesthesiology, Perioperative and
Pain Medicine,
Stanford University School of Medicine,
Stanford, California, USA

Nicholas Chrimes
Consultant Anaesthetist
Department of Anaesthesia
Monash Medical Centre
Melbourne, Australia

Tim Cook
Consultant in Anaesthesia and Intensive Care
Medicine,
Department of Anaesthesia and Intensive Care,
Royal United Hospitals Bath NHS Foundation Trust,
Bath, UK and
Honorary Professor of Anaesthesia
University of Bristol,
Bristol, UK

Richard Cooper
Professor Emeritus,
University of Toronto,
Toronto General Hospital,
Department of Anesthesia,
Toronto, Ontario, Canada

Audrey De Jong
Specialist Intensivist,
Department of Critical Care & Anaesthesiology (DAR B),
Saint Eloi University Hospital and Montpellier School of Medicine,
Montpellier, France

Pierre Diemunsch
Head of Anesthesiology, Intensive Care and Perioperative Medicine
Faculté de Médecine,
de l'Université de Strasbourg,
Strasbourg, France

Laura V. Duggan
Associate Professor,
Department of Anesthesiology and Pain Medicine,
University of Ottawa,
Ottawa, Ontario, Canada

Dietmar Enk
Prof. Dr. med.,
University Hospital Münster (UKM),
Department of Anesthesiology, Intensive Care and Pain Medicine
Münster, Germany

Andrew D. Farmery
Professor of Anaesthetics,
Head of the Nuffield Department of Anaesthetics,
University of Oxford and
Fellow & Dean,
Wadham College,
Oxford, UK

Daniela Godoroja
Department of Anaesthesia and Intensive Care,
Ponderas Academic Hospital,
Regina Maria,
Bucharest, Romania and
Assistant Professor,
University of Medicine and Pharmacy 'Carol Davila',
Bucharest, Romania

Keith Greenland
Honorary Associate Professor,
Department of Anaesthesiology,
The University of Hong Kong,
Hong Kong

Carin A. Hagberg
Chief Academic Officer,
Division Head, Division of Anesthesiology, Critical Care and Pain Medicine,
Bud Johnson Clinical Distinguished Chair
Department of Anesthesiology and Perioperative Medicine,
The University of Texas MD Anderson Cancer Center,
Houston, Texas, USA

Thomas Heidegger
Head,
Department of Anaesthesia,
Grabs, Switzerland;
Professor,
University of Bern,
Bern, Switzerland and
Faculty Professor, Difficult Airway Society, UK

Andy Higgs
Consultant in Anaesthesia & Intensive Care Medicine,
Department of Critical Care,
Warrington & Halton Teaching Hospitals NHSFT,
Warrington, Cheshire, UK

Iljaz Hodzovic
Senior Lecturer/Consultant,
Department of Anaesthetics, Intensive Care and Pain Medicine,
Welsh School of Medicine,
Cardiff University,
Cardiff, UK and
Royal Gwent Hospital,
Newport, UK

Johannes M. Huitink
Airway Management Academy,
Olympic Stadium 24–28,
Amsterdam, the Netherlands

Narasimhan Jagannathan
Vice Chair & Interim Division Head, General Anesthesia,
Department of Pediatric Anesthesiology,
Ann & Robert H. Lurie Children's Hospital of Chicago and
Professor of Anesthesiology,

Northwestern University Feinberg School of
Medicine,
Chicago, Illinois, USA

Brian Jenkins
Senior Lecturer/Hon. Professor in Anaesthetics
and Intensive Care Medicine,
Cardiff University,
Cardiff, UK

P. Allan Klock, Jr
Professor,
Univeristy of Chicago,
Chicago, Illinois, USA

Michael Seltz Kristensen
Department of Anaesthesia,
Center of Head and Orthopaedics,
Rigshospitalet,
University of Copenhagen,
Copenhagen, Denmark

Jeremy A. Langton
Associate Postgraduate Dean,
Health Education South West,
Plymouth, UK

J. Adam Law
Professor and Associate Head,
Department of Anesthesia, Pain Management and
Perioperative Medicine,
QEII Health Sciences Centre,
Dalhousie University,
Halifax, Nova Scotia, Canada

Richard Levitan
Visiting Professor,
Department of Emergency Medicine,
University of Maryland Medical Center,
Baltimore, MD and
Adjunct Professor, Geisel (Dartmouth) School of
Medicine,
Lebanon, New Hampshire, USA

David Lockey
National Director,
Emergency Medical Retrieval and Transfer Service,
Wales and
Consultant in Intensive Care Medicine and
Anaesthesia,
North Bristol NHS Trust,
Bristol, UK

Pierre-Olivier Ludes
Department of Anaesthesiology, Intensive Care and
Perioperative Medicine,
Strasbourg Hautepierre University Hospital,
Strasbourg, France

Adrian Matioc
Staff Anesthesiologist,
Department of Anesthesiology,
William S. Middleton VA Medical Center and
Clinical Adjunct Professor,
Department of Anesthesiology,
University of Wisconsin School of Medicine and
Public Health,
Madison, Wisconsin, USA

Brendan McGrath
Consultant in Anaesthesia and Intensive Care
Medicine,
Wythenshawe Hospital,
Manchester University NHS Foundation Trust,
Manchester, UK and
Honorary Senior Lecturer,
University of Manchester,
Manchester Academic Health Science Centre,
Manchester, UK

Barry McGuire
Consultant Anaesthetist,
Department of Anaesthesia,
Ninewells Hospital and Medical School,
Dundee, UK

Alistair McNarry
Consultant Anaesthetist,
NHS Lothian,
Edinburgh, UK

Viki Mitchell
Consultant Anaesthetist,
University College London Hospitals NHS
Trust,
London, UK

Mary C. Mushambi
Consultant Anaesthetist and Associate Medical
Director,
Leicester, UK and
DAS Professor of Anaesthesia and Airway
Management,
London, UK

Sheila Nainan Myatra
Professor,
Department of Anaesthesia, Critical Care and Pain,
Tata Memorial Hospital,
Mumbai, India

Jerry P. Nolan
Professor of Resuscitation Medicine,
Warwick Clinical Trials Unit,
University of Warwick,
Warwick, UK and
Consultant in Anaesthesia and Intensive Care
Medicine,
Royal United Hospital,
Bath, UK

Anil Patel
Consultant Anaesthetist,
Royal National Throat Nose & Ear Hospital, UCLH,
London, UK and
DAS Professor of Anaesthesia and Airway
Management,
London, UK

John Picard
Honorary Consultant Anaesthetist,
Imperial College NHS Trust and
Honorary Senior Lecturer,
Imperial College of Science and Medicine,
London, UK

Mansukh Popat
Consultant Anaesthetist (retired).
The John Radcliffe Hopsital,
Oxford, UK

Subrahmanyan Radhakrishna
Consultant Anaesthetist,
University Hospitals of Coventry and Warwickshire,
UK

Mridula Rai
Consultant Anaesthetist,
Nuffield Department of Anaesthetics,
Oxford University Hospitals NHS Trust,
Headington,
Oxford, UK

Lars S. Rasmussen
Department of Anaesthesia,
Center of Head and Orthopedics,
Rigshospitalet,
University of Copenhagen,
Copenhagen, Denmark and
Institute of Clinical Medicine,
University of Copenhagen,
Copenhagen, Denmark

Mikael Rewers
Consultant Anaesthetist,
Copenhagen Academy for Medical Education and
Simulation (CAMES),
Centre for Human Resources,
Copenhagen, Denmark

Leif Rognås
Lead Clinician (HEMS Base Skive) and Research
Lead,
Danish Air Ambulance and
Consultant Anaesthesiologist,
Department of Anaesthesiology,
Aarhus University Hospital,
Aarhus, Denmark

William Rosenblatt
Professor of Anesthesiology and Surgery,
Department of Anesthesiology,
Yale University School of Medicine,
New Haven, Connecticut, USA

Charlotte Vallentin Rosenstock
Consultant, Associate Professor,
Department of Anaesthesiology,
Copenhagen University Hospital-Nordsjællands
Hospital,
Hillerød, Denmark

Marie Louise Rovsing
Bispebjerg University Hospital,
Bispebjerg Bakke,
Copenhagen, Denmark

Søren Steemann Rudolph
Senior Consultant Anaesthetist & Traumemanager
Dept of Anaesthesia and Traume Center
Centre of Head and Orthopedics
Copenhagen University Hospital Rigshospitalet
Copenhagen, Denmark

Jasmeet Soar
Consultant in Anaesthesia and Intensive Care
Medicine,
Southmead Hospital,

North Bristol NHS Trust,
Bristol, UK

Massimiliano Sorbello
Consultant in Anesthesia and Intensive Care,
AOU Policlinico San Marco,
Catania, Italy

Mark R.W. Stacey
Consultant Anaesthetist,
Cardiff and Vale NHS Trust and
Associate Dean HEIW,
University Hospital of Wales,
Heath,
Cardiff, UK

Wendy H. Teoh
Private Anaesthesia Practice,
Singapore

Lorenz Theiler
Anesthesia, Emergency and Intensive Care,
Cantonal Hospital of Aarau,
Aarau, Switzerland

Richard Vanner
Private Anaesthetic Practice,
Gloucestershire, UK

Rasmus Winkel
Department of Anaesthesia,
Center of Head and Orthopaedics,
Rigshospitalet,
University of Copenhagen,
Copenhagen, Denmark

Michiel W.P. de Wolf
Maastricht University Medical
Centre,
Maastricht, the Netherlands

Gang Zheng
Associate Professor,
Department of Anesthesiology and Perioperative
Medicine,
The University of Texas MD Anderson Cancer
Center,
Houston, Texas, USA

Foreword

Sixteen years have passed since we began recruiting the contributors to the first edition of *Core Topics in Airway Management* (2005). We are delighted that a third edition has been deemed useful and even more delighted with the editors appointed.

It is not surprising that opinions and techniques have changed, but the extent of the change is remarkable (videolaryngoscopy was covered in two lines in the first edition). It is also true that patients have changed, being often fatter and older and having more co-morbidities.

Problems with the airway are almost uniquely distressing and dangerous, and everybody involved wants to know the best way to ensure safety. We wrote in the first edition that there was 'an uneasy combination of art and science' in management of the airway. The contributors to this edition have done a great deal to solidify the evidence for best practice.

We dedicated the first edition to Dr Archie Brain, so we got something right all those years ago.

Adrian Pearce

Ian Calder

Preface to the Third Edition

The Essence of Airway Management – and Why You Should Read This Book

It is a great honour and pleasure for us to have been asked to take over editing the third edition of this book, so successfully previously edited by Ian Calder and Adrian Pearce. It is now almost 10 years since the last edition of the book was published and it is clearly time for an update.

In this new third edition we have updated only a small number of chapters – most have been completely rewritten to ensure they are up to date and relevant. While a few chapters have been combined we have added several new ones to ensure the book fully covers the range of challenges encountered during modern airway management. There are new full chapters on the epidemiology of airway complications, ultrasonography, videolaryngoscopy, combined techniques, expiratory ventilatory assist, airway management for robotic surgery, during CPR, for the bloody and bleeding airway and during pre-hospital emergency medicine.

We have strived to make this book clinically useful and globally applicable, not too dependent on national strategies or regional cultural or even legal considerations. In order to achieve that almost all chapters are co-authored by two or three individual expert authors with different backgrounds from different countries and often different continents. We are proud that the authors represent institutions from close to 20 different countries including from Europe, North America and Asia. Writing a chapter for a textbook is a labour of love and not one done for reward. We thank every single author for their expertise, knowledge, communication skills and for their patience in enabling us to produce this book.

From the cutting of the umbilical cord and for the rest of a human's life, the airway – from the tip of the nose and mouth to the lungs – must be kept open or within minutes the human will die or suffer irreversible damage. Airway management therefore is the essence of anaesthesia and without getting it right all that follows is arguably futile. The book covers all important topics in airway management and strikes a balance between focussing on the elective patient, routine and specialist settings and emergency airway management. It does not include excessive focus on airway equipment itself but rather emphasises the practicalities of use, suitable techniques and their limitations.

Throughout medicine it is increasingly recognised that understanding equipment and learning techniques is but one part of delivering safe medical care. For that reason, the book starts with several new chapters examining the epidemiology of airway complications, airway assessment both clinical and virtual, airway planning and strategies. The importance of training, human factors/ergonomics and crisis management is mentioned in almost all chapters but each of these topics has a chapter bringing the topic together towards the end of the book.

We hope the book will appeal to and inform everyone who directly manages the airway irrespective of their parent specialty. It is also written for all those who work with airway managers and care for patients who have undergone airway procedures. The book is written with patient safety and comfort as central goals in care.

We hope that readers will understand the broader goals of airway management by a team and become confident in mastering the strategies and techniques described. We hope you will be able to introduce those relevant to your own practice. In the future it will be you who we must trust to manage our airways, and the airways of our loved ones, should it become necessary.

Tim Cook, Bath, UK

Michael Seltz Kristensen, Copenhagen, Denmark

Chapter

1

Anatomy

John Picard

Individual flowers may be pretty. But in a bouquet, it's their relation to each other which makes the arrangement beautiful: context is key. The same is true of topological anatomy: context makes for clinical relevance. This chapter offers a selective account of the functional adult head and neck anatomy as it applies to anaesthetic clinical practice.

Mouth Opening and the Temporomandibular Joint

Cooking and cutlery both evolved after us; while our ancestors lived without tools or open fires, biting hard and opening the mouth wide were both advantageous.

A strong bite and a wide gape may seem to be conflicting ambitions. A firm bite, for instance, depends on a single, fused mandible, and on muscles inserting some way from the joint to gain greater leverage, as in humans. (In snakes, in contrast, each of the two halves of the mandible and the maxilla move independently from the skull and from each other, and their muscles insert close to the relevant joints, to give an enormous gape, but a weak bite.) An adequate gape is nevertheless achieved in most humans by subluxation. When the jaw is closed, the head of the mandible rests in the mandibular fossa in the temporal bone. But as the jaw opens, the head of the mandible is pulled out of the fossa by the lateral pterygoids (Figure 1.1). Rather than turning on its head, the mandible swivels on an axis which runs through the mandibular foramina (i.e. close to the insertion sites of temporalis and masseter).

This shift in the axis of rotation allows both strong bite and wide gape: at the limit of closure, as the molars meet, the jaw is turning on the temporomandibular joint, and masseter and temporalis are working with leverage. But at the jaw's widest opening, it turns about the muscles' insertion sites; they are not so passively stretched, and the bones of the joint do not so impinge on one another.

Overenthusiastic openers of the mouth may sometimes find their jaw becomes stuck in subluxation (during assessment for anaesthesia, for example). The patient is left phonating like a distant gargle, with the mouth wide open; to return the jaw to its joint, it suffices to push firmly on the mandible's molars posteriorly and inferiorly.

Gape may be reduced by abnormal skin around the mouth (e.g. scleroderma), by excessive tone in masseter (e.g. induced by a neighbouring abscess) or by disease in the temporomandibular joint itself (e.g. rheumatoid arthritis).

Mouth opening ability also depends on craniocervical flexion and extension. Head extension facilitates opening. Normal humans extend about 26° from the neutral position at the craniocervical junction to achieve maximal mouth opening. If cervical extension, from the neutral position, is prevented a subject can be expected to lose about one third of their normal interdental distance. Patients with poor craniocervical extension therefore suffer a 'double whammy' in terms of airway management.

The Oral Cavity and Oropharynx

The oral cavity is dominated by the tongue, and for anaesthetists, little else counts but its size. It may be swollen acutely (as in angioneurotic oedema) but is also susceptible to disproportionate enlargement by trisomy 21, myxoedema, acromegaly, tumours and glycogen storage diseases, among others.

Angioneurotic oedema can cause such swelling as to fill the entire pharynx, preventing both nasal and mouth breathing and making a front of neck airway necessary for survival. Less dramatically, a large tongue (relative to the submandibular space) can hinder direct laryngoscopy. That is, manoeuvred with reasonable force, the laryngoscope blade should squeeze the posterior tongue so as to achieve a direct view of the glottis. If the tongue is too large, or the jaw

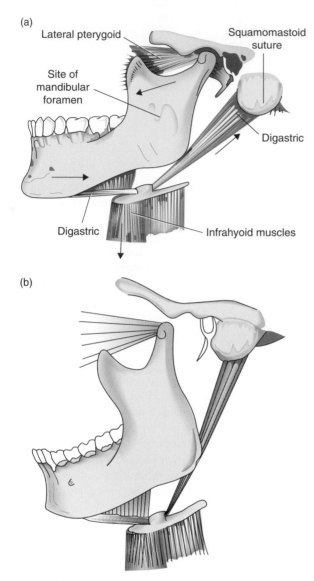

Figure 1.1 (a) Mandible and muscle actions. (b) Mandibular movement for opening the mouth wide.

hypotrophied, it may not be possible directly to see the glottis over the compressed tongue.

Within the oral cavity, the tongue is like a thrust stage in a theatre. It is surrounded by two tiers of teeth (stalls and royal circle), and a series of wings and flies (Figure 1.2).

Each tooth consists of calcified dentine, cementum and enamel surrounding a cavity filled (if the tooth is alive) with vessels and nerves. Each tooth is held in its socket in the jaw by a periodontal ligament. If a tooth is inadvertently knocked out, the sooner it is returned to

its socket the better. If the root is clean, the tooth can simply be put back in; if dirty, the root should first be rinsed with saline or whole milk. A dentist will then be able to splint the tooth in place. If a displaced tooth cannot be immediately replaced, whole milk is the best storage medium; a dental cavity exposed too long to saline, or worse water, dies. Calcification of the periodontal ligament is then inevitable, and the tooth will become brittle and discoloured, and may fracture, loosen or fall out again.

The stage's side wings are formed by mucosal folds running over palatoglossal and palatopharyngeal muscles (from anterior posteriorly). Between the two folds on each side lie the tonsils (which may be invisible in adults, but in children may be so large as to meet, 'kiss', in the midline, hampering laryngoscopy). The glossopharyngeal nerve runs under the mucosa of the base of the palatoglossal arch (towards the posterior tongue) and can be blocked there. Just as in the theatre, so in the oral cavity: confusion surrounds the wings. Properly called the palatoglossal and palatopharyngeal arches, they are also commonly called fauces and pillars. They are all the same thing.

Access to the stage's flies is controlled by the soft palate, a flap of soft tissue which can move up to separate the nasopharynx from the mouth and oropharynx (during swallowing), or move down to separate/shield the pharynx from the mouth (during chewing).

The soft tissues which surround the pharyngeal airway are themselves contained by bony structures (the maxilla, the mandible, the vertebrae and the base of the skull). When awake, tone in the pharyngeal musculature maintains airway patency. But once a patient is asleep, sedated or anaesthetised, muscular tone falls, and airway patency may depend on the relative sizes of these bones and of the soft tissues within them. Patients with more soft tissue, a shorter mandible or squatter cervical vertebrae may be at particular risk of obstructive sleep apnoea.

The Nose and Nasal Cavities

The nasal cavities have evolved to humidify and warm air before directing it to the pharynx and thence towards the lungs; all roles likely to be subverted by anaesthetists. Nevertheless, the anatomies of both inside and outside of the nose have anaesthetic relevance.

The nose encases the two nasal cavities which each lead from nostril to nasopharynx. Each cavity is lined by a mucous membrane of peculiar vascularity; luxuriant perfusion limits local cooling and desiccation despite

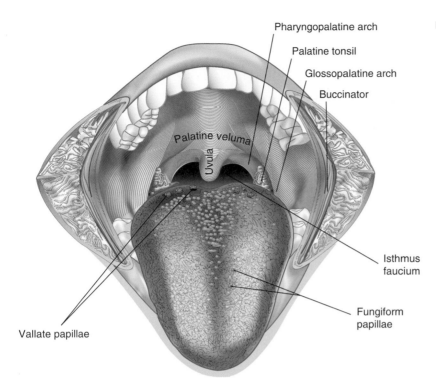

Figure 1.2 The mouth.

Pharyngopalatine arch

Palatine tonsil

Glossopalatine arch

Buccinator

Palatine veluma

Uvula

Isthmus
faucium

Fungiform
papillae

Vallate papillae

evaporation. It also means minimal trauma can cause profuse bleeding.

The mucosa's innervation is so complex as to make topical anaesthesia the most practical option for even the most ardent regional anaesthetist (no less than nine nerves innervate each cavity). That said, simply pouring a local anaesthetic solution down the nostrils of a supine anaesthetised patient is profoundly unanatomical: the medicine can be directed to its target by gravity. Before functional endoscopic sinus surgery, for example, if the solution is to reach the cephalad reaches of the nasal cavity, the head must be tilted back (with Trendelenburg tilt and a pillow below the shoulders). To direct solution along the projected path of an optical bronchoscope, less Trendelenburg is necessary. Moreover, some sensory fibres pass through the contralateral sphenopalatine ganglion. It is therefore sensible to apply local anaesthetic to both nostrils, even if only one is to be subjected to a foreign body.

Each nasal cavity is divided by three turbinates (more properly conchae) which extend medially from the cavity's lateral wall (Figure 1.3). The space between the floor of the nasal cavity and the inferior concha is larger than that between inferior and middle conchae. Furthermore, the ostia (holes) through which the sinuses drain into the nose are all cephalad to the inferior concha. For both reasons, a tracheal tube which runs through the nasal cavity may be best placed along its floor, being less likely to cause damage, or to obstruct drainage and cause sinusitis. On the other hand, an optical bronchoscope advanced between middle and inferior conchae may execute a gentler turn inferiorly toward the glottis.

The damage that can be done by tubes passed blindly through the nose is remarkable; entire conchae have been amputated, and tubes passed into the brain through fractures in the skull base. Clearly tracheal tubes should be of as small a diameter as possible, while bleeding diatheses and basal skull fractures are important relative contraindications to nasal intubation. If a tracheal tube is nevertheless to be directed through the nose, using a flexible optical bronchoscope may reduce the risk of damage.

The nose's external profile also determines how tightly a face mask can fit. Given too large a nasal bone, gas escapes around the mask's sides, and too small, gas escapes at the midline.

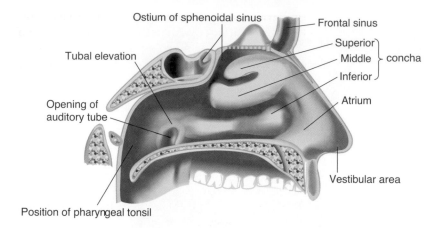

Figure 1.3 The lateral nose.

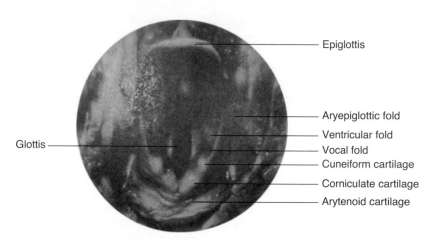

Figure 1.4 Anatomical specimen of adult human larynx.

Glottis and Epiglottis

The human larynx is often declared the organ of speech (Figure 1.4). More extraordinary still, it allows singing. Its intrinsic musculature is accordingly complex, but not always relevant to the anaesthetist simply aiming for the cavity the muscles surround. That said, a naming of the parts seen on laryngoscopy allows accurate description of abnormality. Just as for a glutton before fancy chocolates, only a few details of the box are relevant; the key is to get in, past the epiglottis and past the cords themselves, without doing undue damage on the way.

The epiglottis has evolved to shield the glottis not from anaesthetists, but from nutrients headed towards the oesophagus. It works like the flexible lid of a pedal bin. Generally, it is half open, to allow breathing. But on swallowing the epiglottis and larynx come together. Like the lid closing on the bin, the larger and more flexible the epiglottis, the better it can fit the glottis, but the more it can frustrate direct laryngoscopy. Given adequate anaesthesia, the tip of a laryngoscope placed in the vallecula and drawn anteriorly will generally also pull the epiglottis sufficiently far anteriorly to reveal the glottis. But if an anaesthetised patient is in the supine position, and the epiglottis is long and flaccid, it may fall to hide the cords unless it too is scooped above the laryngoscope's blade (Figure 1.5). Alternatively, the tip of a McCoy laryngoscope blade can be deployed to apply anterior pressure at the root of the epiglottis. Conversely, if the tissue around the epiglottis is incompliant (after radiotherapy, for instance), deploying the McCoy blade's tip may simply push the laryngoscope's blade posteriorly, hindering direct laryngoscopy rather than making it easier (see Chapter 14). A Miller straight blade can be placed posteriorly to a flaccid epiglottis to lift it out of the way.

A hypertrophied lingual tonsil or a tumour at the root of the tongue may also push the epiglottis

4

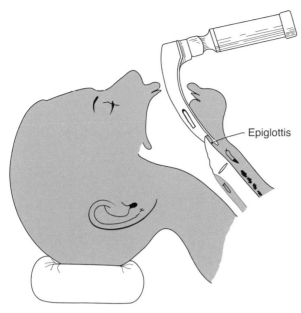

Epiglottis

Figure 1.5 The laryngoscope.

posteriorly to obstruct the glottis, just as a bin's lid may be pushed down. While asymptomatic and imperceptible during a standard examination, such an enlarged tonsil may severely hamper airway control (see Chapter 14).

The mucosa of the larynx above the cords is supplied by the internal laryngeal nerve, which branches off the superior laryngeal nerve just lateral to the greater cornu of the hyoid bone. It then plunges deep to the thyrohyoid membrane. It can be blocked by local anaesthetic injected through a needle gingerly walked off the hyoid and then passed through the perceptible resistance of the membrane. As it is purely sensory, it can be blocked without fear of attendant paresis.

But below the cords, the mucosa is innervated by the recurrent laryngeal nerve, which also supplies almost all the intrinsic muscles of the larynx. Transection of the recurrent laryngeal nerve partially adducts the cord, and – worse – less extreme surgical damage of the nerve can cause the cord to adduct more extremely, across the midline. So, anatomy dictates that the mucosa below the cords is anaesthetised topically, if at all.

The ends of the vocal cords themselves are fixed anteriorly to the thyroid cartilage. But their posterior ends each attach to an arytenoid complex which moves like a cam on the cricoid cartilage. A few degrees' turn tightens the cord to raise the voice's pitch; more extreme movements adduct the cords

(in laryngospasm) to protect the trachea from aspiration or to thwart the anaesthetist. With force, an arytenoid may be knocked off the cricoid cartilage – a remediable hoarse voice and sore throat are the results.

Subglottic Airway: Cricothyroid Puncture and Tracheostomy

'If you cannot go through it, go round it': if teeth, tongue, epiglottis or glottis obstruct the path to the cords, then it may be easier to reach the trachea directly through skin, either by cricothyroid puncture or by tracheostomy.

As the trachea must run posteriorly from the glottis to reach the carina in the mediastinum, it is most superficial at its start. Indeed, the defect between the thyroid and the cricoid cartilages is easily palpable in a slim normal neck, and is covered only by skin, loose areolar tissue and the fibrous cricothyroid membrane (Figure 1.6). So, in theory, a needle or cannula can be passed into the trachea here without risk of haemorrhage from anterior structures. The cricoid cartilage is the only ring-shaped cartilage in the upper airway and the posterior part is broader than the anterior part, thus to some extent preventing a needle or scalpel from penetrating into the oesophagus at the level of the cricothyroid membrane.

More caudally a larger tube can be passed into the trachea without undue force (either surgically or with a percutaneous technique). But again, the oesophagus runs directly behind the trachea, where the cartilages are C-shaped instead of complete rings, and can be damaged through the posterior wall in a percutaneous approach. Moreover, the trachea is far from subcutaneous as it approaches the sternum: the thyroid isthmus lies over the second, third and fourth tracheal rings; from there the inferior thyroid veins drain the gland, running close to the midline towards the chest – and in a short neck, the left brachiocephalic vein and artery may poke above the sternum as they cross the trachea. The position of these vessels, and indeed the trachea and the cricothyroid membrane, can usefully be identified by ultrasound before cricothyroidotomy or tracheostomy.

Trachea and Bronchial Tree

Like a jetliner's wing, the trachea's apparent simplicity belies its complexity. It is held open by the tracheal cartilages. These are shaped like a C, with the curve

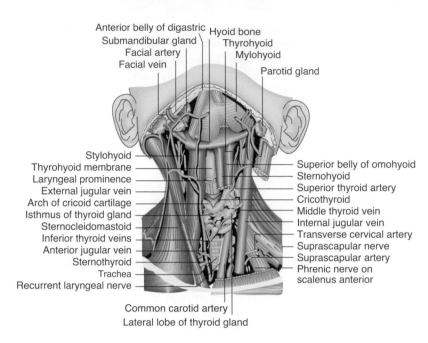

Anterior belly of digastric
Submandibular gland
Facial artery
Facial vein
Hyoid bone
Thyrohyoid
Mylohyoid
Parotid gland

Stylohyoid
Thyrohyoid membrane
Laryngeal prominence
External jugular vein
Arch of cricoid cartilage
Isthmus of thyroid gland
Sternocleidomastoid
Inferior thyroid veins
Anterior jugular vein
Sternothyroid
Trachea
Recurrent laryngeal nerve

Superior belly of omohyoid
Sternohyoid
Superior thyroid artery
Cricothyroid
Middle thyroid vein
Internal jugular vein
Transverse cervical artery
Suprascapular nerve
Suprascapular artery
Phrenic nerve on
scalenus anterior

Common carotid artery
Lateral lobe of thyroid gland

Figure 1.6 Thyroid gland and the front of the neck.

facing anteriorly; their corrugations distinguish the trachea from the smooth oesophagus. Not only do the rings help disorientated bronchoscopists, it also enables the tracheal bore to vary. The two ends of each C are joined by the trachealis muscle, which forms the posterior wall of the trachea. If the muscle tightens the trachea's radius is reduced (as the points of the C are drawn together), airway resistance rises and the volume of the dead space falls; conversely, airway resistance falls and the dead space swells as the muscle relaxes. So, just as in a wing, the trachea's shape can be optimised for different flow rates.

As the bronchial tree ramifies beyond the trachea (Figure 1.7), its initial divisions are crucially asymmetric. The carina itself is on the left of the midline; the left main bronchus is narrower and runs off closer to the horizontal than the right; all conspire to send aspirated material towards the right main bronchus. Moreover, in an adult the left main bronchus is some 4.5 cm long while the right main bronchus runs just 2.5 cm, or less, before giving off the bronchus to the right upper lobe. Clearly a larger target is easier to hit. It is therefore easier to isolate the lungs without occluding a lobar bronchus, if the left rather than the right main bronchus is the target (see Chapter 27).

The trachea is shortened by cervical flexion and lengthened by cervical extension. If a tracheal tube is anchored at the mouth, and rests above the carina when the neck is in the neutral position, it may

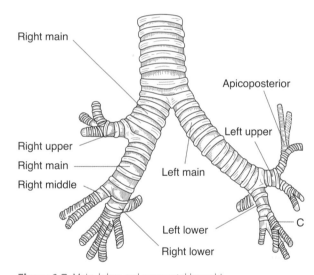

Right main
Apicoposterior
Right upper
Left upper
Right main
Left main
Right middle
Left lower
Right lower
C

Figure 1.7 Main, lobar and segmental bronchi.

stimulate the carina or even pass into a bronchus if the neck is flexed.

Cervical Spine

As in owls, so in humans: our two eyes face in the same direction, so our cervical spines have evolved particular mobility and strength to bear the heavy head, and allow it to turn relative to the body, while protecting the spinal cord within.

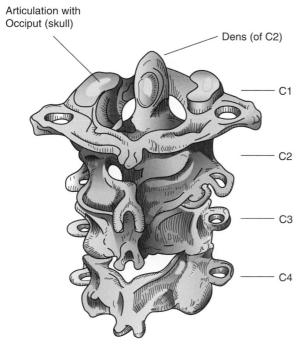

Articulation with
Occiput (skull)

Dens (of C2)

C1

C2

C3

C4

Figure 1.8 Atlas and axis.

Both the mobility and strength are crucial to anaesthetic practice: if pathology limits mobility, management of the airway is typically hampered; if the cervical spine is weakened, inappropriate management of the airway may catastrophically damage the cord.

The three most cephalad bones together form the occipito-atlanto-axial complex (Figure 1.8). Most of the neck's movement occurs between these three bones, both in normal life and during direct laryngoscopy.

Working caudad, the occipital condyles rest on the lateral masses of atlas like the rails of a rocking chair stuck in tram tracks: the head can flex forward at the joint (until the odontoid hits the skull) and extend backwards; some abduction is possible, but rotation is not. Atlas, however, turns around the axial odontoid peg which occupies the anterior third of the space within the axis. Posterior movement of atlas over axis is limited by the axial anterior arch impinging on the peg.

Otherwise ligaments are responsible for the stability of the joints:

- The alar ligaments run from the sides of the peg to the foramen magnum – depending on which way the head is turned, one or other tightens and so limits rotation.

- The transverse band of the cruciform ligament – said to be the strongest ligament in the body – runs behind the peg from one side of atlas to the other – it stops atlas moving anteriorly over axis.
- The tectorial membrane runs as a fibrous sheet from the back of the body of the peg to insert around the anterior half of the foramen magnum – running anterior to the axis around which the head nods, it tightens as the head is extended.

Below the axis, in the 'subaxial' spine, the vertebrae assume a more conventional form. They articulate at the zygoapophyseal joints ('facet joints') between each bone's facets. Flexion is limited by the ligaments between the posterior parts of the vertebrae; extension by the anterior longitudinal ligament and the intervertebral disc capsules.

Direct laryngoscopy is classically facilitated by bringing oral, pharyngeal and laryngeal axes into line. In practice, that means extension at the occipito-atlanto-axial complex and very moderate flexion in the subaxial cervical spine. A normal spine and cord will typically tolerate the forces applied by a gentle anaesthetist.

But after trauma, or with disease or malformation, the cervical spine may be either fixed or abnormally mobile. Ankylosing spondylitis, surgical fusion, or fixation may (for example) all frustrate the anaesthetist hoping to align the oral, pharyngeal and laryngeal axes, and so indicate the need for more artful management of the airway.

At the other extreme, trauma or ligamentous laxity may make the cervical spine so especially mobile as to jeopardise the spinal cord or medulla. Here anatomy is paramount, determining which manoeuvres are safe, and which dangerous. For example, in rheumatoid arthritis, the cruciform ligament may become lax; flexion of the occipito-atlanto-axial complex is then especially dangerous (atlas may move anteriorly on axis, impaling the cord between the peg and the posterior arch of atlas). But if the peg is fractured at its base, atlas is freer to move relative to axis, and both extension and flexion of the occipito-atlanto-axial complex will be dangerous.

Similarly, turning a patient from the supine position to prone will expose the patient to different dangers according to anatomy. Generally, the volume of the vertebral canal is increased in flexion, easing pressure on a cord compressed by, for example, ligamentous hypertrophy. But in bilateral facet fracture dislocation, flexion can precipitate anterior subluxation of the cephalad vertebra, disastrously guillotining the cord.

Summary

Gentle subluxation of the temporomandibular joint facilitates passive mouth opening. Direct laryngoscopy entails extension of the intricate occipito-atlanto-axial joint. Passage through the cricothyroid membrane offers the easiest percutaneous access to the airway in an emergency. The oesophagus lies behind the trachea at this level, and it may be punctured by a needle or scalpel passed posteriorly through the trachea, though the posterior arch of the cricoid cartilage may protect at the level of the cricothyroid membrane. Anatomy determines what manoeuvres will be especially dangerous in cervical instability.

Acknowledgements

Christian Ulbricht and Peter and Ellie Clarke nobly and generously improved an earlier draft; all remaining mistakes are mine alone.

Chapter 2

Physiology of Apnoea, Hypoxia and Airway Reflexes

Andrew D. Farmery and Jeremy A. Langton

Hypoxia

Humans are adapted to tolerate oxygen pressures which range from what might be called 'sea-level normoxia', down to the modest hypoxia of high-altitude living. Humans are not adapted to hyperoxic conditions and these are increasingly recognised as harmful. Why then should the airway specialist be concerned about hypoxia, and seek to counter it with hyperoxic exposure?

Classification of Hypoxia

'Cellular respiration' occurs at the level of the mitochondria, when electrons are passed from an electron donor (reduced nicotinamide adenine dinucleotide (NADH)) via the mitochondrial respiratory cytochromes to 'reduce' molecular oxygen (O_2). The energy from this redox reaction is used to phosphorylate adenosine diphosphate (ADP), thereby generating the universal energy source, adenosine triphosphate (ATP), which powers all active biological processes. If molecular oxygen cannot be reduced in this way, this bit of biochemistry fails and cellular hypoxia occurs. Based on Barcroft's original classification, four separate causes of cellular hypoxia can be considered. Three of these four factors affect oxygen delivery to the tissues ($\dot{D}O_2$), which is described mathematically by the equation in Box 2.1. Derangements of each of the terms on the right-hand side of this equation will reduce oxygen delivery to tissues.

The fourth cause of cellular hypoxia in our classification is *histotoxic hypoxia*. An example of this is cyanide or carbon monoxide poisoning. In histotoxic hypoxia, there is not (or there need not be) any deficit in oxygen delivery. Cellular and mitochondrial partial pressure of oxygen (PO_2) may be more than adequate, but the deficit lies in the reduction of molecular oxygen due to a failure of electron transfer. In order to fully understand the classification of hypoxia, it is useful to consider the example of carbon monoxide poisoning.

What Is the Mechanism of Death in Severe Carbon Monoxide Poisoning?

Let us consider each of the factors of Barcroft's classification.

Hypoxaemic hypoxia is not likely to be the cause. Assuming no lung damage has occurred, this patient's arterial oxygen (P_aO_2) is likely to be normal if breathing air, or elevated if breathing supplemental oxygen. P_aO_2 is determined by the gas-exchanging properties of the lung and is unaffected by haemoglobin concentration or by the nature of the haemoglobin species present.

Anaemic hypoxia. The presence of carboxyhaemoglobin, which has no oxygen-carrying capacity, will certainly reduce the amount of normal oxygen-carrying haemoglobin. But normal oxyhaemoglobin will still be in the majority, and the $\dot{D}O_2$ will be more than adequate. Counter to popular understanding perhaps, the presence of carboxyhaemoglobin is not the problem here.

Stagnant hypoxia is unlikely to be a cause, since the cardiac output is likely to be elevated as a compensatory mechanism.

So, what is the cause of death? The underlying mechanism of cellular death in this case is *histotoxic hypoxia*. Just as carbon monoxide has a high affinity for the haem group in haemoglobin, it also has a high affinity for the iron-containing haem flavoproteins in mitochondrial respiratory cytochromes. Once bound, electron transfer is interrupted and tissue oxygen, albeit in abundant supply, cannot be reduced and bioenergetic failure supervenes. In carbon monoxide poisoning, the presence of carboxyhaemoglobin merely serves as a marker of carbon monoxide exposure. It is not usually part of the mechanism of death.

Differential Effects of Deficits in Oxygen Delivery

The equation in Box 2.1 shows that $\dot{D}O_2$ is simply proportional to the product of the three 'Barcroft

9

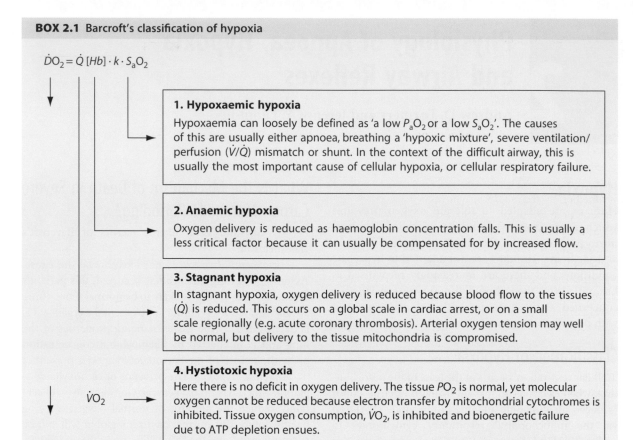

BOX 2.1 Barcroft's classification of hypoxia

$$\dot{D}O_2 = \dot{Q}\,[Hb] \cdot k \cdot S_aO_2$$

1. Hypoxaemic hypoxia

Hypoxaemia can loosely be defined as 'a low P_aO_2 or a low S_aO_2'. The causes of this are usually either apnoea, breathing a 'hypoxic mixture', severe ventilation/perfusion ($\dot{V}/\dot{Q}$) mismatch or shunt. In the context of the difficult airway, this is usually the most important cause of cellular hypoxia, or cellular respiratory failure.

2. Anaemic hypoxia

Oxygen delivery is reduced as haemoglobin concentration falls. This is usually a less critical factor because it can usually be compensated for by increased flow.

3. Stagnant hypoxia

In stagnant hypoxia, oxygen delivery is reduced because blood flow to the tissues ($\dot{Q}$) is reduced. This occurs on a global scale in cardiac arrest, or on a small scale regionally (e.g. acute coronary thrombosis). Arterial oxygen tension may well be normal, but delivery to the tissue mitochondria is compromised.

4. Hystiotoxic hypoxia

$\dot{V}O_2$

Here there is no deficit in oxygen delivery. The tissue PO_2 is normal, yet molecular oxygen cannot be reduced because electron transfer by mitochondrial cytochromes is inhibited. Tissue oxygen consumption, $\dot{V}O_2$, is inhibited and bioenergetic failure due to ATP depletion ensues.

$\dot{Q}$ is the cardiac output, $[Hb]$ is the haemoglobin concentration and S_aO_2 is the arterial oxyhaemoglobin saturation. The constant, k, can be ignored in this analysis. Deficiencies in $\dot{Q}$, $[Hb]$ and S_aO_2 produce *stagnant, anaemic and hypoxaemic* hypoxia, respectively.

variables'. It would, therefore, appear that any given deficit in $\dot{D}O_2$ should cause identical degrees of cellular hypoxia regardless of whether the deficit is due to hypoxaemia, anaemia or low blood flow. We shall see below that whereas $\dot{D}O_2$ deficits due to anaemic and stagnant hypoxia have virtually identical consequences, $\dot{D}O_2$ deficits due to hypoxaemic hypoxia are very distinct and uniquely important.

Anaemic and Stagnant $\dot{D}O_2$ Deficits

Experimental and theoretical models show that the variables $[Hb]$ and $\dot{Q}$ are not uniquely independent variables; it is merely the product, $\dot{Q}\,[Hb]$, which determines oxygen delivery and cellular oxygenation. For example, if haemoglobin concentration is halved and blood flow doubled, oxygen delivery and cellular oxygenation

remain unchanged. This is because these variables simply determine the flux of oxygen to the tissues, and they have no other significance beyond this point.

Hypoxaemic $\dot{D}O_2$ Deficits

Reductions in $\dot{D}O_2$ due to hypoxaemia are much more impactful than if an equal $\dot{D}O_2$ reduction were due to anaemic or stagnant causes. This seems counterintuitive if considered in terms of Barcroft's classification, because this focusses on oxygen delivery (bulk oxygen flux) to the tissue capillaries.

From the lung to the capillary, oxygen transport is by *convection*, whereas from capillary to cell/mitochondrion, oxygen transport is by *diffusion*. It is the PO_2 in the capillary which drives the diffusion of oxygen from capillary to cell. So, the effects of hypoxaemia are twofold:

not only does it reduce oxygen flux along the arterial tree (via a reduced S_aO_2), but it also impairs oxygen delivery beyond the tissue capillary (via a reduced PO_2).

The PO_2 at the cellular level is around 3–10 mmHg (0.4–1.3 kPa), and at the mitochondrion it is around 1 mmHg (0.13 kPa). The PO_2 in tissue capillaries may be around 40 mmHg (5.3 kPa) and this PO_2 gradient drives oxygen from capillary to mitochondrion according to Fick's law of diffusion. Figure 2.1 shows the effect of reducing $\dot{D}O_2$ on the cell's ability to take up and consume oxygen ($\dot{V}O_2$), and how this differs depending on whether the fall in $\dot{D}O_2$ is achieved via anaemic/stagnant or hypoxaemic mechanisms. It can be seen that as $\dot{D}O_2$ falls, $\dot{V}O_2$ remains constant until a critical $\dot{D}O_2$, $\dot{D}O_{2crit}$, is reached, below which cellular oxygen uptake and utilisation are diminished. $\dot{D}O_{2crit}$ represents the oxygen delivery at which cellular hypoxia begins. In normal tissue (bold lines), cellular hypoxia is seen to begin when $\dot{D}O_2$ falls to 0.4 L min^{-1} for hypoxaemic hypoxia, whereas the cell can tolerate a lower $\dot{D}O_2$ if the mechanism is anaemic or stagnant. In other words, cells are more vulnerable to hypoxaemic hypoxia.

According to Fick's law, diffusive oxygen flux depends not only on the partial pressure gradient, but also on the distance between capillary and cell, and this may be increased in oedematous states (where the interstitium occupies a greater volume, separating capillary from cell), and in capillary de-recruitment due to shock (where, if a cell's nearest capillary is de-recruited, its new nearest patent capillary will now be a greater distance away). This may explain why the difference between stagnant/anaemic and hypoxaemic hypoxia on cellular oxygen uptake is exaggerated in states of reduced diffusive conductance. This effect is also shown in Figure 2.1 (feint curves).

The Rate of Arterial Desaturation in Apnoea

We have seen that hypoxaemic hypoxia is of particular importance in the development of cellular hypoxia and clearly in the context of the difficult airway, the principal cause of hypoxaemia is airway obstruction. It is important to understand the mechanisms by which hypoxaemia develops, and the factors which determine the rate of this process.

As soon as apnoea (with an obstructed airway) occurs, alveolar and hence pulmonary capillary PO_2 begins to fall. In apnoea, the process of gas exchange between alveolus and pulmonary capillary becomes non-linear. The rising partial pressure of carbon

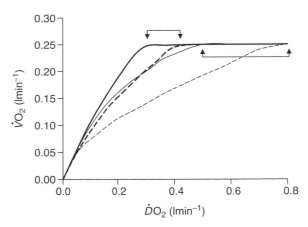

Figure 2.1 Plot of cellular O_2 consumption ($\dot{V}O_2$) vs. bulk O_2 delivery ($\dot{D}O_2$). Solid lines represent stagnant/anaemic hypoxia. Broken lines represent hypoxaemic hypoxia. Bold lines show normal relationship for tissue without significant barrier to O_2 diffusion from capillary to cell. Feint lines represent tissue with significant diffusional resistance, as in oedema or shock. As $\dot{D}O_2$ falls, $\dot{V}O_2$ initially remains constant and satisfies the normal metabolic requirement (0.25 l min^{-1}). When $\dot{D}O_2$ falls to a critical value, $\dot{D}_{crit}$ (shown by arrows), cellular O_2 consumption falls and cellular hypoxia begins. The difference in $\dot{D}_{crit}$ between hypoxaemic and stagnant/anaemic hypoxia is shown to increase when a diffusional barrier exists. (Redrawn from Farmery and Whiteley (2001).)

dioxide (PCO_2) and falling pH associated with carbon dioxide accumulation continually shifts the oxygen–haemoglobin dissociation curve adding yet more non-linearity to the process of arterial desaturation. The time lag between changes in PO_2 feeding through into changes in mixed venous PO_2 enhances the complexity of the mathematical model further. Figure 2.2 shows the effects of six different physiological derangements on the rate of arterial desaturation in obstructed apnoea. Figure 2.2(a) shows that desaturation is exaggerated in small lung volumes (as might occur in supine anaesthetised patients). Figure 2.2(b) shows that the value of the initial alveolar oxygen concentration at the onset of apnoea is also important. Due to the various mathematical non-linearities in the system, the lower the initial alveolar oxygen tension, the greater the rate of desaturation. This has important implications for patients who have periods of partial airway obstruction (and hence diminished alveolar PO_2 (P_AO_2)) before obstructing completely. It also underpins the value of thorough pre-oxygenation before procedures where there is a significant risk of obstructed apnoea. Figure 2.2(c) shows that while shunt diminishes the value of S_aO_2 at any given time during apnoea, the rate of desaturation is unaltered. Figure 2.2(d) shows that increased

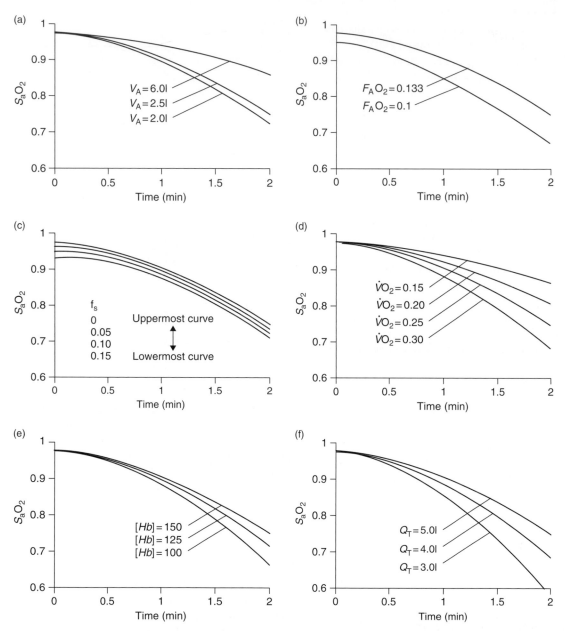

Figure 2.2 (a) Effect of lung volume (V_A in litres) on the time course of S_aO_2 in apnoea. (b) Effect of initial F_AO_2 on the time course of S_aO_2 in apnoea. (c) Effect of shunt fraction (f_s) ranging from 0% to 15% on the time course of S_aO_2 in apnoea. (d) Effect of O_2 consumption rate ($\dot{V}O_2$) ranging from 0.15 to 0.3 litre min^{-1} on the time course of S_aO_2 in apnoea. (e) Effect of haemoglobin concentration ([Hb] in g litre^{-1}) on the time course of S_aO_2 in apnoea. (f) Effect of total blood volume (Q_T) on the time course of S_aO_2 in apnoea. (Reproduced with permission from Farmery and Roe (1996).)

metabolic rates (as may occur in sepsis, or when struggling to breathe in severe airway obstruction) increases the rate of arterial desaturation, and this effect is exaggerated as desaturation proceeds. Figure 2.2(e) and (f) show how both diminished cardiac output and reduced haemoglobin concentrations increase the rate of arterial desaturation in apnoea. This is partly because haemoglobin acts as an oxygen reservoir. The effect of cardiac output is complex. So, not only does arterial hypoxaemia have a unique importance in terms of cellular hypoxia (as discussed above and in Figure 2.1), but in apnoea, anaemia and

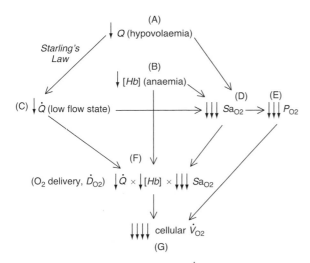

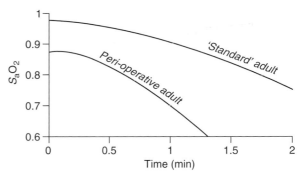

Figure 2.4 Rate of arterial oxyhaemoglobin desaturation with combination of small derangements in pathophysiological variables as might be seen in a peri-operative adult. Haemoglobin = 10 g dl^{-1}, cardiac output = 4 l min^{-1}, initial P_AO_2 = 10 kPa, initial P_ACO_2 = 8 kPa, alveolar volume = 2.0 litres, shunt fraction (f_s) = 0.1. (Reproduced with permission from Farmery and Roe (1996).)

Figure 2.3 Reductions in both [Hb] and $\dot{Q}$ as shown in (A) not only reduce oxygen delivery (B) directly (path A–B), but also indirectly via path A–C–B during apnoea because the rate of arterial desaturation during apnoea is increased by anaemia and low output. The combination of this direct and indirect effect is to produce an exaggerated reduction in oxygen delivery (B). The reduction in oxygen delivery may reduce cellular oxygen uptake (path B–D), as predicted by the solid lines in Figure 2.1. In addition, the hypoxaemic conditions (point C) contribute independently to exaggerating the reduction of cellular oxygen uptake (via path C–D) as predicted by the broken lines in Figure 2.1.

low flow states *compound* the reduction in S_aO_2 and also markedly exaggerate the reduction in oxygen delivery, which is the product of all three of these terms. The interplay of these factors is depicted in Figure 2.3.

Also of note is the fact that small derangements in each of the physiological factors in Figure 2.2 combine to produce a larger overall effect on the rate of arterial desaturation. An example of this might be a 'typical' sick patient about to undergo induction of anaesthesia. This is shown in Figure 2.4.

Pre-oxygenation and Hyperoxia

The use of supplemental oxygen, and particularly high flow, high fraction oxygen is commonplace in anaesthesia. In addition to its use in the anaesthetic room and operating theatre it is routinely used in awake patients in the recovery room and sometimes on the wards post-operatively. Such practice is often regarded as a hallmark of high quality medical care. Recent provocative evidence, however, suggests that hyperoxia is associated with adverse outcomes in stroke, myocardial infarction and cardiac arrest. Although there is no good evidence to support discontinuation of this

practice in the perioperative setting, there are good reasons to consider reserving pre-oxygenation for only those cases who are at increased risk of difficult airway management and desaturation.

Classic pre-oxygenation aims to increase body oxygen stores to their maximum, so that periods of apnoea are tolerated for longer before critical hypoxia occurs. Hyperoxia is an unavoidable consequence of it, rather than its aim. The body store which can be most increased is the lung and airways, whose nitrogen can be exchanged for oxygen. This store holds oxygen at high partial pressures and can release most of it at usefully high partial pressures. The second most significant oxygen store, which is often overlooked, is the arterial and venous blood, which comprise a store which is almost half that of the (denitrogenated) lung. This store (mainly the venous blood) can be increased by almost 20% by pre-oxygenation. Unlike the lung store, the blood store is filled at normoxic partial pressures. It requires moderately hypoxic conditions for the store to be unloaded. As such it buffers the speed of hypoxic decline at these modestly hypoxic levels.

The necessary evil of pre-oxygenation is analogous to the practice of feasting before a period of fasting. An assessment of the risks and benefits dictate that the risks of gluttonous feasting are probably justified by the increased likelihood of surviving prolonged starvation immediately following. This risk–benefit analysis is only valid, however, if the risk of starvation is real and appreciable. Likewise, pre-oxygenation should be undertaken after careful consideration of the risks imposed by not doing so.

13

There are two elements within the practice of pre-oxygenation:

- *Supplying 100% inspired oxygen*: efficient pre-oxygenation involves a close-fitting face mask to avoid air entrainment. Correct face mask application can be confirmed by seeing a full reservoir bag which moves with respiration. The bag is an essential component of the circuit because it provides the reservoir necessary when the patient's peak inspiratory flow (> 30 L min^{-1}) exceeds the fresh gas flow. The fresh gas flow should be high enough to minimise any rebreathing of nitrogen. A small amount of rebreathing of carbon dioxide is not relevant here, since it makes little difference to the oxygenation, so circle systems are no better than a Bain system in this respect. In fact, the larger circuit volume of the circle system means that nitrogen elimination is slower than a Bain system for the same fresh gas flow.

- *Time required for effective denitrogenation with 100% oxygen*: at the end of a quiet expiration the lung volume at functional residual capacity (FRC) may be 2000–2500 mL. This will be affected by patient position or disease processes and may be much reduced by obesity, pregnancy or a distended bowel. On breathing 100% oxygen, the wash-in of oxygen is exponential. The time constant (τ) of this wash-in process is the ratio of FRC or alveolar volume to alveolar ventilation ($V_A/\dot{V}_A$). Given an alveolar minute ventilation of 4 L min^{-1} and FRC volume of 2.0 L we can estimate the time constant to be $2.0/4 = 0.5$ minutes.

Exponential wash-in of oxygen during pre-oxygenation (typical values)

- Time constant (τ) of exponential process = $V_A/\dot{V}_A$

  = 2.0/4

  = 0.5 minutes

- After one time constant (0.5 minutes) pre-oxygenation is 37% complete
- After two time constants (1.0 minutes) pre-oxygenation is 68% complete
- After three time constants (1.5 minutes) pre-oxygenation is 95% complete

It is, therefore, reasonable to continue pre-oxygenation for at least three time constants to ensure maximal pre-oxygenation. It should be noted that patients with a small FRC will pre-oxygenate more quickly than normal but the oxygen store contained in the FRC will be reduced. Increasing alveolar minute ventilation (four to eight deep or vital capacity breaths) increases the rate of increase in P_AO_2 and is extremely useful when time for pre-oxygenation is limited. Administering opioids such as fentanyl before pre-oxygenation may lengthen the time required to achieve a high P_AO_2. Pre-oxygenation is also discussed in Chapter 8.

In any particular patient, the magnitude of the alveolar minute ventilation and FRC is unknown. It is, therefore, useful to monitor the process of denitrogenation by measuring end-tidal FO_2. An end-tidal FO_2 of 90–91% indicates maximal pre-oxygenation and a store of oxygen in the FRC of approximately 2000 mL. The overall increase in oxygen stores in the blood and lungs with pre-oxygenation is from 1200 mL (air) to 3500 mL.

Desaturation following the Use of Suxamethonium

The American Society of Anesthesiologists (ASA) difficult airway algorithm recommends that if initial attempts at tracheal intubation after the induction of general anaesthesia are unsuccessful, the anaesthetist should 'consider the advisability of awakening the patient'. 'Awakening' more realistically means allowing return to an unparalysed state that permits spontaneous ventilation. This is considered to be safe practice. However, to what level might arterial saturation fall before spontaneous ventilation resumes? Using a combination of clinical data and a theoretical model, Benumof demonstrated that during complete obstructive apnoea, and in the 'cannot intubate, cannot ventilate/oxygenate' situation, critical haemoglobin desaturation occurs before the time to functional recovery for various patients receiving 1 mg kg^{-1} of intravenous suxamethonium.

Figure 2.5 shows that in all but the 'normal' adult, critical desaturation occurs long before recovery of even 10% of neuromuscular function.

From this analysis, it is clear that in a complete cannot intubate, cannot ventilate/oxygenate situation, it is not appropriate to wait for the return of spontaneous ventilation, but rather a rescue option should be pursued immediately. Benumof points out that this

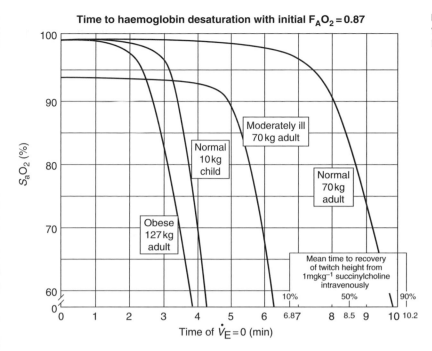

Figure 2.5 S_aO_2 vs. time of apnoea for various types of patients. (Reproduced with permission from Benumof et al. (1997).)

analysis ignores the central respiratory depressant effects of the concomitantly administered general anaesthetics, and so this should be regarded as an underestimation of the time to functional recovery.

The Final Common Pathway of Cellular Hypoxia: Membrane Potential and Cell Death

Venous PO_2 is a reasonable indicator of *capillary* and hence *tissue* PO_2. In many respects, measuring venous PO_2 (either mixed venous, or organ-specific venous such as jugular venous) is more useful in evaluating tissue oxygenation than measuring P_aO_2. Experimental and clinical evidence suggests that consciousness is lost when jugular venous PO_2 (and hence 'tissue PO_2' in the watershed of this drainage) falls below 20 mmHg (2.7 kPa). It is this PO_2 which drives diffusion of oxygen to its final destination in the mitochondria, where the PO_2 may be a fraction of a mmHg. With this degree of mitochondrial hypoxia, electron transfer cannot proceed (there is insufficient available molecular oxygen to accept electrons). This redox reaction falters and there is insufficient energy production to power the generation of ATP. We discuss the events which follow the onset of cellular bioenergetic failure.

Tissues vary in their sensitivity to hypoxia, but cortical neurones are particularly sensitive. They (along with the myocardium) are perhaps the most clinically important and are therefore the most studied. It is said that 'hypoxia stops the machine and wrecks the machinery'. As far as neurones and the myocardium are concerned this aphorism means that hypoxia initially arrests cellular function. For a period the integrity of the cell and its viability remain intact. If hypoxia is reversed, function will resume. However, sustained hypoxia wrecks the machinery. Via numerous and complex mechanisms, and in neurones particularly, an accelerating series of destructive events ensues, which results in cell death. The length of this process is highly variable depending on the tissue, the metabolic rate, blood flow and many other factors. However, it may be as short as 4 minutes for some neurones.

Anoxia and Membrane Potential

In general, living cells can be characterised by possession of a resting membrane potential whereas dead cells have no resting membrane potential. The effect of anoxia on resting membrane potential depends on the nature of the anoxic insult. In ischaemia (as in stroke), the tissue is deprived of oxygen and blood flow, whereas in airway obstruction, hypoxaemia occurs while blood flow (and glucose supply) continues, and this may have more deleterious effects.

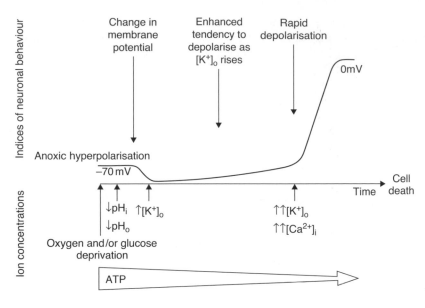

Figure 2.6 Membrane potential changes induced by cellular hypoxia. Intra- and extracellular pH changes are the first to be observed. Changes in membrane potential occur between 15 and 90 seconds. This is usually hyperpolarisation due to increased K^+ channel conductance. K^+ then leaks from within the cell. This causes an increase in extracellular $[K^+]$, especially if perfusion is limited (as in ischaemia), since the extracellular space is not washed out of ions and metabolites. The increasing extracellular $[K^+]$ causes gradual membrane depolarisation which in turn activates voltage-sensitive Ca^{2+} channels, contributing further to the depolarisation. The increasing acidosis and increasing depolarisation triggers Ca^{2+} release from intracellular stores, which in turn triggers synaptic release of glutamate. The release of this massive amount of glutamate stimulates ligand-gated cation channels whose opening coincides with a very rapid phase of membrane depolarisation. At this point, the Na^+–K^+-ATPase pump has ceased to operate and membrane potential is lost irretrievably.

One of the first metabolic features of mitochondrial bioenergetic failure is the depletion in ATP and accumulation of NADH. Small amounts of ATP can be generated from the glycolytic pathway, but this requires oxidised nicotinamide adenine dinucleotide (NAD^+), which is in short supply. However, the necessary NAD^+ can be generated by converting pyruvate to lactate, thus facilitating limited ATP production anaerobically. The intracellular acidosis which results from anaerobic metabolism is one of the first changes to be detected following cellular anoxia. If the nature of the hypoxia is *hypoxaemic hypoxia*, then blood flow will be preserved and there will be an abundant supply of glucose which will exacerbate the acidosis. Hyperglycaemic patients are particularly at risk.

Shortly after the onset of intracellular acidosis, the membrane potential of neurones begins to change. This is shown in Figure 2.6. The effect is variable, but the majority hyperpolarise. It is thought that this is due to an increase in K^+ channel conductance. The mechanisms are not clear, but possibilities include activation of ATP-sensitive K^+ channels (increased conductance in low ATP states), activation of direct oxygen-sensitive K^+ channels or activation of pH-sensitive K^+ channels. Hyperpolarisation of neurones renders them less susceptible to synaptic activation, and this may manifest as loss of consciousness (i.e. 'the machine stops').

From this point, membrane potential changes from hyperpolarisation to slow depolarisation. The mechanism of this is thought to be that the increased K^+ conductance (which initially hyperpolarised the membrane) enables K^+ efflux out of the cell down its concentration gradient. This escaped K^+ is normally removed from the extracellular space by the Na^+–K^+-ATPase, but as this pump begins to fail, extracellular $[K^+]$ increases and, as can be predicted by the Nernst equation, resting membrane potential begins to depolarise. As the membrane potential depolarises further, Ca^{2+} channels are activated and Ca^{2+} influx contributes to an acceleration of the depolarisation.

At this point, these electrophysiological effects are reversible if oxygenation is restored. If not, a cascade of irreversible events ensues.

Within a short time, membrane depolarisation becomes very rapid. This coincides with a number of cellular events: the failure of the Na^+–K^+-ATPase pump, massive release of Ca^{2+} from intracellular stores triggering massive release of excitatory neurotransmitters (principally glutamate) from synaptic vesicles, which in turn stimulate glutamate receptor-linked ion channels triggering further cation influx into the cell. Beyond this point, cell survival is unlikely. The machine is wrecked.

The time course for these events is variable. It is quickest for neurones exposed to ischaemia (arrested flow) under hyperglycaemic and hyperthermic conditions, where the process may be a matter of only 1 to 4 minutes. Under hypoxaemic conditions with preserved flow and normoglycaemia, the process may take between 4 and 15 minutes depending on the degree and abruptness of the insult.

Summary: Hypoxia

Tissue hypoxia can be fatal despite normoxaemia (cyanide and carbon monoxide poisoning). Hypoxaemic hypoxia (airway obstruction) is more damaging to cells than anaemic or stagnant hypoxia. Oxygen saturation will fall more quickly in an apnoeic sick patient. Waiting for spontaneous ventilation to return may not be a sensible option. An end-tidal oxygen fraction of > 90% indicates maximum pre-oxygenation. Pre-oxygenation achieves its end by increasing the store of oxygen in the lung and the blood. Initial hyperoxia is an unwanted consequence.

Airway Reflexes

Upper airway reflexes are important to anaesthetists, as a clear airway enables safe ventilation of the lungs and oxygenation of the patient. It also provides a means by which the depth of inhalation anaesthesia can be rapidly altered. An increase in the sensitivity of airway reflexes during induction of anaesthesia increases the likelihood of laryngeal spasm and coughing. This may impair the smooth administration of inhalation anaesthesia and when severe may be life-threatening. During recovery from anaesthesia the larynx plays a primary role in the protection of the lungs from aspiration of foreign material.

Reflexes from the Nose

The nasal mucosa receives sensory innervation from the trigeminal nerve (cranial nerve V) via branches of the anterior ethmoidal and maxillary nerves. There are not clearly structurally identified sensory end organs in the nose; however, it is thought that non-myelinated nerve endings in the sub-epithelium mediate the nasal reflexes. Airborne chemical irritants cause discharges in the trigeminal nerves and these responses may be responsible for nasal reflexes such as sneezing and apnoea. The apnoeic reflex is part of the complex diving response, caused by the physiological stimulus of water being applied to the face or into the nose. Apnoea can also be induced by odours

or irritants and this response has been identified in all mammalian species. Apnoea is associated with cardiovascular changes and complete laryngeal closure, which occurs as part of the diving response.

Chemical, mechanical stimuli and mediators such as histamine can cause sneezing when applied to the nasal mucosa. Local application of capsaicin, which depletes substance P-containing nerves of their neuropeptide, can prevent the sneeze due to the inhaled irritants, suggesting that non-myelinated nerves may be the receptors. Positive pressure applied to the nose and nasopharynx can stimulate breathing in humans and experimental animals. In addition, nasal irritation can cause bronchoconstriction or bronchodilation by two afferent pathways.

Anaesthetic vapours stimulate the nasal mucosa and elicit nasally mediated reflexes. Enflurane may produce the most marked influence on the breathing pattern. Following the start of insufflation of enflurane or isoflurane into the nose, there is a decrease in tidal volume with a prolongation in the expiratory time. Halothane has the least effect. Inhalation induction of anaesthesia using the volatile agents may be associated with breath-holding, coughing and laryngospasm. It is likely that these reflexes arise from stimulation of upper airway receptors. The nose is an important reflexogenic area, and stimulation of the nasal mucosa may cause some of the most frequently seen airway problems during anaesthesia.

Reflexes from the Pharynx and Nasopharynx

The nasopharynx is supplied by the maxillary nerve (V), and the glossopharyngeal (IX) nerve via the pharyngeal branch provides sensory innervation to the mucous membrane below the nasopharynx. Stimulation of the pharynx and nasopharynx may cause powerful reflexes including hypertension and diaphragmatic contraction.

Reflexes from the Larynx

The innervation of the larynx is by the superior laryngeal nerve (X) and to a lesser extent by the recurrent laryngeal nerves (X). The internal branch of the superior laryngeal nerve contains afferent fibres from the cranial portion of the larynx. The recurrent laryngeal nerve provides afferent innervation to the subglottic area of the larynx. There are many nerve fibres which are thought to be sensory in almost all areas of the laryngeal mucosa and also in some deeper structures. There have been various types of nerve ending identified in the laryngeal mucosa, including myelinated and non-myelinated fibres in the mucosa and submucosa. The posterior supraglottic region has the highest density of free nerve endings, with the afferent fibres being transmitted via the superior laryngeal nerve. Laryngeal afferent neurones with receptive fields in the epiglottis can be activated by a range of stimuli, including water, but mechanical stimuli are the most effective. The sensory units are thought to consist of free nerve endings that lie between the mucosal cells of the airway epithelium.

Laryngospasm

Laryngospasm is a common and potentially dangerous complication of general anaesthesia. It is defined as 'occlusion of the glottis by the action of the intrinsic laryngeal muscles' and is considered to be present when inflation of the lungs is hindered or made impossible by unwanted muscular action of the larynx.

Laryngeal spasm is essentially a protective reflex to prevent foreign material reaching lower down into the lungs. The laryngeal muscles are striated, the most important muscles involved in the production of laryngeal spasm being the lateral cricoarytenoid, thyroarytenoid (adductors of the glottis) and the cricothyroid (tensor of the vocal cords).

During laryngeal spasm in a human, either the true vocal cords alone or the true and false cords become apposed in the midline and close the glottis. There are thought to be two initiators of laryngeal spasm during general anaesthesia. First, direct irritation of the vocal cords may be caused by a sudden increase in concentration of irritant anaesthetic vapour or direct contact with blood or saliva, and second, by traction on abdominal and pelvic viscera. There are many reports in the literature of the inhalation of irritant vapours producing laryngeal spasm, coughing and bronchospasm. Anaesthetic agents may sensitise the receptors.

This complication is not uncommon and may be life-threatening. In a large study of 156,064 general anaesthetics the overall incidence in all patient groups was 8.7/1000 patients. The incidence was high in children aged between 0 and 9 years, with a peak incidence of 27.6/1000 in infants aged 1–3 months. Animal work has demonstrated laryngeal adductor

hyperexcitability in early life and a similar developmental neuronal imbalance may occur in humans.

Other risk factors are a history of asthma or of upper respiratory tract infection (URTI) and smoking. In children with a history of recent URTI the incidence of laryngeal spasm was increased to 95.8/1000

Factors Affecting the Sensitivity of Upper Airway Reflexes

Using low inspired concentrations of ammonia vapour as an irritant chemical stimulus allows study of the upper airway in a repeatable and reliable manner by measuring inspiratory flow patterns. The lowest concentration of ammonia required to elicit a response is termed the threshold concentration (NH3TR). A low value of NH3TR indicates sensitive or reactive airways, whereas a higher NH3TR value represents a reduced upper airway reflex sensitivity and a depression of airway reflexes. Studying the sensitivity of upper airway reflexes in subjects suffering with, and recovering from, a URTI showed increased sensitivity until day 15 (Figure 2.7). This coincided with the presence of symptoms. Upper respiratory tract infections cause acute mucosal oedema followed by shedding of epithelial cells. Loss of airway epithelium can extend down to the basement

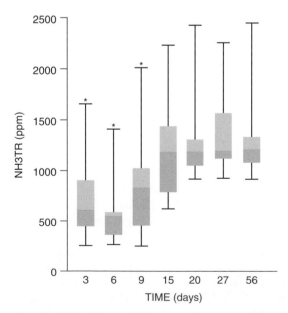

Figure 2.7 The effect of a URTI on upper airway reactivity. Ammonia threshold concentration (NH3TR) in volunteers with an upper respiratory tract infection (URTI) showing the median, interquartile range and the 10th and 90th percentiles **$P < 0.01$ (Wilcoxon). (From Nandwani et al. (1997).)

membrane and may persist for up to 3 weeks. The mechanism for upper airway hyper-reactivity following viral infection may be due to increased exposure of intraepithelial sensory receptors to inhaled irritants. Bronchial reactivity to experimentally inhaled histamine is also increased during a URTI and persists for up to 7 weeks. The high incidence of laryngospasm during inhalation anaesthesia is likely to be due to a direct effect of irritant gases and vapours on the airways. In a cross-sectional study of inhalation anaesthesia the incidence of laryngeal spasm was 12/1000 cases but during iso-flurane anaesthesia was 29/1000.

Cigarette smoking also has an effect on the sensitivity of upper airway reflexes (Figure 2.8). Following abstinence, sensitivity is unaltered after 24 hours but then increases over the next 48 hours achieving a consistent change by day 10. It is known that chronic cigarette smokers develop dysplasia of the respiratory epithelium, which may disrupt the integrity of the respiratory epithelium. In addition, smokers have depressed production of salivary epidermal growth factor, which is known to stimulate epithelial prolifera-tion. The evidence for epithelial injury or inflammation causing increased airway sensitivity comes from work on the lower airway reflexes after damaging epithelium mechanically or chemically. Both ozone and acute

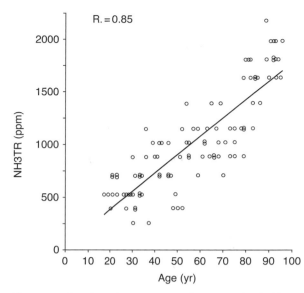

Figure 2.9 Correlation between age and ammonia threshold. Correlation coefficient +0.85. (From Erskine et al. (1993).)

smoke exposure have been shown to increase tracheal mucosal permeability with increased airway respon-siveness. Nebulised lidocaine administered preopera-tively, prior to induction of anaesthesia, significantly improved the quality of induction of anaesthesia in smokers.

Age affects laryngeal reflexes, with reactivity reducing with advancing age (Figure 2.9). Laryngeal reflexes in the elderly are less active, both during induction of anaesthesia and in the recovery room, compared to a younger patient, sug-gesting that airway protection may be impaired in the elderly: sensitivity of airway reflexes decreases by a factor of three between the third and ninth decade of life.

Anaesthetic Agents and Laryngeal Reflexes

Inhalation Anaesthetic Agents

The respiratory tract is hypersensitive to stimuli arising during light general anaesthesia. The historical volatile agents ether and halothane produced laryngeal spasm and isoflurane was also irritant. In modern practice desflurane is the most significantly irritant volatile agent, with sevoflurane being the least irritant.

Sevoflurane does not elicit the cough reflex and is the preferential agent for inhalation induction of anaesthesia.

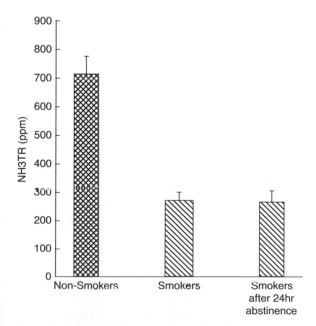

Figure 2.8 Mean (SEM) ammonia thresholds in 20 non-smokers and in 20 smokers before and after 24hr abstinence. ***P =< 0.001. (From Erskine et al. (1994).)

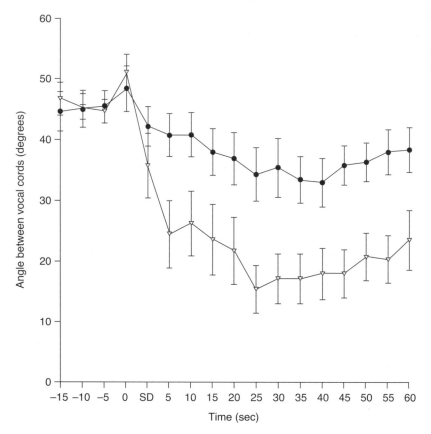

Figure 2.10 Angle between vocal cords after induction of anaesthesia with propofol or thiopentone (mean, SEM). Time 0 = start of the injection of thiopentone or propofol. SD = syringe drop. Circles: propofol; open triangle: thiopentone. (From Barker et al. (1992).)

Intravenous Anaesthetic Agents

Thiopentone

Early work with thiopentone conducted in an animal model found that most of the animals would cough, sneeze or hiccup during thiopentone anaesthesia. Inspection of the glottis in these animals revealed hyperactive adducted vocal cords and lifting the epiglottis elicited complete closure of the glottis. The administration of large doses of atropine (3–5 mg kg^{-1}) would lead to relaxation of the vocal cords and it was concluded that the closure of the glottis following intravenous barbiturates was probably mediated via the parasympathetic nervous system. Following induction of anaesthesia with thiopentone vagal reflexes or increased nerve sensitivity can cause closure of the glottis and a hyperactive state of the laryngeal reflex.

Propofol

Propofol is associated with minimal airway reflex activation. Indeed, the vocal cords may remain abducted enabling tracheal intubation using propofol alone, in contrast to thiopentone after which the vocal cords of > 50% of subjects are closed). Airway manipulation, insertion of airways and laryngeal mask insertion are more easily tolerated following induction of anaesthesia with propofol than other induction agents (Figure 2.10).

Opioids

These depress airway reactivity. Fentanyl has been shown to depress airway reflex responses in a dose-related manner and to reduce desflurane-induced airway irritability. Remifentanil improves the intubating conditions in children during sevoflurane anaesthesia. There have also been many studies showing that remifentanil and alfentanil improve conditions for laryngeal mask insertion and during awake intubation.

Benzodiazepines

Benzodiazepines are widely used to produce short-term sedation and anxiolysis to facilitate endoscopy and minor surgical procedures. However, it is known that these drugs reduce the sensitivity of upper airway reflexes. This may impair the ability of the patient to protect their lower airway from aspiration. Using ammonia challenges, it has been shown that diazepam

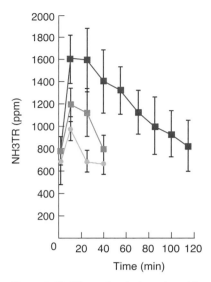

Figure 2.11 Effects of topical vocal cord lignocaine, nebulised lignocaine and oral benzocaine lozenges, on upper airway threshold response to ammonia stimulation (NH3TR) (mean, 95% CI). Black squares represent directly applied lidocaine, grey squares nebulised lidocaine and light grey circles benzocaine lozenges. (From Raphael et al. (1996).).

(0.2 mg kg^{-1}) and midazolam $(0.07 \text{ mg kg}^{-1})$ produce significant depression of upper airway reflex sensitivity within 10 minutes of administration, with baseline values regained within 60 minutes. This is significantly reversed by flumazenil (300 μg) administered 10 minutes after midazolam. Oral diazepam has a similar impact on upper airway reflexes from 30 to 150 minutes after administration. Benzodiazepines also impair airway maintenance by reducing the tonic contraction of genioglossus, whose activity is essential to keep the tongue away from the posterior pharyngeal wall. Benzodiazepines should not be considered safe agents in airway obstruction.

Local Anaesthetic Agents

Local anaesthetic agents may be applied to the airway to facilitate awake intubation or to reduce the reflex physiological effects during tracheal intubation and extubation. Benzocaine lozenges produce a significant effect within 10 minutes returning to normal within 25 minutes. Directly applied lidocaine produces

a significant effect lasting 100 minutes and nebulised lidocaine lasts 30 minutes.

Intravenous lidocaine 1.5 mg kg^{-1} (when plasma concentrations were $> 4.7 \text{ μg mL}^{-1}$) reduced responses to tracheal irritation to only brief apnoea, and other reflex responses were completely suppressed.

Summary: Reflexes

Upper airway reflexes are important to anaesthetists. Anaesthetic agents produce changes in the sensitivity of upper airway reflexes. Propofol is associated with depression of upper airway reflexes. Ageing leads to a gradual reduction in sensitivity of upper airway reflexes. Cigarette smoking increases the sensitivity of upper airway reflexes, a change which persists for up to 2 weeks following cessation of smoking.

Further Reading

Benumof JL, Dagg R, Benumof R. (1997). Critical hemoglobin desaturation will occur before return to an unparalyzed state following 1 mg/kg intravenous succinylcholine. *Anesthesiology*, **87**, 979–982.

Farmery AD, Roe PG. (1996). A model to describe the rate of oxyhaemoglobin desaturation during apnoea. *British Journal of Anaesthesia*, **76**, 284–291.

Farmery AD, Whiteley JP. (2001). A mathematical model of electron transfer within the mitochondrial respiratory cytochromes. *Journal of Theoretical Biology*, **213**, 197–207.

Langton JA, Murphy PJ, Barker P, Key A, Smith G. (1993). Measurement of the sensitivity of upper airway reflexes. *British Journal of Anaesthesia*, **70**, 126–130.

Nandwani N, Raphael J, Langton JA. (1997). Effect of an upper respiratory tract infection on upper airway reactivity. *British Journal of Anaesthesia*, **78**, 352–355.

Nishino T. (2000). Physiological and pathophysiological implications of upper airway reflexes in humans. *Japanese Journal of Physiology*, **50**, 3–14.

O'Driscoll BR, Howard LS, Davison AG. (2008). BTS guideline for emergency oxygen use in adult patients. *Thorax*, **63**(Suppl 6), 1–68.

Olsson GL, Hallen B. (1984). Laryngospasm during anaesthesia. A computer aided incidence study in 136,929 patients. *Acta Anaesthesiologica Scandinavica*, **28**, 567–575.

Chapter 3

The Epidemiology of Airway Management Complications

Johannes M. Huitink and Tim Cook

Overview

Anaesthetists and others who manage the airway are trained airway specialists who strive to prevent harm to our patients, but airway management complications may still occur. Sometimes these happen because of patient factors, sometimes because management is suboptimal and, most often, because of a combination of these two. Recent developments and technology should have made anaesthesia safer but complications during airway management still lead to consequences such as cancelled operations, unplanned intensive care admission, airway trauma, brain damage or even death. Modern anaesthesia has become considerably safer with mortality attributable to anaesthesia falling at least 10-fold in the last few decades. Improvements in airway safety almost certainly contribute to this.

How much airway complications contribute to anaesthesia-attributable mortality and morbidity is unknown and will vary considerably according to the location. In well-resourced environments mortality is low: a Japanese study reported anaesthesia-related deaths in a low-risk population to be 10 per million, 40% of which were airway related. In contrast, in a low-resource environment, in Togo, post-operative mortality rate was 1 in 38 at 24 hours; 93% of deaths were judged avoidable with half attributed to anaesthesia including 30% due to respiratory management. It is likely that much airway-related morbidity and mortality is avoidable, but only with availability of trained personnel and sufficient equipment. Airway complications related to airway management performed outside the operating room (OR) environment are several-fold more common than in the OR. Consequently, although only a modest proportion of airway management takes place in the intensive care unit (ICU) up to a quarter of major events occur in that location.

Details of many specific complications, avoidance strategies and management plans are included in other chapters, so this chapter provides an overview of complications occurring during airway management, focussing particularly on epidemiology and patterns.

Despite almost universal concern amongst anaesthetists about avoidance of airway complications the reality is that serious complications are infrequent enough that individual practitioners will only encounter complications infrequently. For that reason, databases likely provide the most reliable sources of information on complications. In this chapter we will focus on information from clinical practice databases including

- the UK 4th National Audit Project: major complications of airway management (NAP4)
- a Dutch prospective database of airway complications (mini-NAP)
- data from litigation databases including that of the UK National Health Service NHS Litigation Authority (NHSLA) and the USA American Society of Anesthesiology Closed Claims Project (ASACCP).

Common Airway Complications – Difficulty and Failure

Incidences of airway management failure will vary depending on definitions, operator experience and the patient population examined: difficult laryngoscopy occurs in 1 in 16 unselected elective patients but this rises to 1 in 5 in patients having cervical spine surgery. Failure and complications occur disproportionately commonly in ICU and in the emergency department (ED) where failure may be 10-fold higher than during anaesthesia.

Common complications of airway management are listed in Table 3.1. Difficulty and failure of a primary airway procedure should be considered complications, especially as they inevitably precede the vast majority of airway complications leading to

Table 3.1 Estimates of rates of airway procedural failure derived from the literature. None of these rates are 'hard and fast': rates may be much higher in selected groups, in emergency settings, in the hands of inexperienced airway managers or in low-resource settings

Complication	Location or setting	Approximate incidence
Difficulty		
Face mask ventilation	Anaesthesia	1 in 50–100
Ventilation via SGA	Anaesthesia	1 in 10
Intubation (low-risk group)	Anaesthesia	1 in 18
Intubation (high-risk group)	Anaesthesia	1 in 5
Face mask ventilation and laryngoscopy	Anaesthesia	1 in 250
Intubation	ED	1 in 12
Intubation	ICU	1 in 3
Failure		
Face mask ventilation	Anaesthesia	1 in 600
Ventilation via SGA	Anaesthesia	1 in 50
Intubation	Anaesthesia	1 in 200–1500
	ICU	>1 in 100
	ED	>1 in 100
CICO	Anaesthesia	1 in 5000
Front of neck airway	Anaesthesia	1 in 50,000
	ED	1 in 400

CICO, cannot intubate, cannot oxygenate; SGA, supraglottic airway.

patient harm. Failed tracheal intubation likely occurs at some point in almost every airway-related fatality.

Risk factors for failure of airway management and complications are described in Table 3.2.

Procedural difficulty is also associated with secondary complications – including airway swelling, trauma, pulmonary aspiration and development of airway obstruction and the cannot intubate, cannot ventilate/oxygenate (CICV/CICO) situation. Avoidance of primary difficulty is therefore at the heart of complication avoidance.

'Composite Airway Failure'

It is essential to understand that in a patient in whom one airway technique fails, the risk of failure of other techniques is increased – so called 'composite failures'.

- After failed face mask ventilation intubation failure increases more than 10-fold.
- After failed intubation, face mask ventilation fails in approximately 1 in 10.
- After SGA insertion the risk of difficult mask ventilation rises threefold.

To minimise the risk of complications, when one technique is predicted to be difficult it is important to focus carefully on assessing the likely ease of other techniques that may be used for rescue.

National Level Complications: Lessons from NAP4

NAP4 examined major complications of airway management in the UK. This lengthy document cannot be adequately summarised here and is signposted in the Further Reading.

The aims of NAP4 were:

- To examine the extent of major complications of airway management
- To characterise these problems
- To capture recurrent themes and causes
- To make recommendations to improve airway management at national, organisational and individual levels. The former two are the basis of *institutional preparedness* and the latter of *personal preparedness*.

Key Points from NAP4

NAP4 was a 1-year national registry of major airway complications during anaesthesia and in ICU or ED. It only included cases leading to

- death
- brain damage
- emergency front of neck airway (eFONA)
- ICU admission or prolongation of ICU stay

23

Table 3.2 Risk factors for airway complications

Factor	Note
Difficult airway	While seemingly obvious that a difficult airway is a cause of complications it is more complex. Approximately half of difficult intubations are not predicted. Tests have low sensitivity. Previous difficult intubation is the best predictor of future difficult intubation and should never be ignored. Most airway complications, however, occur in patients who are not predicted and may not have anatomically difficult airways
Obesity	Obesity is repeatedly identified as a risk factor for difficulty for all types of airway management in all settings. Increased risk likely starts as low as BMI 35 kg m^{-2}. Reduced safe apnoea time and progression to severe hypoxaemia is the greatest factor
Emergency	Urgency of airway management and factors such as use of cricoid force increase risk of failure and complications up to 10-fold
Outside OR	All locations outside the OR are associated with a marked increase in risk of failure and complications. Multiple reasons are described in the text
Head and neck surgery	The combination of airway abnormality due to disease and treatment increases risk many-fold. The need for a shared airway and blood in the airway at extubation add further difficulty
Reduced mouth opening	Decreases access for laryngoscope, SGA and airway adjuncts
Reduced neck movement	Reduces mouth opening. Increases difficulty in optimal positioning for FMV and intubation. Hyperangulated videolaryngoscopy is useful to overcome the problem
Previous radiotherapy	Increases difficulty in optimal positioning for FMV and intubation. Often associated with reduced neck movement. Hinders anatomical recognition and performance of eFONA
Repetition of failing technique	Repetition of the same airway technique that has already failed is illogical – after a failed attempt at intubation subsequent attempts have an approximately 80% failure rate – but is consistently seen in airway disasters. Also termed 'failure to transition' to describe the failure to move to the next step of the airway algorithm
Lack of strategy	Safe airway management requires a series of plans each consequent on the failure of the preceding plan. A lack of a strategy, communicated to all, leads to repetition of failing techniques and chaotic airway management
Communication issues	Common in airway disasters. Failure to ensure a strategy is understood by all involved, including the transition points
Poor decision making	This often involves choosing a poor primary plan and lacking a strategy for failure. During difficulty, a combination of repetition, missing algorithm steps and using unfamiliar techniques is often seen
Untrained personnel	Training and knowledge are fundamental prerequisites for avoidance of airway complications. Training is not the same as seniority – seniors are more commonly involved in airway mismanagement than junior staff

BMI, body mass index; eFONA, emergency front of neck airway; FMV, face mask ventilation.

As such it only captured the airway events with the worst outcomes, the very 'tip of the iceberg' – lesser complications or 'rescued events' were not captured.

A concurrent denominator survey enabled a national incidence of events to be calculated (Table 3.3). NAP4 studied the complications of approximately 3 million anaesthetics. There were 133 anaesthesia events, 36 in ICU and 15 in ED.

Amongst ≈3 million general anaesthetics, there were 16 airway-related deaths and 3 cases of persistent brain damage. Incidences are reported in Tables 3.3 and 3.4 according to the degree of

injury. The rarity of such events is noteworthy and is a key reason why assessing safety in airway management is so difficult – no individual's or department's practice is likely to shed light on high level safety and this is also true for almost any randomised clinical trial (RCT).

Important themes identified in NAP4 included:

- Omitting an assessment of potential airway difficulty and risk of aspiration, and the failure to tailor the anaesthetic technique appropriately, contributed to poor outcomes.

- Poor planning and 'failure to plan for failure' were common in events. Responses to unexpected

Table 3.3 Point estimates for anaesthesia airway complications in NAP4

	Risk of event	
Included event	46 per million	1:22,000
Death	5.6 per million	1: 180,000
Death and brain damage	6.6 per million	1: 150,000

Table 3.4 Point estimates of risk of complications by airway device in NAP4

Primary airway device	Events	Death and brain damage
Any	1:22,000	1:150,000
Tracheal tube	1:12,000	1:110,000
Supraglottic airway	1:46,000	1:200,000
Face mask	1:22,000	1:150,000

difficulty and failure were unstructured. Airway managers started with only a single plan. Airway *strategies* were advocated; a logical sequence of plans, designed to manage failure at each step and to achieve oxygenation, ventilation and prevent aspiration.

- Difficult or failing techniques were regularly managed with repeated attempts, especially tracheal intubation. This was associated with deterioration from a 'cannot intubate, *can* oxygenate' to a 'cannot intubate, *cannot* oxygenate' (CICO) situation. NAP4 strongly advocates adopting a limited number of attempts as part of any strategy.
- Decisions made and techniques chosen were sometimes illogical, including using routine care in cases of known difficulty and avoiding awake intubation when strongly indicated. Lack of judgement, skills, experience, confidence and equipment all contributed.
- Anaesthetists often used 'their usual technique' when this was not in the patient's interest. Best care may require involvement of colleagues with other skill sets.
- Quality of care was judged to be 'poor' or 'good and poor' in three quarters of cases. In a secondary

study, human factors were identified in all cases (mean of four factors per case). Poor judgement, education and training were the most common contributory factors.

- Delayed, difficult or failed intubation was the primary event in almost half of reports and intubation difficulty and failure likely occurred at some point in all cases.
- SGAs (most often first generation) were used in the face of high aspiration risk or marked obesity and aspiration followed. Use by junior doctors and accepting a poorly functioning airway were themes in non-aspiration SGA events. Use of an SGA to avoid anticipated difficult tracheal intubation, without a rescue plan or strategy, was followed by problems: unstructured management of difficulty followed and some of these patients died. Fatalities would likely have been avoided by an awake intubation technique or tracheal intubation through the SGA (see Chapter 13).
- Obese and morbidly obese patients were over-represented throughout NAP4. This finding has been replicated and reinforced in other important studies (see Chapter 24).
- Head and neck cases accounted for 40% of all anaesthesia cases and the need for multidisciplinary communication and senior anaesthetic and surgical involvement was emphasised.
- Many reported cases involved the obstructed airway. CICO was common in these. Human factors were plentiful including poor planning, communication, equipment, teamwork and situation awareness. Awake tracheostomy was too infrequently considered. When problems occurred transition to eFONA was often slow, even when part of the strategy.
- Transition to eFONA when required was often delayed and eFONA often failed.
- In anaesthesia events aspiration was the commonest cause of death (51% of reports of death or brain damage). Half of these cases involved tracheal intubation. Poor judgement and ignoring risk assessment were causative in many cases.
- Unrecognised oesophageal intubation occurred in all locations and accounted for 1 in 16 cases. It was emphasised that harm from oesophageal intubation is preventable by capnography, even in cardiac arrest. (This is discussed further below.)

25

- One quarter of events took place during emergence and recovery: all were associated with airway obstruction and many with post-obstructive pulmonary oedema. Blood in the airway and a suboptimal airway during maintenance were common precipitants.

ED and ICU

- A quarter of airway events occurred in the ICU or ED. Estimates are that the rate of events leading to death or brain damage were, compared with anaesthesia, 35-fold higher in ED and 55-fold higher in ICU.
- Permanent harm or death followed 61% of ICU reports, 33% of ED reports and 14% of anaesthesia reports.
- In the ICU, much morbidity and mortality followed airway displacement, especially of tracheostomy and in obese patients. Delayed recognition and lack of a structured plan for such an event was prominent (see Chapter 28).
- In the ED, most complications followed rapid sequence induction.
- Suboptimal care, including preventable deaths, was especially common in ICU and ED reports. Issues included not recognising at-risk patients; poor planning; inadequate or inaccessible skilled staff and equipment; slow recognition of problems; unstructured responses; and poorly prepared institutional and individual strategies for managing predictable airway complications.
- Failure to use capnography in ventilated patients or to interpret it correctly (and consequent failure to identify airway displacement or misplacement) contributed to more than 70% of ICU-related deaths.

Lessons from Databases and Registries

Airway-related databases and registries (whether permanent or short term as part of a trial) are sources of useful information but differ from routine databases that generally gather data about a large number of routine cases. Registries more often collect smaller datasets relating to a focussed area, e.g. patient populations, diseases, procedures or complications. There is a degree of overlap between databases and registries. Both can provide useful information about patterns of airway complications and in some cases detailed information.

Databases that include information from routine cases are useful as they generally create a complete dataset and this puts rarer complications into context and provides a denominator enabling calculation of incidences. However, they need to be very large to gather sufficient numbers of cases of interest to be useful. Limitations include: the effort required to collect such a volume of data; that the data is often collected for other purposes (e.g. for financial or administrative purposes) so that clinical information may be of secondary purpose, leading to omissions or perverse associations; databases from a single or atypical institution may not be generalisable. Selective databases and registries are more focussed, and a greater proportion of cases are likely relevant to those interrogating the dataset. This provides economy of effort in collection and analysis. Their limitations include that: they lack denominators so cannot (by themselves) provide incidences; and the methods by which cases are captured may lead to uncertainty over whether all cases are included.

A range of airway-related databases have been established in the last decade and they are now starting to provide important data about rates of complications and identifying risk factors for harm and insight into the efficacy of various rescue techniques. Some examples are listed in Table 3.5.

For both databases and registries, the expansion of digital capacity over the last decade has been a huge benefit but with this comes responsibility for protection of personal data and effective information governance.

Notable findings from these databases (in some cases contradicting findings from RCTs and meta-analyses) are the identification of higher rates of airway difficulty than previously reported and the poor predictability of difficult tracheal intubation (NAP4), the clinical importance of avoiding multiple intubations (Sakle's group and APRICOT) and the value of videolaryngoscopy for airway rescue in children (PeDI and APRICOT).

Lessons from Fatalities and Sentinel Cases

Airway complications leading to fatality are often reviewed at multiple levels from local, regional, coronial, legal or even at a national registry level. They may appear in media or academic publications. Other than registries and national audits, such reviews are

Table 3.5 A selection of useful airway databases providing information on the epidemiology and patterns of airway complications and their management

Database or registry	Area of practice and year started	Data source	Notes
DAD The Danish Anaesthesia Database	Anaesthesia (Denmark) 2012	Routine data from > 70% of cases nationally	Detailed data on > 600,000 cases. Useful incidences and risk factors of e.g. difficult mask ventilation, difficult intubation and eFONA
NAP4 4th National Audit Project	Anaesthesia, ED, ICU (UK) 2009	One-year registry of all UK hospitals	Captured complications of 2.8 million anaesthetics. Contemporaneous denominator survey enabled incidence and risk factor determination https://www.nationalauditprojects.org.uk/NAP4_home
APRICOT (Anaesthesia PRactice In Children Observational Trial: European prospective multicentre observational study: Epidemiology of severe critical events)	Paediatric anaesthesia (Europe) 2014	One-off collection of routine data from > 30,000 paediatric anaesthetics in 250 hospitals	A large database trial exploring the incidence of severe critical events during and immediately after anaesthesia http://www.esahq.org/apricot
ASACCP American Society of Anesthesiologists Closed Claims Project	Anaesthesia (USA) 1984	Rolling database of closed litigation cases from USA	Database covers perhaps 50% of litigation claims, with considerable temporal delay. Not restricted to airway topics https://www.aqihq.org/ACCMain.aspx
University of Arizona College of Medicine registry	ED (USA) 2007	Single centre database of all ED intubations	Run by Drs J Sakles and J Moiser. Well reported and comprising > 6000 cases.
NZEMN-ANZEDAR New Zealand Emergency Medicine Network-Australian New Zealand Emergency Department Airway Registry	ED (Australia/New Zealand) 2015	Database of all intubations in ED 40 + contributing units	http://www.thesharpend.org/airway-registry
NEAR National Emergency Airway Registry	ED (USA, Canada, Singapore) 2003	Database of all intubations in ED in > 20 contributing units	Including data on 30,000 intubations http://www.nearstudy.net
NEAR4KIDS National Emergency Airway Registry for Children	Paediatric ICU (USA, Canada) 2010	22 specialised paediatric hospitals	Collecting data on all tracheal intubations and analysing risk and incidence of difficulty and including > 2000 difficult intubations http://www.near.edu/near4kids/welcome.cfm

Table 3.5 (cont.)

Database or registry	Area of practice and year started	Data source	Notes
PeDI Pediatric Difficult Intubation registry	Paediatric anaesthesia (USA) 2012	13 children's hospitals in the USA	North American registry of difficult intubation in specialised centres with data on > 1000 difficult intubations
PeAR (PaEdiatric Airway Registry)	Paediatric anaesthesia (Europe) 2019	UK initially, expanding to Europe	A recently established registry of difficult airway management (focussing on laryngoscopy) in paediatrics https://w3.abdn.ac.uk/clsm/pear/home.aspx
The Airway App	*Specific to FONA* Anaesthesia/ED/ICU/PHEM (Global) 2016	Self-reported cases	A novel open platform for reporting anonymised data on eFONA either on-line or using a smartphone app. Currently with approximately 200 cases http://www.airwaycollaboration.org/
RCoA-DAS FONA database	*Specific to FONA* Anaesthesia/ICU/ED (UK) 2020	Self-reported cases	Due 2020

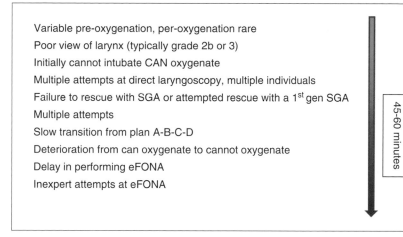

Variable pre-oxygenation, per-oxygenation rare

Poor view of larynx (typically grade 2b or 3)

Initially cannot intubate CAN oxygenate

Multiple attempts at direct laryngoscopy, multiple individuals

Failure to rescue with SGA or attempted rescue with a 1st gen SGA

Multiple attempts

Slow transition from plan A-B-C-D

Deterioration from can oxygenate to cannot oxygenate

Delay in performing eFONA

Inexpert attempts at eFONA

45-60 minutes

Figure 3.1 A typical timeline for the development of a major complication of airway management. Notable features include an airway that initially appears manageable, repeated attempts at the same procedure, failure to progress through an airway algorithm and development of the CICO situation. (Reproduced with permission from Wiley from Cook TM. Strategies for the prevention of airway complications – a narrative review. *Anaesthesia* 2018; 73: 93–111.)

usually single cases analysed by individual clinicians. Learning may or may not be of value. Through systematic collection of these cases and analysis common themes can be identified (as illustrated in Figure 3.1): NAP4 was an example of such a process.

Occasionally cases arise of such prominence that their analysis fosters national or international learning and those of Elaine Bromiley (https://emcrit.org/wp-content/uploads/ElaineBromileyAnonymousReport.pdf) and Gordon Ewing (https://www.scotcourts.gov.uk/search-judgments/judgment?id=328 e86a6-8980-69 d2-b500-ff0000d74aa7) are two such cases where the analyses of their deaths have learning potential for all airway managers.

A limitation of 'fatal case review' is that as much or more may be learnt from reviewing cases of difficulty that were resolved with a favourable outcome. This rarely happens.

Lessons from Litigation

Another source of knowledge about major complications of airway management is from litigation databases and analyses of these are available from the USA, UK and Denmark. The strength of these analyses is that they focus on events that are important enough to patients to initiate litigation. There are several major weaknesses to such analyses: cases are often at least a decade old; the trigger for litigation may be unrelated to severity of injury or negligence; there is no denominator so incidences of events cannot be calculated. Providing these limitations are understood the data may be of significant value.

Anaesthesia is a low-litigation specialty (with claims some 40-fold less than against surgeons and obstetricians) and airway-related claims account for fewer than 10% of all anaesthesia claims. However, they are especially important because amongst anaesthesia claims they are among those strongly associated with the greatest patient harm and the greatest medicolegal costs and they often affect young patients, many of whom do not have predicted difficult airways. Understanding the claims illustrates avoidable harm within cases and teaches avoidance strategies (see Further Reading).

Table 3.6 provides a comparison of the distribution of litigation related to airway trauma in the American and UK legal systems.

Lessons from a Departmental Level: 'Mini-NAP4'

Even a moderately large hospital will only deliver approximately 15,000–20,000 anaesthetics per year and most anaesthetists will anaesthetise in the range of 250–500 patients per year. This means that local data collection systems are unreliable for collecting data on the most serious and uncommon events. However, it also means they are well placed to collect data on more frequent and so-called 'minor events': these are often minor in the opinion of anaesthetists but are of potential interest because they are the precursors of more serious events, are important to patients and may have health economic importance. There is surprisingly little published in this area.

Table 3.6 Comparison between claims of airway trauma reported in the American Society of Anaesthesiologist Closed Claims Project (ASACCP) in 1991, in 1999 and those notified to the UK National Health Service Litigation Authority (NHSLA)

	ASACCP 1991	ASACCP 1999	NHSLA 1995–2007
Percentage of all anaesthesia claims	5%	6%	3%*
Deaths	12%	8%	14%
Payments to claimant	60%	54%	61%
Laryngeal injury	33%	33%	36%
Pharyngeal injury	14%**	19%	32%
Oesophageal injury	14%**	18%***	14%****
Difficult airway	42%	39%	9%*****

* Denominator adjusted to exclude dental damage (as per ASACCP).

** Pharyngeal and oesophageal injuries were 28% combined, but were not subdivided: a 50:50 split is assumed.

*** 90% were perforations.

**** All were perforations.

***** Likely an underestimate of true incidence due to methodology.

From Cook TM, Scott S, Mihai R. Litigation following airway and respiratory-related anaesthetic morbidity and mortality: an analysis of claims against the NHS in England 1995–2007. *Anaesthesia* 2010; 65; 556–563. Reproduced with permission from Wiley

The 'mini-NAP4' study (see Further Reading) is an example of a study that collected such data. All cases were studied prospectively: researchers interviewed all anaesthetists at the end of every day to identify any problems and all cases where hypoxia occurred (identified in the central theatre monitoring system) led to investigation of the cause. Episodes were divided into airway problems (unavoidable events not leading to harm) and complications (avoidable events with the potential for or causing actual harm). Degree of harm was graded, with 'serious' harm equivalent to NAP4 entry criteria. The results are shown in Table 3.7, which includes potential changes that might be made to mitigate these complications. Events such as hypoxia in 1 in 64 cases, intubation difficulty in > 1 in 100 cases, accidental oesophageal intubation and airway obstruction in 1 in 561 cases and CICO in 1 in 2803 case are all notable. Twenty-four events (0.9%) would have triggered inclusion in NAP4 including 1 death, 1 CICO, 2 eFONAs and 12 unplanned ICU admissions. Intubation difficulty accounted for 23% of events, failed mask ventilation 3%, aspiration 1.8% and laryngospasm for 7%. Of note events were most common in healthy patients and in males, those aged > 40 or < 10 years and in patients with an elevated body mass index (BMI) (half of events in patients with BMI > 26 kg m^{-2}). More than two thirds (69%) of events occurred at induction, 12% during maintenance and 14% after surgery.

This is an important study and similar studies are underway in other countries. In an ideal world every department, and perhaps every airway manager, would know their own rate of such events.

Timing of Complications

More than half of airway problems and complications occur during induction of anaesthesia. However, up to one in five major airway complications occur during emergence and recovery and this period requires due care, especially in higher-risk patients including patients with blood in the airway. Post-operative complications are less frequent but for example late airway swelling may be difficult to manage and should not be underestimated.

Specific Complications

Oesophageal Intubation

If there is one complication above all that airway managers should seek to avoid it is perhaps unrecognised oesophageal intubation. When an intended tracheal tube is inadvertently placed in the oesophagus, this will result in severe hypoxaemia, followed by brain injury or death if it is not recognised and corrected within 3–5 minutes. In modern healthcare many would think such an event would be inconceivable,

Table 3.7 Incidence of airway management problems and complications derived from a continuous prospective 2-month study of 2803 patients at an academic teaching centre in the Netherlands

Event (N=2803)	Occurrence	Incidence (%)	Incidence (odds)	Potential solutions
Desaturation < 93%	44/2803	1.57%	1:64	HFNO
Unanticipated intubation problems	29/2803	1.03%	1:97	Triage
Bronchospasm	12/2803	0.43%	1:234	–
Unanticipated ICU admission because of airway complications	12/2803	0.43%	1:234	Triage
Laryngospasm	11/2803	0.39%	1:255	–
No seal with SGA	6/2803	0.21%	1:467	Second generation SGA
Accidental oesophageal intubation	5/2803	0.18%	1:561	–
Airway obstruction	5/2803	0.18%	1:561	–
Cannot mask ventilate	5/2803	0.18%	1:561	Triage
Aspiration	3/2803	0.11%	1:934	Triage, second generation SGAs, gastric ultrasound
Emergency surgical airway	2/2803	0.07%	1:1402	CICO kits
Blood clots in airway	2/2803	0.07%	1:1402	–
Epistaxis	1/2803	0.04%	1:2803	–
Death	1/2803	0.04%	1:2803	Triage
Cannot intubate, cannot oxygenate	1/2803	0.04%	1:2803	CICO kits
Dental injury	1/2803	0.04%	1:2803	–

HFNO, High flow nasal oxygen.

but in NAP4 unrecognised oesophageal intubation accounted for 6% of reports and eight deaths. Such deaths continue to be reported.

Most clinical tools to detect a misplaced tracheal tube are unreliable and this includes tube 'misting' and auscultation of the chest. However, capnography is close to 100% sensitive, such that whenever the capnograph trace is flat the tube should be assumed to be in the oesophagus until this possibility has been actively excluded. Importantly, even during cardiac arrest ventilation via a correctly placed tracheal tube will lead to a visible (attenuated) capnograph trace. In the UK a 'no trace wrong place' campaign has been launched to highlight the role of capnography in detecting oesophageal intubation (https://www.youtube.com/watch?v=t97G65bignQ&t=15s). Use of waveform capnography in all settings where intubation is performed, allied with appropriate training, has the potential to eliminate this complication. In skilled hands ultrasonography can also be used to rapidly detect oesophageal intubation (see Chapter 7).

Pulmonary Aspiration of Gastric Contents

In NAP4 (in line with previous historical reports) pulmonary aspiration was the commonest primary cause of anaesthesia reports, of deaths and of brain damage. Most cases included avoidable harm and were contributed to by poor judgement or educational deficit. Approximately half of the cases involved tracheal intubation (often involving inadequate preparation for management of the full stomach) and half involved SGAs (including use in the morbidly obese, in patients with full stomachs and a preponderance of cases were with first generation SGAs).

Avoidance of aspiration starts with assessment of the risk of aspiration and where such risk is identified it is essential that the anaesthetic technique chosen is appropriate. The advent of gastric ultrasound may prove to be an opportunity to make an important impact on this complication. The subject is discussed in Chapters 7 and 11.

High-Risk Patient Groups

Obesity

NAP4 shed a bright light on obesity as a risk factor for major airway complications. Both the obese and morbidly obese were significantly over-represented (two- to fourfold) in the incidence of complications and in all locations. Numerous other studies have confirmed these findings. Obese patients may have distortion of the oropharynx, limited neck extension and a higher incidence of co-morbid conditions: obesity is a risk factor for difficult mask ventilation, SGA insertion, intubation and eFONA procedures. While the difficulty of individual airway procedures likely increases with obesity, the overriding risk in obese patients is from increased likelihood of airway obstruction and the dramatically increased rate of hypoxia during apnoea. All airway managers should treat obese patients with a heightened caution. This is discussed further in Chapter 24.

Head and Neck Surgery

NAP4 also highlighted head and neck surgery as a key area of increased risk, accounting for more than 40% of all reported cases. Chapters 25 and 26 discuss this topic in detail.

Complications Related to Specific Airway Devices

Face Mask Ventilation

Failure is the greatest complication here, though poor technique may also precipitate gastric inflation, regurgitation and aspiration of gastric contents. When mask ventilation fails it may start a spiral of hypoxaemia and other airway failures. Where difficulty occurs, there is convincing evidence that muscle paralysis improves ease of mask ventilation.

Supraglottic Airways

The rate of complications from SGAs is low. Soft tissue injuries from the SGA include tongue ischaemia and neuropathies including unilateral and bilateral recurrent laryngeal, hypoglossal and lingual nerve injuries. These neuropraxias manifest as vocal cord paralysis, hemitongue paralysis and tongue anaesthesia, respectively. Most resolve over several weeks to months. The mechanism is likely to be direct mechanical compression of the nerve by the SGA. While it is logical that reduced SGA cuff pressures will reduce these events, they are so rare that this is not practical to test. Nitrous oxide diffuses into the SGA cuff, particularly if it is silicone.

Best practice is to

- select the appropriate size of SGA
- monitor SGA cuff pressure and avoid cuff pressures > 60–70 cmH$_2$O
- when using nitrous oxide, routinely measure cuff pressure after 20 minutes and again if the concentration of nitrous oxide is increased
- avoid extreme neck positions, especially extension
- use extreme caution if surgery is very prolonged, opinions differ as to whether 3 or even 8 hours are safe limits

Direct Laryngoscopy

A single attempt at direct laryngoscopy is rarely injurious. However, multiple attempts lead to airway swelling and may progress to development of a CICO situation (see Figure 3.1). Tracheal intubation should be undertaken with great care. Direct vocal cord injury and arytenoid dislocation are injuries that can permanently damage the patient's voice, which may have significant implications for them. Use of a small tube (e.g. 6.0–6.5 mm ID), with an atraumatic tip, and placement first time with an optimal view of the larynx will logically reduce these complications, the latter perhaps being an argument for routine use of videolaryngoscopy. Vocal cord granulomas have been reported to be as common as 1% after tracheal intubation, but it is hoped this is of historical relevance.

Bougies, Exchange Catheters and Stylets

When bougies and stylets are used for tracheal intubation, the risk of injury is increased. Perforation of the pharynx, oesophagus and trachea are all described (see Table 3.6). These may lead to mediastinitis and can be fatal. Use of soft and non-rigid bougies, avoidance of use of the hold-up sign and ensuring a rigid stylet never enters the glottis are all important precautions to prevent such wholly avoidable complications.

When bougies and exchange catheters (Aintree intubation catheters, airway exchange catheters) are used it is important that they are not inserted beyond the carina (23–25 cm from the lips). This is particularly important if oxygen is administered via these devices (though that is generally not necessary) as there is a major risk of barotrauma if the exchange catheter wedges in the bronchial tree (see Chapter 15).

It is possible for plastic particles to be sheared off intubation catheters during railroading, especially if a large exchange catheter is used with a smaller tracheal tube. The clinical relevance of this is unknown but it is undesirable and avoidable.

Videolaryngoscopy

The most common complication specific to videolaryngoscopy is injury to the soft palate or posterior pharynx.

The mechanism of injury with the videolaryngoscope differs from that with traditional intubation; with videolaryngoscopy a hyperangulated blade or the styletted tube may be advanced without direct observation into a 'blind spot' in the posterior pharynx where it is not seen directly or by video and leads to tissue trauma. Such injury is reduced (or eliminated) by directly watching the blade or tube enter the airway as far as is possible and then immediately switching to the video screen to watch its further progress. Ensuring the styletted tracheal tube runs along the blade of the hyperangulated videolaryngoscope will not only reduce the risk of injury to posterior structures but also facilitate successful intubation (see Chapter 17).

If lacerations do occur, mild ones can be managed conservatively, whereas more substantial injuries may benefit from haemostasis and primary repair.

Double-Lumen Tube

Because of their size and relative difficulty in placement double-lumen tubes (DLTs) are associated with a greater risk of complications. Airway trauma, including vocal cord damage, dental damage, cuff damage or airway bleeding, is a particular issue.

Videolaryngoscopy and DLTs with an integrated camera within the DLT both have the potential to reduce complications but more studies are needed to confirm this.

Tracheostomy

Tracheostomies are perhaps the airway with the greatest risk of complications. Complications may occur at placement, but this is perhaps overstated. More important is the risk of complications during use with displacement (especially in critical care and in patients whose lungs are ventilated) and obstruction (especially on the wards) being prominent problems in critical airway events. These are discussed in Chapter 29.

Emergency Front of Neck Airway (eFONA)

eFONA is the final common pathway of all airway algorithms. When a needle-based technique is used the greatest procedural risks of harm are from failure and from barotrauma during high-pressure source ventilation and this increases dramatically in an emergency setting (see Further Reading). When a scalpel-based technique is used the greatest procedural risks are failure and bleeding. However, by far the commonest complication is hypoxaemic brain damage or death due to delay: whether outside or in hospitals, patients do not die from eFONA but from delay or failure to perform it.

Complications by Anatomical Location

Mouth and Oropharynx

Dental injury during laryngoscopy, often due to pressure on the maxillary incisors, is one of the most common complaints against anaesthetists: however, in a recent prospective study dental injury occurred in only 1:2803 cases. A careful history and documentation of the condition of dentition preopcratively, communication of risk and appropriately gentle care are all essential.

Minor bruising and lacerations to the lips, buccal mucosa, floor of mouth, palate, uvula and tongue are all relatively common, caused by direct tissue trauma from airway devices, especially the laryngoscope or tracheal tube. Careful technique during airway manipulations should reduce the incidence of injuries. Injuries should be documented and discussed with the patient.

Hyperangulated videolaryngoscopes enable an easier view of the larynx with lesser force exerted on soft tissues; whether this translates to lesser minor soft tissue injury is unknown.

Nasal Cavity

Epistaxis during nasotracheal intubation or instrumentation is relatively common (30–50%) and vasoconstrictors are recommended. It is usually self-limiting but severe blood loss has been reported. With forceful

33

intubation, turbinate fracture or avulsion or posterior pharyngeal lacerations may occur. Prolonged nasal intubation is associated with self-limiting sinusitis.

Complications are minimised by use of lubricants, nasal vasoconstrictors, use of small, warmed tracheal tubes, avoidance of force and even guiding placement with a flexible optical bronchoscope (FOB).

Mucosal abrasions, tears and haematomas resolve with conservative management, such as nasal humidification and pressure. Large septal haematomas are a risk for septal perforation. Pharyngeal lacerations may heal without sequelae, but should be observed for development of retropharyngeal haematoma or abscess which can cause airway compromise

Larynx and Pharynx

Temporary laryngeal injury is common with tracheal intubation: 97% of intubations, however brief, may lead to some degree of microscopic laryngeal injury including vocal cord erythema, granulomas, ulcers or vocal cord immobility. Transient dysphagia, sore throat, hoarseness, throat clearing and aspiration are common. The vast majority of symptoms, however, settle within a few days. Up to 1% of patients continue to experience dysphonia related to chronic vocal cord injury. Sore throats after SGA placement are approximately sixfold less common, are less severe and resolve more promptly.

Vocal fold paralysis is thought to occur in 0.033–0.07% of intubations. Though rare, this accounts for 4–7.5% of cases of unilateral vocal cord immobility and 9–25% of cases of bilateral vocal cord immobility. Surgery (carotid endarterectomy, anterior approaches to the cervical spine and thyroid surgery) account for much higher proportions (24–56%).

The recurrent laryngeal nerve runs in the tracheo-oesophageal groove lateral to the cricoid cartilage and its internal branch enters the larynx between the cricoid and thyroid cartilages near the cricoarytenoid joint. This endolaryngeal segment is especially vulnerable to compression between a tracheal tube cuff and the internal thyroid lamina, particularly if the cuff sits too high and if the cuff pressures exceed capillary perfusion pressure, compromising blood flow and causing nerve injury. Stretching of the nerve during tube manipulation or intubation has also been proposed as a mechanism of injury. During robotic-assisted laryngectomy the robot larynx retractors should be released every 2 hours, to prevent oedema

and nerve damage (see also Chapter 33). When unilateral vocal fold immobility is suspected, otolaryngology examination with visualisation of the larynx can confirm the diagnosis.

Neuropraxias may recover spontaneously but after 6–12 months or if electromyography shows signs of denervation, recovery is unlikely. Midline unilateral paralysis rarely requires intervention. However, patients who have glottic insufficiency related to a paramedian or lateral position of the paralysed vocal fold may benefit from medialisation of the immobile vocal fold so that glottic closure and function (voice and protection from aspiration) is improved.

Arytenoid Dislocation and Subluxation

Unilateral vocal cord immobility can also occur due to mechanical disruption (total dislocation) of the cricoarytenoid joint. Cricoarytenoid joint trauma can cause haemarthrosis, joint adhesion and fixation of the arytenoid in an abnormal position. During intubation, posterior dislocation is the commonest consequence, though more rarely anterior dislocation is caused by direct forward pressure on the posterior arytenoid, by the laryngoscope or tracheal tube.

Cricoarytenoid dislocation presents like true vocal cord paralysis with hoarseness, breathlessness and vocal fatigue. Direct laryngoscopy under general anaesthesia may help differentiate the diagnoses as joint palpation enables assessment of passive joint mobility.

Late Complications of Intubation

Non-immediate (> 1 to < 7 days) and long-term complications (> 7 days) are uncommon.

Acquired tracheomalacia may be caused by cuffed tracheal or tracheostomy tubes. The tracheomalacia arises from a combination of pressure necrosis caused by elevated cuff pressures, mechanical erosion due to tube movement, chronic inflammation, infection and perhaps hypotension reducing tissue perfusion. These lead to thinning and destruction of the tracheal cartilages. Clinical manifestations range from mild dyspnea, chronic cough and wheezing to stridor, airway compromise and eventual respiratory failure. Management includes tracheostomy, stenting and surgical resection of the affected area.

Tracheo-innominate artery fistula is a rare but devastating complication of tracheostomy and prolonged intubation. Pressure necrosis of the anterior tracheal wall can cause a fistulous communication between the trachea and the innominate artery as it passes anterior to the trachea. The fistula presents as a sentinel bleed followed by massive haemoptysis. Immediate hyperinflation of the tracheostomy cuff, if present, may be lifesaving. If this fails the tracheostomy tube should be replaced by a tracheal tube through the tracheostoma: the cuff can be inflated distal to the bleeding site to protect the airway and digital pressure is applied with a finger inserted through the stoma compressing the anterior tracheal wall and innominate artery against the sternum. Immediate transfer to the OR for definitive surgery is paramount.

Tracheal stenosis is a rare long-term consequence of prolonged intubation, usually in the ICU. While textbooks quote figures as high as 1–21% after a week of intubation, the reality is that clinically important stenosis is rare. Modern tracheal tubes and nursing practices to maintain cuff pressures below 30 cmH$_2$O, and < 20 cmH$_2$O where possible, may have been beneficial. Management of symptomatic cases includes balloon or rigid bronchoscopy dilation, laser or surgical tracheal resection.

Tracheo-oesophageal fistula is an equally rare complication of prolonged intubation with a mechanism similar to tracheomalacia and tracheainnominate fistula. Erosion of the posterior tracheal wall leads to fistula between it and the oesophagus behind. Risk factors include diabetes, infection and the presence of a nasogastric tube. The fistula results in aspiration of food, coughing during feeding, recurrent aspiration pneumonia, a positive cuff leak, or gastric distention. Diagnosis is confirmed radiologically or endoscopically and treatment is surgical.

Avoidance of Complications

Avoidance of complications of airway management is a huge topic and has recently been reviewed – see Further Reading. Here we only highlight some 'high level' principles.

1. As all airway management modes not infrequently fail individually, and composite failure increases with every failure, every anaesthetic needs a strategy that is communicated to all the team members (see Chapter 4). This requires personal and organisation preparedness (see Chapter 34). Failure often follows failure to prepare for failure!

Table 3.8 Complexity factors

- Procedural airway difficulty
- Low apnoea tolerance
- Time stress
- Cardiovascular instability
- Non-theatre location
- Unfamiliar teams
- Low skill set
- Fatigue of the team
- Patient factors, e.g. prior history of difficult airway, medical syndrome, high ASA classification, low oxygen saturation at start of procedure
- Technical problems with equipment

2. Assessment and triage are the cornerstones of preparation. Assessment should aim to identify increased risk of

   a. Procedural difficulty
   b. Aspiration risk
   c. Complexity.

   The techniques (strategy) chosen should be compatible with the risks identified.

3. Triage appropriately. Huitink has developed the concept of 'airway complexity' as a means of triaging. Using this approach, a number of complexity factors (see Table 3.8, Box 3.1) in patients' airway management are identified and the clinicians' approach to airway management is guided by the overall degree of complexity. In a prospective study there was a strong correlation between the number of complexity factors and the occurrence of severe adverse events. Evidence from litigation and from NAP4 and mini-NAP4 also support this concept. When complexity and the context indicate higher risk, this triggers the need for advanced airway management techniques and more senior staff. This approach is discussed in detail in sources in Further Reading.

4. Ensure the right team is present. First, airway management generally requires a team rather than individual performance. When it is complex, specific skill sets may be required and the team may need to be changed or enlarged to ensure appropriate skill sets are covered. The most senior clinician will not always be the individual with the right skill set. See Chapters 34 and 36.

5. Make efforts to maintain oxygenation at all times. Airway management is merely a means to an end, that being adequate oxygenation and ventilation. Oxygen supplementation should occur both

---

Box 3.1 The importance of complexity factors

- Airway management under time pressure in patients with low apnoea tolerance often requires urgent intervention, without adequate time to obtain a thorough patient history or airway assessment.
- Time stress may be an important factor in increasing mistakes.
- Critically ill and emergency patients are also more likely to be haemodynamically unstable, which contributes to the complexity of airway management in this setting.
- The location of airway management may impact care, for example whether patients are intubated in the ED, ICU or operating theatre. Different teams undertake different airway procedures and the context of all these procedures is important.
- The skill level of the provider who performs the intubation has been studied as a risk factor for airway complications. Skill level inversely correlates with number of attempts at laryngoscopy, with higher skill levels correlating with fewer attempts.
- Senior supervision during emergency intubation also lowers complication rates by up to fourfold: this is the source of much debate because the presence of a second anaesthesia provider, regardless of experience level, may facilitate intubation.
- Risk of severe complications is high when more than two complexity factors are present in patients with advanced airways.

---

before *and during* airway procedures, especially in high-risk and already hypoxic patients. See Chapter 8.

6. Do not intubate when it is not indicated. Intubation per se is associated with more complications than other modes of airway management. Intubation should not be a 'thoughtless default' but rather an active decision.

7. Do intubate when it is indicated. There are many circumstances when intubation *is* indicated. In these circumstances avoidance of intubation simply because it may be difficult is unwise, particularly when a different technique is used without a backup strategy for when it fails.

8. Do not repeat failing techniques. Limiting the number of attempts at a given technique is a fundamental aim during difficult airway events. If a technique fails once it is likely to fail again if repeated unchanged and there is clear evidence from adult and paediatric anaesthesia, critical care and emergency medicine that such repetition is unsuccessful and harmful. Repeated failures waste precious time and oxygen reserves and cause minor airway trauma that progresses to oedema and airway obstruction (Figure 3.1). This compromises not only the success of the technique being tried but also of subsequent rescue techniques. In general

techniques should not be repeated unless something active is changed (device type, device size, approach etc.). Simply changing the individual doing the procedure is rarely enough unless the new operator brings a significant uplift in skill set. Where a 'best effort' has failed there is no need or benefit to repeating this.

9. If mask ventilation is difficult, during intubation and before resorting to eFONA, muscle paralysis is clearly indicated and may rescue a failed airway.

10. Get the human factors right. This is the topic of Chapter 36 but is also part of many other chapters. Personal and organisational preparation, equipment governance, planning, communication, leadership and teamwork all contribute. Well-designed and implemented use of checklists and cognitive aids is likely to both prevent and aid in the management of airway difficulty and complications.

Conclusion

Although rare, acute or chronic injuries can occur during airway management. A full understanding of not only mechanisms of complications but the settings, contributory and mitigating factors is essential for all advanced airway practitioners.

Further Reading

Cook TM. (2018). Strategies for prevention of airway complications – a narrative review. *Anaesthesia*, **73**, 93–111.

Cook TM, Scott S, Mihai R. (2010). Litigation related to airway and respiratory complications of anaesthesia: an analysis of claims against the NHS in England 1995–2007. *Anaesthesia*, **65**, 556–563.

Domino KB, Posner KL, Caplan RA, Cheney FW. (1999). Airway injury during anesthesia: a closed claims analysis. *Anesthesiology*, **91**, 1703–1711.

Duggan LV, Ballantyne Scott B, Law JA, et al. (2016). Transtracheal jet ventilation in the 'can't intubate can't oxygenate' emergency: a systematic review. *British Journal of Anaesthesia*, **117**, i28–i38.

Cook TM, Woodall N, Frerk C. (Eds.) (2011). *Fourth National Audit Project of the Royal College of Anaesthetists and Difficult Airway Society. Major Complications of Airway Management in the United Kingdom. Report and Findings.* London: Royal College of Anaesthetists. ISBN 978-1-9000936-03-3. Available at: https://www.nationalaudit projects.org.uk/NAP4_home.

Huitink JM, Lie PP, Heideman I, et al. (2017). A prospective, cohort evaluation of major and minor airway management complications during routine anaesthetic care at an academic medical centre. *Anaesthesia*, **72**, 42–48.

Jaber S, Amraoui J, Lefrant JY, et al. (2006). Clinical practice and risk factors for immediate complications of endotracheal intubation in the intensive care unit: a prospective, multiple-center study. *Crit Care Med*, **34**, 2355–2361.

Mort TC. (2004). Emergency tracheal intubation: complications associated with repeated laryngoscopic attempts. *Anesthesia & Analgesia*, **99**, 607–13.

Structured Planning of Airway Management

J. Adam Law and Thomas Heidegger

Introduction

A structured approach to airway management helps optimise patient safety throughout the procedure. With a consistent strategy to assessing the patient, the clinician will be in a position to determine the safest approach to managing the airway and to address whether additional equipment or personnel are needed to implement the chosen approach. During its implementation, should difficulty be encountered, a predetermined, structured approach will help efficiently transition from step to step, thus minimising perseveration and avoiding the morbidity associated with multiple attempts.

Patient Assessment Prior to Airway Management

Important to perform to the extent possible in all patients, airway assessment involves evaluation of the following components:

1. Identification of *anatomical predictors* of significant technical difficulty in managing the airway. In large measure, this will inform the safest approach to airway management.
2. Identification of significant *physiological issues* that may exacerbate or pose danger to the patient during airway management. These may impact or alter the otherwise chosen approach.
3. Identification of *contextual issues* such as the skills and experience of the clinician and team, availability of experienced help or equipment availability. As with physiological issues, contextual factors may also alter the otherwise planned approach.

These are each explored in more detail below.

Anatomical Predictors of Difficulty

The airway exam seeks to determine whether the airway can be successfully managed using normal techniques. It generally begins by seeking predictors of difficulty with the planned primary technique. Thus,

for planned tracheal intubation, the patient might be assessed for predicted difficulty with both direct (DL) and videolaryngoscopy (VL). Fallback options such as face mask ventilation (FMV) or supraglottic airway device (SGA) use should also be assessed for potential difficulty. Similarly, for the case planned with use of an SGA, the patient should be assessed for difficulty with SGA use but secondarily for ease of FMV and tracheal intubation. Although often not routinely done, evaluation of the patient for ease of rapid front of neck airway (FONA) access is advisable. Published predictors of difficult DL and VL, FMV, SGA use, and FONA appear in Table 4.1 and are reviewed in more detail in Chapter 5. Information gleaned from the airway examination should be supplemented by history from the patient, review of old anaesthetic records or, if available, difficult airway management databases.

The patient with obstructing airway pathology warrants additional evaluation. Often invisible to the standard examination of externally visible anatomical features, known or suspected obstructing airway pathology at or above the glottis can be evaluated with preoperative nasendoscopy. Known or suspected subglottic pathology requires review of imaging studies such as CT or MRI. Nasendoscopy and virtual imaging are discussed in Chapter 6.

The clinician must remember that conditions present during awake airway evaluation may not be maintained during general anaesthesia.

Physiological Issues

Numerous physiological issues may pose risk to the patient during airway management (Table 4.2). These may alter the planned approach to airway management (e.g. tracheal intubation after general anaesthesia vs. awake); in others, the approach may not change, but the physiological issue may require additional attention (e.g. pre-existing hypoxaemia requiring additional oxygenation techniques and earlier use

Table 4.1 Anatomical predictors of difficulty with airway management

Predictors of difficult direct laryngoscopy
- Limited mouth opening
- Narrow dental arch
- Limited mandibular protrusion
- Short thyromental distance
- Poor submandibular compliance
- Modified Mallampati class III or IV
- Limited head and upper neck extension
- Increased neck circumference
- Obesity
- Adverse dentition
- Difficult face mask ventilation
- Inexperience with direct laryngoscopy

Predictors of difficult videolaryngoscopy
- Limited mouth opening
- Blood or gastric contents in the airway
- Limited mandibular protrusion
- Short thyromental distance
- History of neck radiation, neck pathology, limited neck mobility, thick neck or previous neck surgery
- Obesity
- Known Cormack and Lehane Grade 3 or 4 during direct laryngoscopy
- Inexperience with videolaryngoscopy

Predictors of difficult face mask ventilation
- Beard or other mask seal issue
- Male sex
- Edentulous
- Age > 50 years
- Limited mandibular protrusion
- Modified Mallampati class III or IV
- BMI > 26 kg m^{-2}
- History of snoring or obstructive sleep apnoea
- History of neck radiation
- Difficult intubation

Predictors of difficult SGA insertion or use
- Limited mouth opening
- Obstructing or distorting pathology in the upper airway
- Fixed neck flexion deformity
- Applied cricoid force
- BMI > 29 kg m^{-2}

Predictors of difficult front of neck airway access
- Female sex
- Age < 8 years
- Thick neck
- Obesity
- Displaced trachea
- Overlying pathology, e.g. radiation or other tissue induration
- Fixed neck flexion deformity

BMI, body mass index.

of rescue techniques). Rarely, severe physiological disturbances may require deferral of airway management pending optimisation of the underlying condition.

Contextual Issues

Contextual issues relate to the clinician or assembled team, the environment or the patient (Table 4.3) and may also alter the optimal airway management technique.

Bedside screening tools for airway assessment have been criticised for low sensitivity and poor positive predictive value. Most of these studies have only addressed predictors of difficult DL, DL-facilitated intubation and to a lesser extent, FMV. Predicted difficulty with VL, SGA and FONA have less evidence one way or the other. Regardless of sensitivity concerns, airway examination will identify overt anatomical issues (e.g. very limited mouth opening or a fixed flexion deformity) best dealt with by awake airway management. Conversely, another approach is to screen for the easy airway: those predicted easy consist of the truly easy – which is the majority – and a small minority who will be unexpectedly difficult. Nevertheless, this small minority of unexpectedly difficult airways still makes up the majority of all difficult airways.

Importantly, even if it predicts no difficulty (or fails to predict difficulty) performing an airway examination is a cognitive forcing strategy that makes the clinician decide how they might approach unanticipated difficulty if encountered. Pragmatically, performing an airway assessment remains a standard of care.

Deciding How to Manage the Anticipated Difficult Airway

Difficulty Predicted: Management Choices

When patient assessment indicates the potential for difficulty, the clinician must decide how best to proceed. In broad terms, the choices are as follows:

1. Despite predicted difficulty, airway management proceeds after induction of general anaesthesia, with extra preparation. This may occur during spontaneous ventilation or apnoea.
2. Awake airway management, facilitated by airway local anaesthesia, with or without sedation. This can occur via nasal, oral or front of neck routes.
3. Avoidance or deferral of airway management.

39

Table 4.2 Physiological issues that may pose risk to the patient during airway management

Physiological issues

- Full stomach
- Intolerance of apnoea:
  - Predicted rapid oxygen desaturation with the onset of apnoea due to reduced functional residual capacity or increased oxygen consumption (e.g. obese, septic or pregnant patients)
  - Large minute ventilation (e.g. compensatory for metabolic acidosis)
- Haemodynamic instability:
  - Shock states, including hypovolaemia and right ventricular failure

Decision Making on How to Proceed When Difficulty Is Predicted

Many published airway management guidelines emphasise management of the unconscious patient in whom difficulty has been encountered. Whilst a recipe for successful management of the patient with predicted difficulty is difficult to provide, what follows at least represents a thought process.

When no technical difficulty is predicted, airway management generally occurs after induction of general anaesthesia. This is more comfortable for the patient (arguably, also the clinician) and delivers optimal conditions, particularly when facilitated by neuromuscular blockade. Although in many cases an SGA is the planned technique, the following discussion chiefly addresses predicted difficult laryngoscopy and tracheal intubation.

General Anaesthesia despite Predicted Difficult Laryngoscopy or Tracheal Intubation

Pragmatically, many patients are managed during general anaesthesia despite having anatomical predictors of difficult laryngoscopy and intubation. There are two general scenarios:

1. General anaesthesia is *chosen* when moderately difficult DL or VL and intubation is predicted but airway management during general anaesthesia is deemed safe. This should only occur after deliberately considering whether the following conditions are met:

   - while laryngoscopy/tracheal intubation is predicted to be *moderately difficult*, it is not predicted to be *impossible* with the clinician's usual laryngoscopy/intubation

     techniques – e.g. there must be a reasonable probability that use of DL and a bougie, or VL (often with a hyperangulated blade) will facilitate successful tracheal intubation
   - fallback options (e.g. FMV, SGA and FONA) to maintain oxygenation between attempts, or as final rescue, are predicted to succeed
   - there are no significant physiological or contextual predictors of hazard to the patient, e.g. a full stomach or likely intolerance of apnoea
   - success is predicted within an acceptable number of attempts – e.g. within three attempts. If predicted difficulty suggests that multiple devices, personnel or attempts will be needed, this suggests the need for an awake approach.
   - the clinician has a strategy for difficulty if or when encountered and all team members have been briefed on the plan *before* induction of general anaesthesia
   - appropriate help is readily available if needed
   - extra attention is paid to the details of implementation of the chosen approach, especially with pre-oxygenation and apnoeic oxygenation during airway management

2. General anaesthesia is *unavoidable* despite predicted difficulty due to lack of patient cooperation with a preferred awake technique or because of urgency, such as resuscitation. Although the former scenario is not uncommon in the paediatric patient, in the adult patient, this should only proceed when:

   - the benefit of proceeding at that time exceeds the risk of deferral
   - informed consent has been obtained from the patient or surrogate, if feasible
   - detailed attention to planning has occurred, including plans for failed tracheal intubation and failed oxygenation
   - help is physically present
   - a briefing has been performed
   - a 'double set-up' for emergency FONA (eFONA) is prepared, with identification of the location of the cricothyroid membrane (by palpation or ultrasound), together with the presence of the necessary equipment and personnel to proceed rapidly with the procedure, if needed

Table 4.3 Contextual issues that may impact the approach to airway management

Issues related to the primary clinician or team

- *Experience and skills*: when difficulty is predicted, the clinician must be sufficiently experienced in the planned technique to achieve acceptable success rates. In the absence of this experience, securing the airway in the awake patient, with the additional safety margin of having the patient maintain their own gas exchange and airway patency during the process, may be a safer approach.
- *Availability of skilled help*: rendering a patient apnoeic when the potential for technical difficulty in securing the airway has been identified can be anxiety-provoking and stressful. Having a colleague stand by during the process or even knowing that such a colleague is nearby and could be called upon should significant difficulty be encountered can alleviate such stress. Skilled help may also help technically. When difficulty is predicted, the absence of readily available help may impact the decision of how to proceed by elevating the advisability of awake intubation.

Issues related to the environment

- *Equipment*: when difficulty is predicted, the lack of the necessary equipment to successfully and expeditiously manage the airway after induction of general anaesthesia may elevate the advisability of awake intubation.

Issues related to the patient

- *Patient cooperation*: on occasion, although awake intubation may have been identified as the safest approach after assessment of anatomical predictors of technical difficulty, this may be precluded by the lack of patient cooperation.
- *High acuity situation*: in similar fashion, a high acuity situation during a resuscitation situation may preclude awake intubation due to the need to rapidly move on to other resuscitation priorities.

In either scenario, induction of general anaesthesia may proceed with *ablation* or *maintenance* of spontaneous ventilation. Although each may have theoretical advantages, neither has a proven outcome benefit compared with the other:

- *General anaesthesia with ablation of spontaneous ventilation*. Intravenous induction of general anaesthesia combined with neuromuscular blockade generally optimises airway management conditions. However, in the apnoeic patient the clinician must control gas exchange and airway patency during efforts to secure the airway.
- *General anaesthesia with maintenance of spontaneous ventilation*. This is usually achieved with volatile anaesthetics but can be achieved with a total intravenous anaesthetic technique or dissociative anaesthesia with ketamine. The theoretical advantage is that the patient will maintain ventilatory efforts and reasonable gas exchange. However, all volatile anaesthetics impair spontaneous breathing in a dose-dependent fashion and neither maintenance of airway patency nor protection against aspiration of gastric contents or blood are guaranteed. Furthermore, airway reflexes are not necessarily suppressed, so that airway instrumentation or secretions may stimulate responses such as regurgitation and laryngospasm, especially during lighter planes of anaesthesia.

Awake Techniques When Difficult Laryngoscopy or Tracheal Intubation Is Predicted

When tracheal intubation is predicted to be significantly difficult, awake intubation provides additional safety because the patient maintains gas exchange, airway patency and protection against aspiration of gastric contents, blood or secretions during the procedure. All routes can be used for awake tracheal intubation. Awake oral or nasal intubation is most often facilitated by use of topical airway anaesthesia. Awake FONA is facilitated by local infiltrative anaesthesia. As sedation is often also provided, the term 'awake intubation' can sometimes be a misnomer.

Clinicians vary in their personal thresholds for use of awake tracheal intubation. Although there are no absolute indications, the following situations may lower the threshold for considering an awake approach:

1. *Laryngoscopy and tracheal intubation is predicted to be impossible* using the clinician's standard tracheal intubation techniques – usually DL and VL. If there is *no* chance these techniques will succeed (e.g. extremely limited mouth opening, or severe cervical spine flexion deformity), then awake tracheal intubation is indicated because:

   - the generally effective and familiar techniques cannot be used
   - anatomical predictors of difficulty overlap (e.g. those of DL with those of FMV), so that if, for example, DL is predicted to be impossible,

41

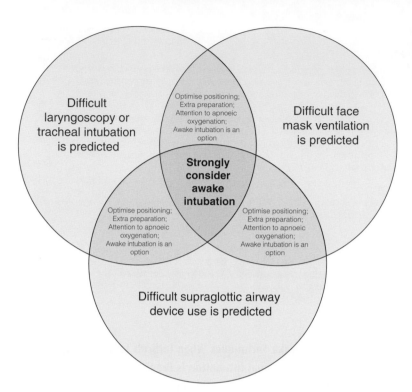

Figure 4.1 The occurrence of predicted difficulty with more than one modality of airway management elevates the need for extra preparation and planning, up to and including the use of awake tracheal intubation, if feasible.

fallback use of FMV or an SGA will likely also be difficult

2. *Laryngoscopy and tracheal intubation is predicted to be difficult (although not impossible) and* fallback techniques (FMV, SGA, FONA) are also predicted to be difficult (Figure 4.1). In this scenario, multiple attempts may be compromised by fallback failure and failure to maintain oxygenation so the advisability of awake tracheal intubation is increased.

3. *Laryngoscopy and tracheal intubation is predicted to be difficult (although not impossible) with* physiological and/or contextual risk factors (Figure 4.2). Even when only moderate technical difficulty is predicted, its coincidence with significant physiological or contextual predictors of risk lowers the threshold for awake tracheal intubation.

4. *Need for skills maintenance or teaching* may warrant proceeding with an awake approach when difficult tracheal intubation is predicted, even if judged potentially safe to manage during general anaesthesia. Naturally this requires patient consent and the chosen technique should maximise patient comfort.

5. *Extreme physiological* disturbances may sometimes be more safely dealt with using awake tracheal intubation even without anatomical predictors of technical difficulty (e.g. significant haemodynamic instability or significant anticipated intolerance of apnoea). If patient cooperation and time allows, awake VL or DL facilitated by topical anaesthesia and minimal sedation is often chosen.

6. *Published departmental protocols* in some locations may mandate the use of awake intubation for certain predictors of difficulty. This addresses variability in personal thresholds for use of awake intubation, may help decrease the incidence of unanticipated difficult intubation and will help maintain department-wide competence in awake intubation.

Difficult Laryngoscopy or Tracheal Intubation Is Predicted: Alternative Paths of Action

When difficult tracheal intubation is predicted, after a risk assessment, an alternative approach may be deemed appropriate:

1. *Using a local or regional anaesthetic technique* instead of tracheal intubation may be safe provided:

   - the regional anaesthetic technique is reliable and suitable for the planned surgery

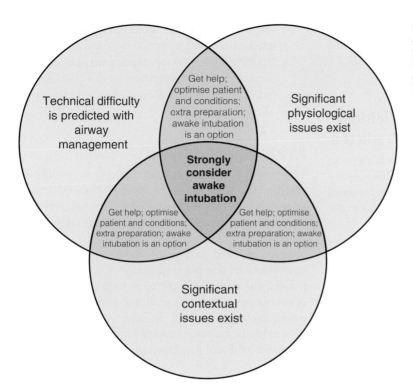

Figure 4.2 When technical difficulty with airway management coincides with significant physiological or contextual issues, extra preparation and planning is warranted, up to and including the use of awake tracheal intubation, if feasible.

- the block is assessed as working before surgical incision
- the team is briefed on the plan for intraoperative failure of the block or other complication
- where the fallback plan requires it, there is good access to the patient's airway intraoperatively

If these conditions are not met, it will be safer to secure the airway definitively before surgical incision.

2. *Use of an SGA or FMV to avoid anticipated difficult tracheal intubation* can be considered with the following caveats:
   - If a surgical case would normally be performed with an SGA, then this approach (even in a patient with known or predicted difficult tracheal intubation) is often successful.
   - If a surgical case would not normally be performed with an SGA, then planning to *electively* use an SGA simply to avoid the difficult tracheal intubation situation is hazardous.

In either situation, it must be recognised that should intraoperative SGA malfunction occur, the usual fallback of tracheal intubation may be difficult or impossible, especially in a now suboptimally positioned patient. Regardless, in some emergencies (e.g. after failed tracheal intubation for a caesarean section for fetal distress) the benefit of proceeding with the case using an SGA may exceed the risk.

3. *Deferring airway management pending arrival of, or transfer to a better-resourced situation.* The availability of better equipment or more experienced and skilled personnel might improve airway management safety despite a delay. The benefit of waiting must be balanced against the risk of deferring airway management until such conditions are obtained.

4. *Deferring airway management to optimise the patient's underlying pathology, or to avoid tracheal intubation completely.* Depending on their presenting pathology, no matter how well managed, some critically ill patients may be at risk of dangerous physiological decompensation during airway management (e.g. due to predictable effects of drugs or the onset of positive pressure ventilation with right heart failure or profound hypovolaemia).

5. *Oxygenation without airway management.* In high-risk cases and where time, equipment and skills permit, oxygenation may be achieved without airway management by extracorporeal membrane

oxygenation (ECMO). Once considered an unusual option, its feasibility has been increased by recent developments in availability, portability and the use of venovenous systems.

Safe Implementation of the Planned Approach When Difficulty Is Predicted

Regardless of the planned airway management approach, it must be implemented safety. This requires optimal patient, clinician and equipment preparation, as well as communication of the planned strategy to the whole team.

Patient and Clinician Positioning

For awake intubation, a sitting or semi-sitting position is optimal. For management during general anaesthesia, the patient is generally supine and positioned to line up the tragus of the ear with the sternal notch (unless contraindicated). Morbidly obese patients may need to be 'ramped' with blankets or a commercial positioner to attain this position. Haemodynamics permitting, a reverse Trendelenburg or back up position delays oxygen desaturation after the onset of apnoea.

Managing Threats to Patient Physiology

Physiological threats can be just as dangerous to a patient as technical difficulties and when anticipated, there must be a plan to manage them.

- Apnoea intolerance:
  - pre- or re-oxygenation before proceeding
  - apnoeic oxygenation during airway management (see Chapter 8)
- Aspiration avoidance:
  - before general anaesthesia, this might include gastric decompression and pharmacological prophylaxis, placing the table in a reverse Trendelenburg position, use of a rapid-sequence induction technique with cricoid force, and ensuring immediate availability of suction
  - for awake intubation, excellent airway anaesthesia is important to help prevent activating the gag reflex, together with avoiding deep sedation
- Haemodynamics:
  - appropriate monitoring
  - good intravenous access, with administration of a fluid bolus if indicated

- use of a vasopressor bolus during or immediately after induction, if indicated
- starting a vasopressor infusion may be required before airway management
- adjustment of induction medication type or dosage, as needed

Airway Equipment

When difficult tracheal intubation is predicted, whether the plan is for an awake or anaesthetised approach, all equipment needed for the primary and alternative airway management techniques (including failed intubation and failed oxygenation) should be present, checked and ready to use. Arranging the equipment in the planned order of usage provides a visual cue as to the next step to be taken if difficulty is encountered. When significant difficulty is anticipated, having a second clinician in attendance is invaluable in helping manage technical aspects, the cognitive load and to offload stress.

Safety Briefing

With predicted difficulty, the whole airway team should be briefed before starting. The brief includes the planned primary and alternate techniques (including plans for failed tracheal intubation and failed oxygenation) and the transition points. Beyond coaching what to expect, this ensures the primary clinician has thought through the situation, and in fact has a plan. 'Bundles', including checklists, may aid the briefing and decrease tracheal intubation-related adverse events (see Chapter 36).

A Structured Approach to Difficult Airway Management Encountered after Induction of General Anaesthesia

All clinicians must be prepared to manage airway difficulty encountered after induction of general anaesthesia. Whether difficulty is predicted or unanticipated, a structured approach is required. Although the algorithms accompanying many published guidelines addressing the unanticipated difficult airway differ in appearance, their underlying messages are broadly similar.

Failed intubation attempts should be avoided wherever possible. Each attempt should be optimised by attention to patient and clinician positioning, performing 'best attempt' laryngoscopy and facilitating tracheal intubation with adjuncts such as stylets or bougies, when needed. 'First-attempt success' is desirable, as published literature suggests increased patient morbidity with as few as two attempts, further increasing with more attempts. While most such evidence is from outside the operating theatre, the guiding principles also apply to the surgical patient. Minimising attempts eliminates unnecessary trauma to the delicate tissues of the oropharynx and larynx. Generally, a failed attempt with one technique should be followed by use of a different technique or device: ideally one which addresses the nature of the difficulty encountered during the previous attempt. *After a failed attempt, further attempts at tracheal* *intubation should only occur if patient oxygenation remains unchallenged.*

Failed Primary Approach

The primary approach to airway management involves use of tracheal intubation, an SGA or FMV. Failure of FMV will usually escalate to use of an SGA or tracheal intubation, and failed SGA use will usually escalate to tracheal intubation, sometimes with interposed FMV (Figure 4.3). Failed FMV and SGA are further considered in Chapters 12 and 13, respectively.

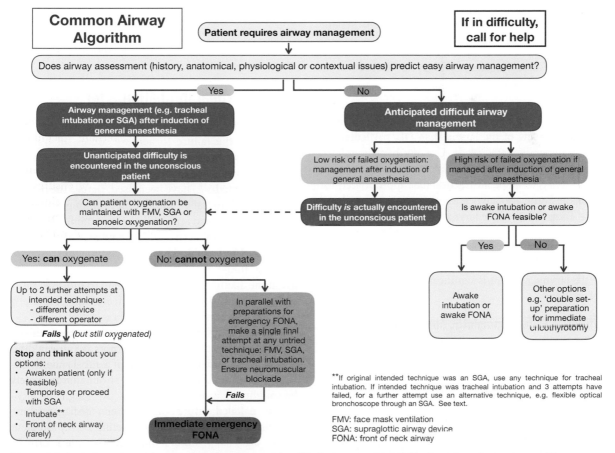

Figure 4.3 A common airway algorithm for management of the difficult airway encountered in the unconscious patient and for management of the anticipated difficult airway. (Adapted with permission from Law JA et al. The difficult airway with recommendations for management – Part 1 – Difficult tracheal intubation encountered in an unconscious/induced patient. *Canadian Journal of Anesthesia* 2013; 60: 1089–1118, and Law JA et al. The difficult airway with recommendations for management – Part 2 – The anticipated difficult airway. *Canadian Journal of Anesthesia* 2013; 60: 1119–1138.)

Difficult or Failed Direct Laryngoscopy-Facilitated Tracheal Intubation

Difficult tracheal intubation with DL generally results from failure to view the glottis or its surrounding structures (failed laryngoscopy) and (provided the patient is positioned correctly and paralysed) is usually caused by patient anatomy not conducive to attaining the needed direct line of sight from the clinician's eye to the patient's larynx (see Chapter 14). Standard technique involves positioning the patient, placing a curved DL blade fully into the vallecula, engaging the underlying hyoepiglottic ligament and lifting along the long axis of the laryngoscope handle. External laryngeal manipulation, head lift or directly elevating the epiglottis with straight or curved blades may also help. Use of a bougie is instrumental to achieving high success rates with DL-facilitated intubation when only the posterior extremity of the larynx or the epiglottis is seen (i.e. a modified Cormack and Lehane Grade 2b or 3a view, respectively).

Difficult or Failed Videolaryngoscopy-Facilitated Tracheal Intubation

VL has been incorporated into several recent airway management guidelines and it often enables a substantially better view of the larynx than DL, particularly if using a hyperangulated blade. Use of a hyperangulated VL necessitates use of a curved airway introducer (most often a stylet) to shape the tracheal tube appropriately for the blade. Some also advocate seeking only a partial and more distant view of the larynx by positioning the blade more proximally in the oropharynx resulting in a wider field of view. Failed intubation during VL generally follows from failure of tube passage, rather than failure to see the larynx, and this is significantly increased by poor technique.

Difficult or Failed Supraglottic Airway Placement

Failed ventilation after SGA placement may reflect the wrong size of device, poor device positioning, failure to inflate the cuff, downfolding of the epiglottis or even laryngospasm. If oxygenation is unchallenged, corrective manoeuvres include gradual withdrawal of the mask, an 'up-down' manoeuvre to release a downfolded epiglottis, reinsertion or changing the SGA size or type. As with tracheal intubation, the total number of attempts at SGA placement should be limited, although reasonable evidence supports attempting a second size or type of SGA. Ongoing difficulty or failure to establish adequate ventilation with an SGA should generally be managed with tracheal intubation, with or without interposed FMV.

Difficult or Failed Face Mask Ventilation

Although often not emphasised in airway management education programmes, effective FMV is crucial to a structured approach to difficult airway management. In many guideline algorithms, success or failure in oxygenation using FMV dictates which pathway to follow subsequently. Success at FMV should be monitored by visible chest rise and an appropriate capnography trace. Difficult or impossible FMV is aided by an oral airway, two-handed mask application, exaggerated jaw lift, additional head extension (if not contraindicated) and application of continuous positive airway pressure. If applied, cricoid force should be eased or released, and the presence of an obstructing foreign body excluded. Especially in the child, gastric decompression may aid FMV after gastric inflation caused by difficult FMV. FMV can generally be expected to become easier with the onset of neuromuscular blockade.

Failed Tracheal Intubation after Multiple Attempts

In general, the failure to achieve successful tracheal intubation after a maximum of three attempts, especially if two substantially different devices (e.g. DL and hyperangulated VL) have been used, signals the need to verbally declare 'failed intubation'. As long as patient oxygen delivery can still easily be maintained by FMV or an SGA, an unhurried plan can be made for what to do next. Most published airway guidelines espouse limiting initial intubation attempts in this way to avoid the 'fixation error' that can lead to multiple futile and potentially harmful intubation attempts, especially with repetitive use of a single device.

In contemporary practice, failure to intubate within a maximum of three attempts is unusual and should be considered indicative of a substantially difficult situation. Additional help should immediately be sought.

Once failed intubation has been declared, some guidelines are prescriptive in directing SGA placement as the next step; others include SGA placement as a temporising option. Regardless, in a failed intubation situation, as long as oxygenation remains unchallenged, most guidelines espouse a 'stop and think'-type reflection and include a number of suggestions on how to proceed next (Figure 4.3). Options include:

1. *Allowing the patient to emerge from general anaesthesia.* Although no outcome benefit has been published on this approach, it is commonly espoused in published guidelines. Once awake, the patient can have their surgery deferred, or immediately be managed with awake tracheal intubation, regional anaesthesia, or rarely, FONA. The following caveats apply:

   - awakening the patient will not be an option for most critically ill patients
   - spontaneous ventilation may not necessarily be restored once neuromuscular blockade wears off or is reversed, if other anaesthetic agents are still acting
   - profound oxygen desaturation may preclude a return to consciousness or spontaneous ventilation

2. *Placement of an SGA* can be followed by one of the following actions:

   - the patient can be allowed to emerge from general anaesthesia with the SGA in place
   - proceeding with surgery under SGA ventilation after failed tracheal intubation, which is warranted only in rare circumstances. The NAP4 report was clear that to do so could be associated with significant morbidity. A careful risk–benefit assessment is required and there should be a plan for the intraoperative failure of ventilation via the SGA.
   - the SGA can be used to temporise until personnel or equipment are obtained for another definitive tracheal intubation attempt
   - tracheal intubation via the SGA (see below)

3. *A further attempt at tracheal intubation*, with the following caveats:

   - oxygen delivery must continue to be non-problematic, and 'bigger picture' issues must be considered, such as maintenance of hypnosis, optimal neuromuscular blockade and avoiding aspiration of gastric contents
   - any go-to technique should be different from those that have already failed, should ideally address the anatomical or equipment constraint(s) that caused these failures, and should have a high likelihood of succeeding without causing further airway trauma

   - further attempts should only take place with the necessary equipment and expertise. Use of a flexible optical bronchoscope (FOB) – alone or in combination with another device – may be helpful.

     o **FOB intubation through an SGA**: several SGAs have an airway tube sufficiently wide to accommodate a tracheal tube (e.g. i-gel, Ambu Aura-i or AuraGain). A well-lubricated tracheal tube is placed into the SGA and the FOB is advanced through the tracheal tube, through the larynx and into the trachea. The tracheal tube is then railroaded over the FOB, after which the FOB and SGA are removed. For SGAs with a narrower calibre (e.g. cLMA, PLMA) an Aintree intubation catheter (AIC) (Cook Medical LLC, Bloomington, IN) is mounted on a slim FOB (maximum 4 mm external diameter) and the combination is passed through the SGA into the trachea. The FOB and SGA are removed before railroading the tracheal tube over the AIC. All techniques rely on the SGA being well placed over the laryngeal inlet, which in patients undergoing difficult airway management is often not the case.

     o **FOB intubation combined with VL**: this combination requires two clinicians, but the two devices work synergistically to make for a highly successful technique. It is described in Chapter 19.

     o **FOB on its own**: in the anaesthetised patient this usually requires assistance in creating a patent lumen through which to advance the FOB. A second person performing jaw thrust or gentle anterior traction on the patient's tongue, or use of an intubating oral airway are options.

4. Although it would rarely occur, *proceeding with FONA* is an option after failed tracheal intubation in the still-oxygenated patient. This would be unlikely to be the correct choice for elective surgery, but might be indicated during an emergency surgical case or resuscitation.

Failed Oxygenation: the 'Cannot Intubate, Cannot Oxygenate' Situation

Failure to oxygenate (or ventilate) the apnoeic patient despite *optimised* attempts at FMV, SGA placement and tracheal intubation defines a 'cannot intubate, cannot oxygenate' (CICO) situation. The default manoeuvre when CICO is encountered is rapid performance of FONA. Recommendations for location and technique of FONA in CICO vary and are discussed in detail in Chapter 20. In brief, most guidelines recommend access via the cricothyroid membrane and use of a scalpel-based cricothyroidotomy for the adult patient. Needle cricothyroidotomy with jet (high-pressure source) ventilation in the emergency, CICO setting is associated with a substantial failure and morbidity rate.

Whilst many guidelines espouse a final attempt at FMV or SGA placement in the CICO situation, the guiding principle is to perform FONA in a timely fashion in a still viable patient. Thus, 'last ditch' attempts at SGA placement or FMV should occur *in parallel* with preparations for FONA and thus not delay proceeding rapidly with FONA. That said, prior to performing FONA an attempt with an SGA should have been undertaken. If not already given or no longer acting, a neuromuscular blocker should be administered.

Because FONA often occurs too late to save a patient from brain damage or death, some recent guidelines have espoused a 'priming' principle when airway management difficulty is encountered in the unconscious patient. Thus, should a primary technique not succeed (e.g. tracheal intubation), a call for help should be initiated, as should consideration of awakening the patient if feasible. If a second modality (e.g. FMV) then also fails, equipment for performing FONA should be obtained and the team briefed on the potential impending need for FONA. Failure of a third modality of airway management (e.g. use of an SGA) would trigger the declaration of a CICO situation and onset of FONA.

After successful eFONA, options in the now re-oxygenated patient include proceeding with unhurried attempts at oral or nasal tracheal intubation, allowing the patient to awaken followed by de-cannulation, or if the requirement for longer term FONA is anticipated, surgical consultation to assess whether conversion from cricothyroidotomy to tracheostomy is warranted.

Extubation of the Difficult Airway Patient

Large-scale studies of airway-related morbidity are consistent in their findings that up to a quarter of events relate to extubation or tracheal tube exchange. Especially when tracheal intubation was initially difficult or might now be, great care must occur upon extubation. Consideration should be given to leaving a small-diameter placeholder airway exchange catheter in the trachea upon extubation. Equally, an airway exchange catheter can be used to aid tracheal tube exchange, if indicated. This topic is explored in more detail in Chapter 21.

Conclusions

A structured step-by-step approach to airway management is essential. Airway planning should address management of both the anticipated and unanticipated difficult airway. Patient assessment prior to airway management, including evaluation of anatomical, physiological and contextual issues, will help optimise patient safety by identifying potentially difficult situations as well as patients in whom no difficulty is anticipated. The unanticipated difficult airway is probably the most common difficult airway situation (because most bedside airway screening tools have low sensitivity), so appropriate preparation is crucial for every airway intervention. Effective airway management is dependent on prior experience with a variety of techniques and devices, equipment availability, teamwork, communication and adherence to guidelines or local standardised protocols.

Further Reading

Amathieu R, Combes X, Abdi W, et al. (2011). An algorithm for difficult airway management, modified for modern optical devices (Airtraq laryngoscope; LMA CTrach): a 2-year prospective validation in patients for elective abdominal, gynecologic, and thyroid surgery. *Anesthesiology*, **114**(1), 25–33.

ANZCA. (2016). *Guidelines for the Management of Evolving Airway Obstruction: Transition to the Can't Intubate Can't Oxygenate Emergency* [cited 2018 January 22]. Available at: http://www.anzca.edu.au/getattachment/resources/profes sional-documents/ps61_guideline_airway_cogniti ve_aid_2016.pdf.

Apfelbaum JL, Hagberg CA, Caplan RA, et al. (2013). Practice guidelines for management of the difficult airway: an updated report by the American Society of Anesthesiologists Task Force on Management of the Difficult Airway. *Anesthesiology*, **118**(2), 251–270.

Chrimes N. (2016). The Vortex: a universal 'high-acuity implementation tool' for emergency airway management. *British Journal of Anaesthesia*, **117**(Suppl 1), i20–i27.

Cook TM, Woodall N, Frerk C; Fourth National Audit Project. (2011). Major complications of airway management in the UK: results of the Fourth National Audit Project of the Royal College of Anaesthetists and the Difficult Airway Society. Part 1: anaesthesia. *British Journal of Anaesthesia*, **106**(5), 617–631.

Cook TM, Woodall N, Harper J, Benger J; Fourth National Audit Project. (2011). Major complications of airway management in the UK: results of the Fourth National Audit Project of the Royal College of Anaesthetists and the Difficult Airway Society. Part 2: intensive care and emergency departments. *British Journal of Anaesthesia*, **106** (5), 632–642.

Duggan LV, Ballantyne Scott B, Law JA, Morris IR, Murphy MF, Griesdale DE. (2016). Transtracheal jet ventilation in the 'can't intubate can't oxygenate' emergency: a systematic review. *British Journal of Anaesthesia*, **117**(Suppl 1), i28–i38.

Frerk C, Mitchell VS, McNarry AF, et al. (2015). Difficult Airway Society 2015 guidelines for management of unanticipated difficult intubation in adults. *British Journal of Anaesthesia*, **115**(6), 827–848.

Heidegger T, Hagberg CA. (2018). Algorithms for management of the difficult airway. In: Hagberg CA, Artime CA, Aziz MF (Eds.), *Hagberg and Benumof's Airway Management*. 4th ed. Philadelphia: Elsevier. pp. 203–214.

Heidegger T, Schnider TW. (2017). 'Awake' or 'sedated': safe flexible bronchoscopic intubation of the difficult airway. *Anesthesia & Analgesia*, **124**(3), 996–997.

Heidegger T, Gerig HJ, Ulrich B, Kreienbuhl G. (2001). Validation of a simple algorithm for tracheal intubation: daily practice is the key to success in emergencies – an analysis of 13,248 intubations. *Anesthesia & Analgesia*, **92** (2), 517–522.

Law JA, Broemling N, Cooper RM, et al. (2013). The difficult airway with recommendations for management – part 1 – difficult tracheal intubation encountered in an unconscious/ induced patient. *Canadian Journal of Anaesthesia*, **60**(11), 1089–1118.

Mosier JM, Joshi R, Hypes C, Pacheco G, Valenzuela T, Sakles JC. (2015). The physiologically difficult airway. *The Western Journal of Emergency Medicine*, **16**(7), 1109–1117.

Norskov AK, Rosenstock CV, Wetterslev J, Astrup G, Afshari A, Lundstrom LH. (2015). Diagnostic accuracy of anaesthesiologists' prediction of difficult airway management in daily clinical practice: a cohort study of 188 064 patients registered in the Danish Anaesthesia Database. *Anaesthesia*, **70**(3), 272–281.

Piepho T, Cavus E, Noppens R, et al. (2015). S1 guidelines on airway management: Guideline of the German Society of Anesthesiology and Intensive Care Medicine. *Anaesthesist*, **64**(Suppl 1), 27–40.

Rosenblatt W, Ianus AI, Sukhupragarn W, Fickenscher A, Sasaki C. (2011). Preoperative endoscopic airway examination (PEAE) provides superior airway information and may reduce the use of unnecessary awake intubation. *Anesthesia & Analgesia*, **112**(3), 602–607.

Pre-anaesthetic Airway Assessment

Chapter 5

Carin A. Hagberg, Gang Zheng and Pierre Diemunsch

Introduction

Recommended by the major anaesthesia societies around the world, pre-anaesthetic airway assessment is essential for all patients undergoing anaesthesia care. An adequate airway assessment provides fundamental information to aid developing airway management strategies. Conventional airway assessment focusses on the patient's airway characteristics to stratify risk factors for a difficult airway, in which the success of direct laryngoscopy and intubation, placement of supraglottic airway (SGA) and face mask ventilation are challenging. The primary goal of airway evaluation is to ensure that potential issues are identified and safety measures are adequately addressed. With the advancement of technology, more advanced airway tools and techniques continue to be added to the toolbox such as transnasal high flow humidified oxygen and the various video-assisted tracheal intubation tools and their corresponding accessories. These new tools are expanding our vision and advancing airway management methodology. The airway assessment should also reflect these changes; and the strategy of risk stratification should be focussed on the clinical feasibility of using available advanced airway tools and techniques and their corresponding risk factors of failure. In practice, failure of airway management is often the escalating result of composite errors. Thus, assessing the impacts of human factors including the influences of environment, team and person in airway management should be a routine practice and is addressed in this chapter as well.

Conventional Airway Assessment Strategies

Conventional airway assessment includes a review of the patient's history, diagnostic imaging and a bedside interactive airway examination. The assessments aim to detect potential risks for difficulty in direct or videolaryngoscopy and tracheal intubation, SGA

insertion, face mask ventilation and increased risk of pulmonary aspiration, intolerance of apneoa and difficulty in oxygen delivery to the lungs. The recommended components of pre-anaesthetic airway assessment are listed in Box 5.1.

History

The patient history should be evaluated for potential risk factors. Clinical conditions associated with a difficult airway may be the result of congenital abnormalities of the face and upper aerodigestive tract; airway pathology such as head and neck trauma, airway infection, tumour or acquired airway defects; and chronic medical conditions or diseases.

Congenital Conditions

Children with congenital syndromes associated with difficult airway management are usually seen in an anaesthesia paediatric clinic. Some of the common clinical features associated with difficult airway management found in these syndromic patients include limited neck mobility and shortness of the neck resulting from fusion of cervical vertebrae in Klippel–Feil syndrome, micrognathia and retraction of the tongue due to mandibular hypodysplasia in Pierre Robin syndrome and Treacher Collins syndrome, and macroglossia and small mouth opening in Beckwith–Wiedemann syndrome and Goldenhar syndrome. Down syndrome (trisomy 21) is associated with multiple airway issues, including macroglossia, short neck and atlantoaxial instability. Multiple dysmorphic features may coexist in the same patient. Predicting airway difficulty is based on assessment of the abnormalities and their impacts on airway management. However, for patients with an abnormal aerodigestive tract such as mucopolysaccharidosis in Hurler syndrome and subglottic stenosis in Down syndrome, prediction of a difficult airway is mainly based on a previous diagnosis, history of airway obstruction such as significant sleep apnea, or findings of bedside flexible endoscopy.

Table 5.1 The TRS airway assessment tool for patients with head and neck tumour

Score	T (Tumour)	R (Radiotherapy)	S (Surgery)
0	Small tumour without respiratory symptoms	Slight skin change without restriction of neck mobility	Uncomplicated neck dissection without involvement of airway
1	Large oropharyngeal tumour with some difficulty breathing but no stridor	Skin discolouration and thickening without impedance of neck motion	Minor surgery in upper aerodigestive track without the need for reconstructive surgery
2	Bulky laryngeal tumour resulting in stridor	Acute or chronic radiation-related complications including microsites, dermatitis, skin sloughing and oedema, or tissue fibrosis with loss of mobility or anatomical landmarks	Extensive upper aerodigestive track resection with complex reconstruction with various flaps

Modified from Truong A et al., 2018.

Box 5.1 The components of airway evaluation

- History of previous airway difficulty
- Medical conditions that could be associated with difficulty
- History of previous surgery or radiotherapy to the head, neck or mediastinum
- External overall assessment
- Bedside interactive tests
- Accessibility of the cricothyroid membrane
- Implications of the presenting disease with regard to airway management
- Review of relevant diagnostic imaging

Airway Pathology

Various airway pathologies or acquired tissue defects from previous surgery are seen in head and neck patients. The major challenges in airway management in these individuals are the results of obstruction of airflow or the intubation path or changes in airway anatomy. A patient's previous airway history is unlikely to be helpful if there has been disease progression. Further, because disease locations vary, conventional airway assessment tools may not be reliable in evaluating the impact of disease on the airway. For those who have disease in the oral cavity or oropharynx, direct visual inspection is often sufficient for forming a management plan. For patients with a lesion in the deep airway, bedside flexible endoscopy (see Chapter 6) and reviewing imaging studies are essential. Assessing the airway in patients with head and neck pathology requires special considerations and methods. An example of

this is the novel *TRS score* for patients with head and neck pathology. In this system, the airway is evaluated with the components of Tumour, Radiation and Surgery (TRS) with each component rated from 0 to 2 to reflect the minimal, moderate and severe impacts of tumour, radiotherapy and surgery to airway management respectively (Table 5.1). The cumulative score not only indicates the potential difficulty of airway management but is also proposed by the authors as an 'airway time-out' tool for the entire team to perform prior to managing the airway.

Computed tomography (CT) is the most commonly used imaging modality in patients undergoing head and neck surgery. The findings of the CT scan are used to delineate the extent of the pathology and how it affects the airway. Because the effects of disease on the airway may be asymmetric, the series of images from all three planes (transverse, coronal and sagittal) should always be reviewed. In addition to various airway pathologies, the tonsils (especially the lingual tonsil), vallecular space and hypopharyngeal volume may be evaluated with CT imaging in a patient with a grossly normal airway. A hypertrophic lingual tonsil imposes a mass effect in the hypopharyngeal space and thus increases the difficulty of laryngoscopy and visualisation of the glottis (Figure 5.1a–c).

However, due to the limits of CT imaging in spatial resolution, variations in imaging methods, and variation in phase of the respiratory cycle at the time of image capture, CT imaging cannot be relied on to accurately measure the calibre of the airway and to adequately estimate the level of tissue oedema of various anatomical sites.

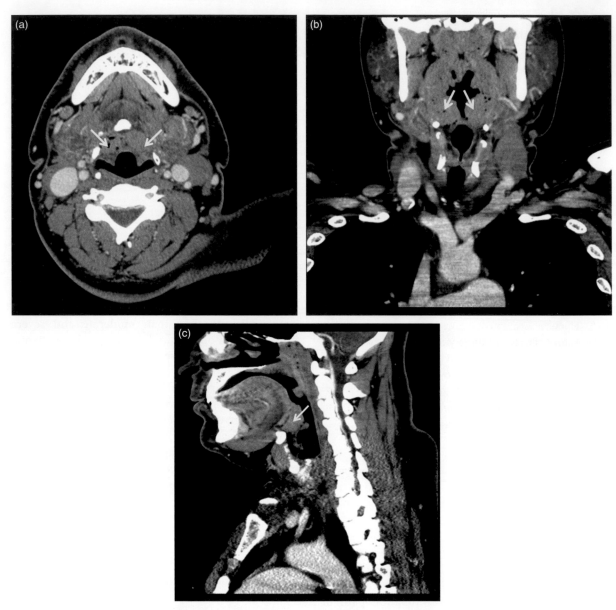

Figure 5.1 (a–c) Computed tomography (CT) imaging of the airway in a patient with grossly normal airway anatomy. Yellow arrows show a significantly hypertrophic lingual tonsil in the transverse (a), coronal (b) and sagittal (c) planes.

Medical Conditions Associated with Difficult Airway

Airway management can be complicated by the effects of chronic diseases. Three conditions with particular relevance are rheumatoid arthritis, ankylosing spondylitis and obstructive sleep apnoea.

Rheumatoid arthritis is characterised by destructive inflammation in the joints, principally affecting the small joints. Involvement of the temporomandibular

and/or cricoarytenoid joints and the cervical spine may impose significant impacts on airway management. In patients with rheumatoid arthritis, the atlantoaxial joint may be affected with attenuation of the transverse ligament and erosion of the odontoid process.

While radiographic evidence of atlantoaxial subluxation is present in up to 40% of patients with rheumatoid arthritis, clinical syndromes are uncommon.

Table 5.2 Subtypes of atlantoaxial subluxation

Subtype	Prevalence (%)	Changes	X-ray presentation	Precaution
Anterior	80	Forward movement of C1 on C2. Destruction of transverse/apical ligaments	> 3 mm gap between odontoid process and arch of atlas	Avoid flexion
Posterior	5	Backward movement of C1 on C2. Destruction of odontoid process	Deficiency of odontoid process on lateral flexion view	Avoid extension
Vertical	10–20	Displacement of odontoid process through foramen magnum. Destruction of lateral mass of C1	> 4.5 mm movement of odontoid process above McGregor line on lateral view	Avoid extension
Lateral/ rotatory	5–10	Lateral or rotational shift of C1 from C2	> 2 mm of misalignment of C1/C2 on open-mouth odontoid view	N/A

Four atlantoaxial subluxation subtypes have been described: anterior, posterior, vertical, and lateral rotatory; anterior is the most common. When subluxation is present neck movement should be minimal during airway management. However, the neck range of motion varies by subtype. Table 5.2 summarises some of the clinical characteristics of atlantoaxial subluxation. A routine preoperative X-ray to rule out cervical joint subluxation is controversial.

Regarding assessment of generalised cervical condition in rheumatoid arthritis, there is poor correlation between radiographic findings and clinical symptoms or risk of harm, so these are of limited value. Scrupulous clinical assessment is the cornerstone of safe care here.

Patients with cricoarytenoid rheumatoid arthritis may present with dyspnoea and hoarseness, resulting in difficult passage of a tracheal tube due to local tissue oedema or the cricoarytenoid joint stiffness. Forceful insertion of an tracheal tube may cause dislocation of arytenoid cartilage from the cricoarytenoid joint. Bedside flexible endoscopy is important to verifying the airway condition. When the temporomandibular joint is involved, limited mouth opening curbs the ability to perform direct or videolaryngoscopy.

Ankylosing spondylitis is a painful chronic inflammatory arthritis affecting the spine and sacroiliac joints which can progress to cause fusion of the spine. The peak age of onset is 20–30 years. It is more prevalent in males. The impact of ankylosing spondylitis on airway management is primarily due to restriction of the range of movement in the cervical spine. In addition, restricted mouth opening may be seen in 10% of patients. The diagnosis of ankylosing spondylitis relies on clinical examination and radiological studies. However, bedside airway assessment often yields adequate information to develop an airway management strategy.

Obstructive sleep apnoea (OSA) is a common and underdiagnosed sleeping disorder. Male sex, advanced age, obesity, alcohol consumption and craniofacial abnormalities are considered predisposing factors. With an increasing elderly population, the population with undiagnosed OSA is growing substantially; as many as 90% of individuals with moderate to severe OSA have not been diagnosed. Definitive diagnosis is made by polysomnography. The severity of the disorder is determined by stratification using the apnoea–hypopnoea index. Routine preoperative testing for OSA is not recommended. Several tools, including the Berlin, STOP-Bang and STOP questionnaire and the Epworth Sleepiness Scale, have been evaluated for their accuracy in diagnosing OSA compared with polysomnography: overall this is suboptimal. Among all the screening tools, the STOP-Bang questionnaire is the most validated and widely accepted tool for preoperative screening in surgical patients (Table 5.3).

Risk assessment for patients at risk of OSA should focus on the factors hindering airway management, the impact of the surgical procedure on airway management and the availability of airway management resources.

Airway Examination

Conventional airway examination consists of external global assessment of facial structures and bedside

Table 5.3 STOP-Bang Questionnaire and scoring for evaluation of obstructive sleep apnoea

Measure	Question	Score	
		No	Yes
STOP			
Snore	Do you snore loudly?	0	1
Tired	Do you often feel tired, feel fatigue, or sleep in the daytime?	0	1
Observe	Has anyone observed you stopping breathing or gasping during sleep?	0	1
Pressure	Do you have or are you being treated for high blood pressure?	0	1
BANG			
BMI	BMI > 35 kg m^{-2}?	0	1
Age	Age of 50 years old or higher?	0	1
Neck	Neck circumference Male > 43 cm? Female > 4 cm?	0	1
Gender	Male gender?	0	1

BMI, body mass index.

Total score: 5–8 = high risk of obstructive sleep apnoea, 3–4 = intermediate risk, 0–2 = low risk.

interactive tests. External global assessment evaluates the gross anatomy of the face, patency of the nares, length of the upper incisors and whether the maxillary teeth are positioned anterior to the mandibular teeth. The bedside interactive tests measure the space availability and feasibility of placement of airway instrumentation. The choice of assessment tests or tools is at the discretion of the anaesthetist. Mallampati classification, assessment of mouth opening, measurement of thyromental distance and assessment of neck mobility are the most commonly performed bedside tests.

Mouth opening is one of the most relevant information for the selection of intubation technique and tool for airway management. It measures the maximal interincisor distance with full mouth opening. It should be measured in centimetres, but in practice, the examiner's fingers may measure the value described as 'finger(s) breadth mouth opening'.

Mallampati classification was initially proposed in 1985. Primarily, this three-score system was used to measure the proportion of the tongue size to the volume of oral cavity and oropharynx by the ability to visualise the faucial pillars, the uvula and soft palate. It was modified into a four point classification by adding visualisation of hard palate only as the highest class in 1987. This modified system is referred to as Modified Mallampati Classification or Samsoon and Young Modified Mallampati Classification. When measuring the Mallampati class, the patient should be in an upright position facing the examiner with maximal mouth opening and tongue protruding.

Thyromental distance (TMD) is used to estimate the size of mandible floor. The importance of this measurement is to estimate the mandibular space for the displacement of the tongue during direct laryngoscopy. When measuring, the patient is instructed to close the mouth and fully extend the neck in order to read the maximal distance between the chin (mentum) and the top of the thyroid notch. In practice, most physicians measure the distance by the fingerbreadth. With varying size of examiners' fingers, the accuracy of the documented measurement is often questionable.

Sternomental distance (SMD) measures the distance between chin and the upper border of sternal notch. When measuring, the patient is instructed to have the mouth closed and to fully extend the neck. The primary aim of this measurement is to examine the ability of neck extension; therefore, its clinical application is partially overlapped with assessing the neck range of motion. In practice, the measurement of SMD is less performed than the assessment of neck range of motion.

Mandibular protrusion test is used to assess the functionality of the temporomandibular joint (TMJ). It is used to estimate the ease of anteriorly lifting the mandible when performing laryngoscopy. When examining, the patient is instructed to place the lower teeth in front of upper teeth, or to bite the upper lip by placing the bottom teeth to bite the upper lip as high as possible. Inability to do so is indicative of decreasing the functionality of the TMJ. Poor mobility of the mandible is suggestive of difficult direct laryngoscopy.

Neck range of motion measures the neck flexion by the ability of chin touching the chest, and the neck extension by measuring the angle between the jaw (with mouth naturally opened) and a horizontal surface such as ground with full extension of the neck. In practice, this examination is usually done by the subjective judgement of the examiner.

Table 5.4 The components of conventional airway assessment

Component of assessment	Findings of the assessment	Significance of the value
Mouth opening	≥ 4 cm or 3 fingerbreadths	Small mouth opening may be indicative of difficult laryngoscopy
Modified Mallampati score	Class I: visualisation of faucial pillars, the uvula and soft palate Class II: visualisation of uvula and soft palate Class III: visualisation of soft palate and the root of uvula Class IV visualisation of hard palate only	Class III or IV is suggestive of increasing the difficulty of glottic opening exposure by direct laryngoscopy
Thyromental distance	≥ 6 cm or 3 fingerbreadths	< 6 cm is considered as a short thyromental distance and indicative of increasing the difficult direct laryngoscopy
Sternomental distance	≥ 12.5 cm	< 12 cm is considered as short sternomental distance and may be suggestive of decreasing the degree of neck extension
Mandibular protrusion	Ease of performing mandibular protrusion or upper lip biting	Inability to prognath increases the risk of difficulty of anteriorly lifting the mandible during direct laryngoscopy
Neck range of motion	Normal atlanto-occipital extension is 35°	Restriction of neck extension correlates with difficulty visualising the glottic opening

In general, the bedside airway assessment tests have low sensitivity, high variability and moderate specificity. Accuracy and reliability of the tests often depend on the patient's efforts and cooperation. Application of multiple bedside tests should be emphasised. Common conventional airway assessment tools and recommended corresponding values are listed in Table 5.4.

An important lesson learned from the NAP4 study was the delay and high failure rate by anaesthetists in establishing an emergency front of neck airway (eFONA). Reluctance and inexperience in performing an eFONA are universal issues in anaesthesia practice. However, assessment of the cricothyroid membrane has not traditionally been included in routine airway assessment. Both clinical experiences and studies showed that inability to identify cricothyroid membrane by palpation is a common issue. In practice, although it should be a last measure, performing an eFONA should be considered routine in airway management and therefore assessment of the potential route of access should also be routine. In this area of practice ultrasound has a major role (see Chapter 7).

With the progress of ultrasound technology, upper airway ultrasound has been used for pre-anaesthetic identification of the cricothyroid membrane, evaluating anatomical distortion, airway trauma and airway pathology. Because it can be used as a point-of-care device, ultrasound enables bedside airway assessment and facilitates airway management. It is likely that the potential for airway ultrasound as a modality for airway assessment and risk stratification will develop considerably in the next decade. The details of ultrasound in airway management are described in Chapter 7.

New Airway Assessment Technology

Conventional airway assessment methods may be augmented by novel tools and technology. Computer-assisted airway analysis with digital three-dimensional models or three-dimensional printed models reconstructed from the patient's CT or magnetic resonance imaging (MRI) data have been used for surgical planning and airway analysis. These models provide the opportunity for onsite measurement of structures of interest and enable the clinicians to analyse facial and airway characteristics in patients with complex airways. They may even enable 'in vitro' practice of proposed airway techniques. These techniques are non-invasive, enable a full assessment of the (static) airway and require minimal patient preparation. Compared with CT or MRI studies requiring interpretation by radiology specialists, three-dimensional airway models are easy to understand, readily used for planning management strategies for patients with pre-existing airway pathology and useful in teaching, research and patient education.

Cone-beam computed tomography (CBCT) is being evaluated for visualisation of airway anatomy, mechanics and pathology. Long-term obstruction of the upper airway often changes respiratory patterns and alters craniofacial structures, resulting in OSA, difficult ventilation and difficult management of airway instrumentation. Such anatomical changes include a narrow maxillary arch, crossbite, mandibular growth rotation and mandibular retrognathia. CBCT may be used to automatically or semi-automatically reconstruct the entire or segmental airway and to evaluate the airway abnormality and mechanics of the obstruction.

Virtual endoscopy involves reconstruction of a virtual model of the patient's airway using digital technology. Like three-dimensional printing it can be used to create a model in which the clinician can do a virtual 'fly through' and practise the airway techniques that might be used in clinical practice. Virtual endoscopy is described in Chapter 6.

Future Directions of Airway Assessment

New airway management techniques and tools continue to emerge. Videolaryngoscopy, including its combination with other techniques, provides solutions to previously unmanageable situations. High flow nasal oxygenation enables us to prolong oxygenation during apnoea for brief surgical procedures, obviating the needs for tracheal intubation or jet ventilation (see Chapter 8). The Tritube and Ventrain (Ventinova, Eindhoven, the Netherlands) (Chapter 18) enable controlled ventilation via a very small-calibre tracheal tube in patients with significant airway stenosis. These new devices are expanding our approach in managing complex airways, and providing new solutions for patients with acquired airway defects from previous surgery, airway trauma or cancer, that have previously challenged anaesthetists and surgeons. This evolution of techniques and technology needs to be integrated into our airway assessment strategies.

Software applications designed to facilitate communication and information sharing will also play a role in improving airway assessment and management. Failure in airway management with adverse patient outcome is invariably the result of a compound error. The traditional way of sharing airway information relies on patient report, or the 'difficult airway letter', which often offers little or no help in understanding the mechanism of difficulty. An advanced information tracking system (with appropriate data protection mechanisms) has great potential for pre-anaesthetic airway assessment. Such a system could enable physicians to share or exchange critical information such as treatment history, imaging, airway models and multimedia records such as video clips of airway instrumentation from previous endoscopic assessment or tracheal intubation.

Summary

The primary goal of airway evaluation is to ensure that potential issues are identified and safety measures are adequately addressed. The conventional airway tests emphasise the patient's airway characteristics; however, failure of airway management is often the escalating result of composite errors. Traditional methods of airway management are evolving all the time: in parallel to this it is important that the new technologies available for assessment are tested and where appropriate integrated into airway assessment to reflect this progress.

Further Reading

Alsufyani NA, Flores-Mir C, Major PW. (2012). Three-dimensional segmentation of the upper airway using cone beam CT: a systematic review. *DentoMaxilloFacial Radiology*, **41**, 276–284.

American Society of Anesthesiologists Task Force on Perioperative Management of Patients with Obstructive Sleep Apnea. (2014). Practice guidelines for the perioperative management of patients with obstructive sleep apnea: an updated report by the American Society of Anesthesiologists Task Force on Perioperative Management of Patients with Obstructive Sleep Apnea. *Anesthesiology*, **120**, 268–286.

Anderson J, Klock Jr AP. (2018). Airway assessment and prediction of the difficult airway. In: Hagberg CA, Artime CA, Aziz MF (Eds.), *Hagberg and Benumof's Airway Management*. 4th ed. Philadelphia: Elsevier. pp. 185–196.

Bradley P, Chapman G, Greenland K. (2016). Part 2. The traditional approach to normal and difficult airway assessment. In: Bradley P, Chapman G, Crooke B, Greenland K, *Airway Assessment*. ANZCA. Available at: www.anzca.edu.au/documents/pu-airway-assessment-2016 0916v1.pdf (Accessed 2 March 2019).

Chrimes N. (2016). The Vortex: a universal 'high-acuity implementation tool' for emergency airway management. *British Journal of Anaesthesia*, **117** (Suppl 1), i20–i27.

Chung F, Abdullah HR, Liao P. (2016). STOP-Bang questionnaire: a practical approach to screen for obstructive sleep apnea. *Chest*, **149**, 631–638.

Cook TM, Woodall N, Harper J, Benger J. (2011). Major complications of airway management in the UK: results of the Fourth National Audit Project of the Royal College of Anaesthetists and the Difficult Airway Society. Part 2: intensive care and emergency departments. *British Journal of Anaesthesia*, **106**, 632–642.

Kapur VK, Auckley DH, Chowdhuri S, et al. (2017). Clinical practice guideline for diagnostic testing for adult obstructive sleep apnea: an American Academy of Sleep Medicine clinical practice guideline. *Journal of Clinical Sleep Medicine*, **13**, 479–504.

Pearce A, Shaw J. (2011). Airway assessment and planning. In: *4th National Audit Project of the Royal College of Anaesthetists and Difficult Airway Society. Major Complications of Airway Management in the United Kingdom. Report and Findings*. Editors Cook TM, Woodall N, Frerk C. London: Royal College of Anaesthetists. pp. 135–142. ISBN 978-1-9000936-03-3. Available at: https://www.nationalauditprojects.org.uk/NAP4_home.

Truong AT, Truong DT, Rahlfs TF. (2018). TRS score: proposed mnemonic for airway assessment and management in patients with head and neck cancers. *Head & Neck*, **40**, 2757–2758.

Woodward LJ, Kam, PCA. (2009). Ankylosing spondylitis: recent developments and anaesthetic implications. *Anaesthesia*, **64**, 540–548.

6

Pre-anaesthetic Airway Endoscopy, Real and Virtual

William Rosenblatt and Imran Ahmad

In Greenland's three column model of the airway (see Chapter 14), the 'middle column' (i.e. the airway passage beyond the oropharynx) is the airspace most of which is beyond the vision of the unaided eye of the airway examiner. Long appreciated and routinely examined by the otolaryngologist, this anatomical and functional region of the airway is too often ignored by the anaesthetist or other clinician planning airway management. Ovassapian identified lingual tonsil hyperplasia (Figure 6.1) as a principal cause of unanticipated difficulty with direct laryngoscopy in patients who appear otherwise normal. Additionally, pathological lesions extending into the middle column from the supraglottic larynx (Figure 6.1), base of tongue and the glottis itself may likewise contribute to failure to see or intubate the larynx. Fortunately, most of the patients harbouring these pathologies will be known at the time of presentation to the operating room. However, uncontrolled data suggest clinicians may be poor at predicting difficulty – in 17% of patients with relevant pathology, the lesions interfere with routine airway management, while in 63% of these patients with an anticipated difficult airway based on clinical examination, no difficulty is encountered.

A thorough examination of the middle column has been shown to reduce the number of patients who are falsely identified as having a difficult- or easy-to-manage airway. A caveat is that this applies to patients without lingual tonsil hypertrophy, as this group has not been studied, though similar results might be anticipated.

Otolaryngologists commonly examine the middle-column region in their initial diagnostic and planning assessments especially when a lesion is known or suspected. This may be by CT, MRI or ultrasound imaging, use of an upper airway mirror or endoscopic examination. While, it might be expected that the description of these examinations would be helpful to the airway manager, the otolaryngologist's interpretation can often be irrelevant and even misleading in this respect. The

otolaryngologist's examination focusses on the extent of disease, the preservation of function and the immediacy of intended surgery, i.e., the level and likely progression of airway obstruction, pathological bleeding, interference with oral nutrition etc. The examination is not concerned with factors that may affect airway management such as the ability to face mask ventilate, place a supraglottic airway or intubate the larynx and trachea. All modalities of imaging may be deceptive in both underestimating the role of significant pathology or because they only capture a single point in time. Further, they are static images, often acquired with the patient only supine (CT, MRI), or only sitting (mirror and nasendoscopy) and with the head and neck in a neutral position, which may not be the position adopted during anaesthesia. Therefore, though these examinations may be helpful to the airway manager, they cannot be conclusive when planning management.

Preoperative Endoscopic Airway Examination with Nasendoscopy

Fortunately, techniques that enable bedside, point-of-care evaluation of the middle column are readily available to the anaesthetist, and in many cases are well within existing skill sets. Endoscopic evaluation of the upper airway can rapidly and safely be performed at the bedside, whether in a preoperative evaluation clinic, holding area or in the operating room. A flexible optical bronchoscope or nasendoscope can be used, and this requires minimal patient preparation. Rosenblatt and colleagues found that preoperative endoscopic airway examination (PEAE) altered the intended airway management plan – developed on clinical data alone – in one quarter of cases. Most examinations were reassuring compared with clinical decision making and prompted routine induction of anaesthesia and airway management. Conversely, in a small group of patients, PEAE revealed significant lesions that were not suspected

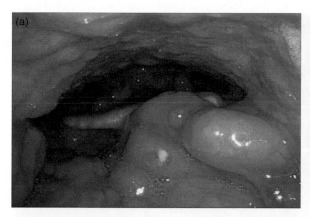
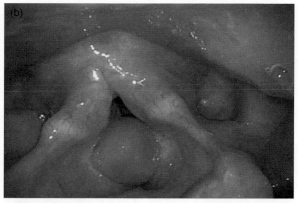

Figure 6.1 Findings causing unanticipated difficult direct laryngoscopy (a) Lingual tonsil hyperplasia and (b) epiglottic cyst.

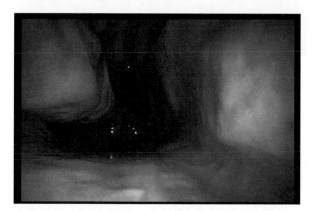

Figure 6.2 Path of flexible intubation scope passing beneath the inferior turbinate.

from patient history and physical examination, and awake management was chosen.

When performing PEAE, a small intubating bronchoscope or nasendoscope is used. A device with an external diameter < 4 mm is most comfortable for the patient. The patient's nares are prepared with a topical vasoconstrictor (e.g. oxymetazoline, phenylephrine) and a topical anaesthesia (e.g. 50 mg of lidocaine as spray, jelly or ointment) is placed using a cotton swab or soft catheter-on-syringe. Some patients will tolerate very small endoscopes without any topical anaesthesia. Anaesthetic preparation beyond the nose (i.e. the pharynx and hypopharynx) is not needed because the endoscope transverses these areas tangential to the sensitive posterior pharyngeal wall and little gag reflex is elicited provided the endoscope is controlled so as to not touch the superior side of the epiglottis. The endoscope is introduced into a naris, and a position below the inferior turbinate is maintained (Figure 6.2). Obstruction or pain should prompt further preparation and/or attempts in the opposite naris. It is common that the patient experiences some discomfort (usually pressure) as the turbinates are passed by the endoscope tip. Once the nasopharynx is reached, the examination should not be disturbing. Fogging of the endoscope objective lens may be resolved with a purposeful touch onto the posterior nasopharyngeal wall. At this position the hinged end of the endoscope is deflected downward and the examination continues. Generally, most information will be gained once the epiglottis is seen. Should the operator need to pass the point at which the glottis is seen, the examination should proceed slowly and deliberately, following the patient's respiratory phases which lift the epiglottis off the posterior pharyngeal wall during inspiration. The arytenoids, false and true vocal cords should not be contacted. Asking the patient to breathe more deeply, protrude their jaw or to repeat the letter 'e' may improve the ease with which the glottis is seen.

Though the examination will likely provide obvious information that will help the clinician's airway management decision making, the authors always seek three distinct pieces of information:

1. Is there a non-obstructed path to the larynx?
2. Is there any finding that would prevent use of a supraglottic airway from seating, should this be used as a rescue device after intubation failure?
3. Is there any anterior sitting structure that might be damaged or caused to bleed should a bladed instrument (e.g. direct or videolaryngoscopy) be used?

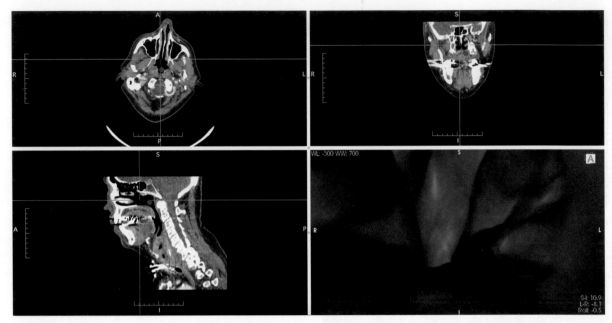

Figure 6.3 CT and virtual endoscopy view of the velopharynx.

Any of these findings should prompt the operator towards an awake approach to airway management.

Virtual Endoscopy

Though endoscopy is a technique familiar to the anaesthetists, and diagnostic nasoendoscopy should be easy to master, other technologies may provide similar information without the potential for patient discomfort and complications such as epistasis. Should the appropriate imaging be available, three-dimensional reconstructed CT data can be used to create a virtual endoscopy.

For a number of years radiologists have been using image navigation and display software to create virtual endoscopy images to aid pathological diagnosis and to guide biopsies of the tracheobronchial tree. Following on from this, virtual endoscopy has been introduced into anaesthetic practice to assess and plan airway management of patients with airway pathology.

Digital Imaging and Communications in Medicine (DICOM) data files from a previously acquired CT examination are imported into software such as the free OsiriX Lite Viewer v5.5 32-Bit (Pixmeo Sari, Bernex, Switzerland) and used to construct a three-dimensional 'fly-through' video of the relevant airway anatomy. The result is an anatomically accurate depiction of the patient's upper airway in a format familiar to all anaesthetists that can contribute to the planning of airway management strategies, even before the anaesthetist meets the patient face to face (Figures 6.3–6.5). Importantly, unlike PEAE, virtual endoscopy can also be used to image deep into the tracheobronchial tree to examine subglottic, tracheal and bronchial lesions that may be of concern.

The preoperative virtual endoscopy video of a patient with head and neck pathology enables better understanding of the airway anatomy and enables planning of the optimal pathway for flexible endoscopic intubation in either an awake or anaesthetised patient. The concept of a 'virtual warm up' on high fidelity bronchoscope simulators before flexible intubation has been shown to improve the clinical performance and time to intubation.

Virtual endoscopy is an emerging and encouraging technology, though the literature supporting its use is only starting to appear. El-Boghdadly and colleagues demonstrated that adding virtual endoscopy videos to review of conventional CT images improved the anaesthetist's diagnostic accuracy of airway pathology by ≈13% and led to changes in airway management in half of cases, 90% of which involved a more cautious plan. Overall, this suggests improved safety.

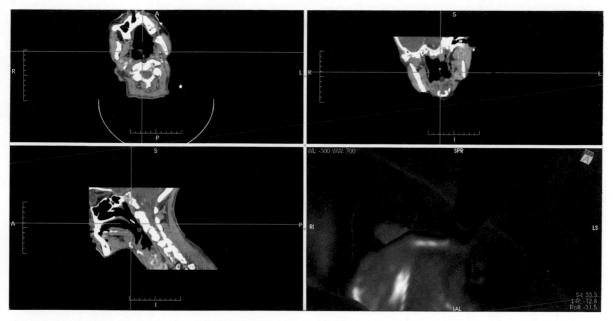

Figure 6.4 CT and virtual endoscopy view of the epiglottis and nasogastric tube.

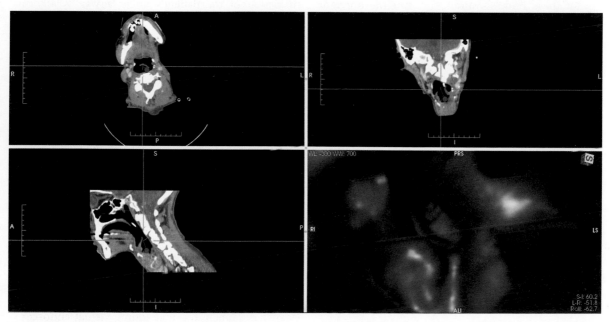

Figure 6.5 CT and virtual endoscopy view of the glottis.

The quality of the fly-through videos is dependent on the quality of the uploaded DICOM data files, natural colour is absent and there is excessive smoothening of the airway walls. Some small lesions may not be reconstructed based on the resolution of the original CT data capture, and the anatomy of three-dimensional fly-though is static, not reflecting the dynamic changes that occur with the respiratory cycle. Many of these limitations of virtual endoscopy technology are likely to be resolved with improved data acquisition and processing technology.

The knowledge that much of a patient's airway is beyond the reach of the anaesthetist's routine examination has prompted an effort to improved access to imaging of the middle column. Preoperative endoscopic airway examination and virtual endoscopy are two promising tools for any airway manager. In the absence of the information made available by these technologies, the anaesthetist must maintain increased vigilance and a high suspicion that obstructive lesions may be present in the patient with head and neck pathology. Alternative plans to routine airway care (e.g. awake intubation) should be given a high priority in such patients.

Further Reading

Ahmad I, Millhoff B, John M, Andi K, Oakley R. (2015). Virtual endoscopy – a new assessment tool in difficult airway management. *Journal of Clinical Anesthesia*, 27, 508–513.

El-Boghdadly K, Onwochei DN, Millhoff B, Ahmad I. (2017). The effect of virtual endoscopy on diagnostic accuracy and airway management strategies in patients with head and neck pathology: a prospective cohort study. *Canadian Journal of Anaesthesia*, 64, 1101–1110.

Ovassapian A, Glassenberg R, Randel GI, et al. (2002). The unexpected difficult airway and lingual tonsil hyperplasia: a case series and review of the literature. *Anesthesiology*, 97, 124–132.

Rosenblatt W, Ianus AI, Sukhupragarn W, Fickenscher A, Sasaki C. (2004). Preoperative endoscopic airway examination (PEAE) provides superior airway information and may reduce the use of unnecessary awake intubation. *Anesthesia & Analgesia*, 112, 602–607. http://doi.org/10.1213/ANE.0b013e3181fdfc1c

Samuelson ST, Burnett G, Sim AJ, et al. (2016). Simulation as a set-up for technical proficiency: can a virtual warm-up improve live fibre-optic intubation? *British Journal of Anaesthesia*, 116, 398–404.

Ultrasonography for Airway Management

Wendy H. Teoh and Michael Seltz Kristensen

Ultrasonography is an indispensable tool in the hands of the anaesthesiologist to identify and mark the trachea and the cricothyroid membrane *before* embarking on further airway management or induction of anaesthesia in patients with predicted difficult airways, morbid obesity or pathology of the neck. Evaluating the ability to identify the trachea and the cricothyroid membrane is a fundamental part of airway examination before induction of anaesthesia, just as identification of predictors for difficult intubation or mask ventilation. We know from the literature that clinical methods have a disappointingly low success rate especially in the morbidly obese and patients with pathology of the neck (8–39%), whereas ultrasonography reaches 80–100% success in these patients, and also improves success with cricothyroidotomy.

In this chapter, we describe in detail a systematic approach that will enable the clinician to identify and mark the trachea and the cricothyroid membrane *before* induction of anaesthesia, thus being prepared to undertake a front of neck airway access should it become necessary during subsequent airway management. This procedure is also beneficial for elective tracheotomy. With ultrasound, we can depict the airway from the tip of the tongue to the mid trachea, and at the pleural level (Table 7.1). There are numerous indications for ultrasonography in the management of the airway (Table 7.2): we describe the most important of these and for the rest we refer to the Further Reading. Ultrasound of the stomach is of increasing interest and is also discussed.

Airway-Ultrasound Technical Aspects

Tissue/Air Border

When the ultrasound wave travels through tissue and reaches air, a strong white line, the *tissue/air border*, appears because air has an extremely high

Table 7.1 Anatomical structures relevant for airway management and visible with ultrasonography

Mouth
Tongue
Oropharynx
Hypopharynx
Hyoid bone
Epiglottis
Vocal cords
Thyroid cartilage
Cricothyroid membrane
Cricoid cartilage
Trachea
Oesophagus
Lungs
Pleurae
Diaphragm
Gastric antrum

Reproduced with permission from www.airwaymanage ment.dk

resistance to ultrasound (Figure 7.1). Everything beyond that line is only artefact. This means that we can depict the tissue from the skin to the anterior luminal surface of the upper airway from the mouth to mid trachea.

Cartilage

Cartilage transmits ultrasound well and thus appears hypoechoic (black). The cricoid cartilage and tracheal rings normally remain cartilaginous throughout one's life (Figure 7.1), whereas the thyroid cartilage starts to calcify early in life, and thus becomes gradually less penetrable for ultrasound waves.

Lung sliding

When the transducer is placed over an intercostal space, the two ribs bordering the intercostal space are visible as two hyperechoic (light) lines with an underlying shadow (Figure 7.2). Lying a bit deeper between the two ribs, a hyperechoic horizontal line is seen representing the visceral and parietal pleura and called the *pleural line*. A horizontal motion of the pleural line, called *lung sliding*, can be seen, synchronous with the patient's breathing or ventilation. The motion represents the movement of the visceral pleura. (See video at http://www

.airwaymanagement.dk/ultrasonography-in-airway-management.) When M-mode scanning is applied, the corresponding characteristic image is called the *seashore sign* because the area under the pleural line looks like a sandy beach and the parallel lines above look like waves.

Lung Pulse

Every heartbeat pushes the lungs a tiny bit; this is visible on ultrasonography as a small double motion at the pleural line synchronous with the pulse. In the breathing or ventilated lung this is difficult to see because the lung sliding will be dominant. But in a lung that is not being ventilated, it becomes easily visible (Figure 7.3).

Localisation of the Cricothyroid Membrane and Trachea

The success rate of anaesthesiologists attempting to perform lifesaving cricothyroidotomy is unsatisfactorily low despite it being the ubiquitously recommended procedure when ventilation and oxygenation with non-invasive methods fail. The inability to identify the cricothyroid membrane by external visualisation or palpation is an important contributor to this low success rate, and misplacement is the most common complication when attempting cricothyroidotomy. In order to improve the success rate of emergency cricothyroidotomy it has been recommended to identify the cricothyroid membrane before induction of anaesthesia in all patients. If identification by inspection and/or palpation is not possible, then it can be performed with the help of ultrasonography,

Table 7.2 Clinical applications for airway ultrasonography

Evaluation of pathology that can affect the management of the airway

Diagnosing sleep apnoea

Determine the nature and volume of stomach contents

Predict the optimal single-/double-lumen-tube-diameter

To guide blockade of the recurrent laryngeal nerve

Identify the cricothyroid membrane for cricothyroidotomy

Identify trachea for tracheotomy

Confirmation of tracheal, endobronchial or oesophageal intubation

Ruling out/diagnosing pneumothorax

Identification of vocal cord palsy

Diagnosing pleural or pulmonary disease

Predicting successful extubation/weaning from ventilator

Major applications for airway ultrasonography. Only those in bold are described in this chapter, for the rest please see Further Reading.

Reproduced with courtesy from www.airwaymanagement.dk

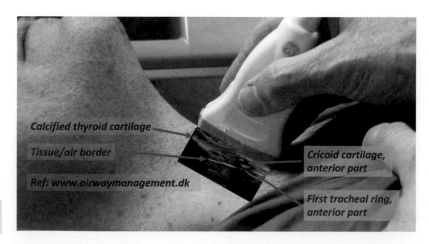

Figure 7.1 This shows the white (hyperechoic) appearance of the tissue/air border, the black (hypoechoic) appearance of cartilage and the white appearance of the calcified part of the thyroid cartilage. (Reproduced with permission from The Scandinavian Airway Management course www.alrwaymanagement.dk.)

Calcified thyroid cartilage

Tissue/air border

Ref: www.airwaymanagement.dk

Cricoid cartilage, anterior part

First tracheal ring, anterior part

LUNG SLIDING

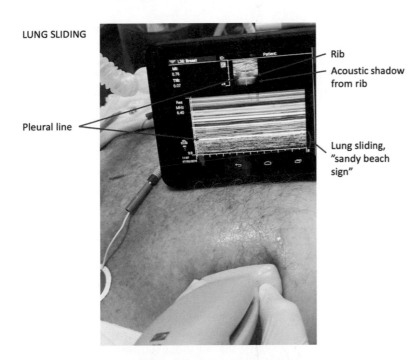

Rib

Acoustic shadow from rib

Pleural line

Lung sliding, "sandy beach sign"

Figure 7.2 Scan of the right lung and pleura with A-mode in the small upper screen image and M-mode visible in the lower larger part of the screen. Transducer is placed so that two ribs are seen with the pleural line just deep to the ribs. Lung sliding is seen, indicating that the lung is in contact with the parietal pleura and is ventilated. (Reproduced with permission from The Scandinavian Airway Management course www.airwaymanagement.dk.)

LUNG PULSE

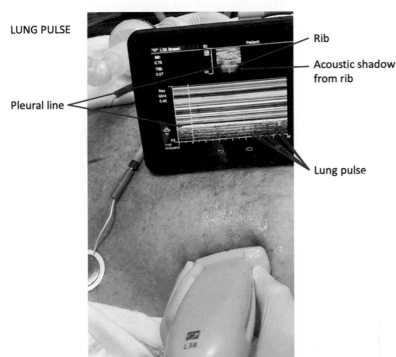

Rib

Acoustic shadow from rib

Pleural line

Lung pulse

Figure 7.3 Scan of the right lung and pleura with A-mode in the small upper screen image and M-mode visible in the lower larger part of the screen. Transducer is placed so that two ribs are seen with the pleural line just deep to the ribs. Lung pulse is seen, but no lung sliding, indicating that the lung is in contact with the parietal pleura but is not ventilated. (Reproduced with permission from The Scandinavian Airway Management course www.airwaymanagement.dk.)

which greatly improves the success rate. Ultrasound guidance not only reveals the location of the cricothyroid membrane, but also the depth of tissue between the skin and the airway lumen. Studies have shown that if the midpoint of the cricothyroid membrane is identified with ultrasonography and marked with a pen, even if the patient's head and neck position changes (e.g. is subsequently manipulated as in a failed intubation attempt), then the original marking will still be accurate and correctly sited after the patient's head is brought back to the original position in which the marking was performed. Ultrasonography has been shown to improve cricothyroidotomy success rate in human cadavers and in clinical case reports.

Two techniques have been described for the systematic, stepwise identification of the cricothyroid membrane:

- The longitudinal *string of pearls* technique
- The transverse TACA – Thyroid–Airline–Cricoid–Airline – technique

The *string of pearls* technique is the most well published and it has proven its superiority over palpation in a cadaveric study that demonstrated its ability to increase success and limit tube misplacement in cricothyroidotomy. The same technique can be used to identify the best interspace between tracheal rings for tracheostomy placement. We recommend the longitudinal technique as the first to learn and as the initial technique to use, such that every anaesthesia department dealing with difficult airways on a regular basis should have the expertise to apply it. On occasions when one encounters a patient with a very short neck, or flexion deformity of the neck, that leaves no space to place the ultrasound transducer in the longitudinal position, the transverse *TACA* technique may be the only successful technique. When both the longitudinal and the transverse techniques are applied in tandem, the cricothyroid membrane can be identified in close to 100% of cases.

Longitudinal, String of Pearls Technique

1. Standing on the patient's right side, the sternal bone is identified and the transducer is placed transversely on the patient's neck just cephalad to the suprasternal notch to visualise the trachea as a horseshoe-shaped dark structure with a posterior white line (Figure 7.4, first row).
2. The transducer is slid towards the patient's right side (towards the operator), so that the right border of the transducer is positioned at the midline of the trachea. The ultrasound image of the tracheal ring is thus truncated into half on the screen (Figure 7.4, second row).
3. The right end of the transducer is maintained over the midline of the trachea, while the left end is rotated 90° upwards into the sagittal plane resulting in a longitudinal scan of the midline of

the trachea. A number of dark (hypoechoic) rings will be seen anterior to the white hyperechoic line (air–tissue border), akin to a string of pearls. The dark hypoechoic 'pearls' are the anterior part of the tracheal rings (Figure 7.4, third row). In patients with a short neck most of the tracheal rings may be behind the sternal bone.

4. The transducer is kept longitudinally in the midline and slid cephalad until the cricoid cartilage comes into view (seen as a larger, more elongated and anteriorly placed dark 'pearl' compared to the other tracheal rings. Further cephalad, the distal part of the thyroid cartilage can be seen as well (Figure 7.4, fourth row). The longitudinal midline of the airway can now be depicted by marking the skin at the midpoint of each end of the transducer with a pen.
5. While still holding the transducer, the other hand is used to slide a needle (as a marker, for its ability to cast a shadow in the ultrasound image) between the transducer and the patient's skin until the needle's shadow is seen midway between the caudal border of the thyroid cartilage and the cephalad border of the cricoid cartilage (Figure 7.4, fourth row).
6. Now the transducer is removed, and the needle marks the centre of the cricothyroid membrane in the transverse plane and this can be marked on the skin with a pen. The midpoint of the cricothyroid membrane is at the cross section of the two lines.

A video of the technique is at http://airwaymanagement.dk/pearls.

Transverse TACA Technique (Thyroid Cartilage, Airline, Cricoid Cartilage, Airline)

1. Estimate where the level of the thyroid cartilage is on the neck and place the ultrasound transducer transversely over it, scanning to identify the thyroid cartilage as a hyperechoic triangular structure (Figure 7.5, first row).
2. Move the transducer caudally until the cricothyroid membrane is identified: this is recognisable as a hyperechoic white line resulting from the echo of the air–tissue border of the mucosal lining on the inside of the membrane, often with parallel white lines (reverberation artefacts) below (Figure 7.5, second row).

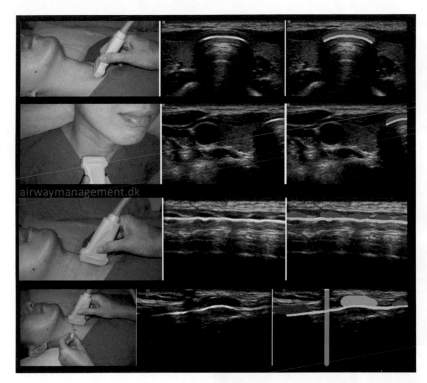

Figure 7.4 The longitudinal *String of pearls* technique for identifying the cricothyroid membrane and the interspaces between tracheal ring: see text for details. Orange-red = tracheal ring, light-blue = tissue-air border, green = cricoid cartilage, purple = distal end of the thyroid cartilage, yellow = shadow from the needle slid in between the transducer and the skin. (Reproduced with permission from The Scandinavian Airway Management course www .airwaymanagement.dk.)

3. Move the transducer further caudally until the cricoid cartilage is identified (a *black lying C* with a white lining) (Figure 7.5, third row).

4. Finally, move the transducer slightly back cephalad until the centre of the cricothyroid membrane is identified again (Figure 7.5, fourth row).

5. Mark the skin at the midpoint of the transducer at both ends and both sides and then connect these four marks after removing the transducer, to create a cross at the midpoint of the cricothyroid membrane. The centre can be marked both transversely and sagittally on the skin with a pen. By identifying both the highly characteristic shapes of the thyroid and the cricoid cartilages, both the cephalad and caudal borders of the cricothyroid membrane can be identified.

A video of the technique is at http://airwaymanage ment.dk/taca.

The combined technique, in which the course of the trachea is identified with the longitudinal technique, verified with the TACA technique followed by marking the midpoint of the cricothyroid membrane and performing a cannula cricothyroidotomy, all in less than a minute, is shown in a video at http://airwaymanagement.dk/US_guided _cannula_cric.

Confirmation of Tracheal, Oesophageal or Endobronchial Intubation

The ultrasound probe is placed transversely on the neck just cranial to the suprasternal notch. A tracheal ring is visualised and the oesophagus is usually seen on the posterior left side of the trachea (Figure 7.6). When the tube is passed into the trachea it will either result in just a brief 'flicker' at the anterior tracheal wall or not be seen at all, whereas an oesophageal intubation will distend the normally collapsed oesophagus and result in the '*double trachea sign*' (Figure 7.6). If the tube is in the oesophagus it can be withdrawn and reinserted before ventilation is started. After intubation, the transducer is placed at a rib interspace bilaterally and bilateral lung sliding (Figure 7.2) confirms correct tracheal intubation. If the tip of the tube is in the right

67

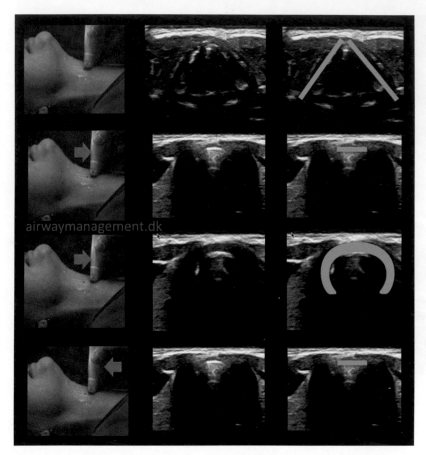

Figure 7.5 The transverse TACA: Thyroid-Airline-Cricoid-Airline technique for identifying the cricothyroid membrane: see text for details. Blue triangle = thyroid cartilage, blue horizontal line = the 'airline' = the cricothyroid membrane, blue 'lying C' = the anterior part of the cricoid cartilage. (Reproduced with permission from The Scandinavian Airway Management course www.airwaymanagement.dk.)

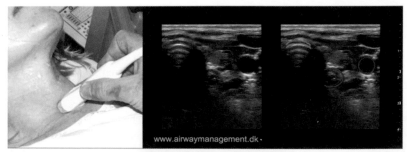

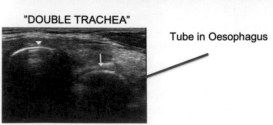

"DOUBLE TRACHEA"

Tube in Oesophagus

Figure 7.6 Ultrasonography during tracheal intubation. The transducer is placed just cranial to the jugular notch. The oesophagus is seen to the posterior left of the trachea (marked in purple). Blue curved lines represent the anterior part of a tracheal ring and the red circle represents the common carotid artery. On the lower image the tube is in oesophagus, this creating the *double trachea* sign. (Reproduced with permission from The Scandinavian Airway Management course www.airwaymanagement.dk.)

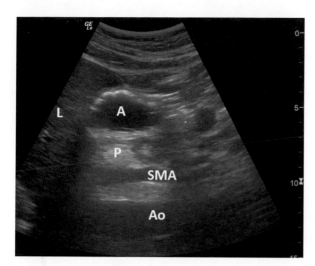

Figure 7.7 A cross-sectional view of the gastric antrum in the epigastric area in the right lateral decubitus position. A = gastric antrum, L= liver, P = pancreas, Ao = aorta, SMA = superior mesenteric artery. (Reproduced with permission from Anahi Perlas, University of Toronto, Canada.)

main-stem bronchus this will result in lung sliding on the right and lung pulse (Figure 7.3) on the left: the tracheal tube can be withdrawn gradually until there is lung sliding bilaterally.

Ruling Out an Intraoperative Pneumothorax

The detection of lung sliding or lung pulse (Figures 7.2 and 7.3) confirms that there is contact between the parietal and the visceral pleura at the point where the transducer is, and thus rules out the presence of a pneumothorax at that point of the thoracic cage. In the supine patient, free air in the pleural cavity will rise against gravity and accumulate just below the anterior chest wall. Hence, when scanning the anterior surface of a supine patient's chest, the presence of lung sliding or lung pulse excludes a pneumothorax on the side that is examined. If there is a pneumothorax typically a *bar code* sign will be seen in M-mode; this consists of only parallel lines indicating that there is no movement taking place as there is no contact between the pleural layers.

Determining the Nature and Volume of Stomach Contents

Gastric ultrasound can determine the nature (empty, clear fluid or solid) and volume of stomach contents. A cross-sectional view of the gastric antrum in the epigastric area is obtained with a curvilinear probe in the supine and right lateral decubitus positions and antral findings correlate with those of the entire organ. The antral findings thus allow the examiner to precisely predict the content of the whole stomach (Figure 7.7). Based on qualitative findings, the type of content is first assessed: no content in an empty stomach, hypo-echoic homogeneous content with clear fluids and heterogeneous and/or hyperechoic content with thick fluids or solid. Identification of an empty stomach or one with solid content has obvious implications for aspiration risk (low vs. high respectively). In the presence of clear fluid content, a volume assessment can help differentiate baseline gastric secretions (Grade 0 or 1 antrum with < 1.5 mL kg^{-1}) with negligible aspiration risk vs. higher than baseline volumes that may increase the risk of aspiration (Grade 2 antrum and/or > 1.5 mL kg^{-1}). If fluid is not visible it indicates a Grade 0 antrum (empty), if fluid is visible in the antrum in right lateral decubitus position only it indicates a Grade 1 antrum. If fluid is visible in both supine and in right lateral decubitus position it indicates a Grade 2 antrum. The gastric volume can be precisely determined by measuring the cross-sectional area (CSA) of the antrum: Gastric volume (ml) = 27 + 14.6 × Right lateral CSA (cm^2) − 1.28 × age. Alternatively, tables and a flowchart can be used to assess gastric volume and starvation status based on measuring the antral area (Table 7.3 and Figure 7.8).

Acknowledgements

Anahi Perlas, MD, Professor, Department of Anesthesia, University of Toronto, Toronto Western Hospital, UHN, Canada. For contribution and figure describing gastric ultrasonography.

Michael Friis-Tvede, MD, Rigshospitalet, University Hospital of Copenhagen, Denmark. For uploading and maintaining the videos on www.airwaymanagement.dk.

Table 7.3 Table used to determine the volume of gastric content from antral ultrasound measured cross-sectional area (CSA).

Right Lat CSA (cm^2)	Age (y)						
	20	30	40	50	60	70	80
2	31	18	5	0	0	0	0
3	45	32	20	7	0	0	0
4	60	47	34	21	9	0	0
5	74	62	49	36	23	10	0
6	89	76	63	51	38	25	12
7	103	91	78	65	52	40	27
8	118	105	93	80	67	54	41
9	133	120	107	94	82	69	56
10	147	135	122	109	96	83	71
11	162	149	136	123	111	98	85
12	177	164	151	138	125	113	100
13	191	178	165	153	140	127	114
14	206	193	180	167	155	142	129
15	220	207	194	182	169	156	143
16	235	222	209	200	184	171	158
17	249	236	224	211	198	185	173
18	264	251	239	226	213	200	187
19	278	266	253	240	227	214	202
20	293	281	268	255	242	229	217
21	307	295	282	269	256	244	231
22	323	310	297	284	271	259	246
23	337	324	311	298	285	273	260
24	352	339	326	313	301	288	275
25	366	353	340	327	315	302	289
26	381	368	355	343	330	317	304
27	395	382	369	357	344	331	318
28	410	397	385	372	359	346	333
29	424	411	398	386	373	360	347
30	439	427	414	401	388	375	363

(Reproduced with permission from gastricultrasound.org.)

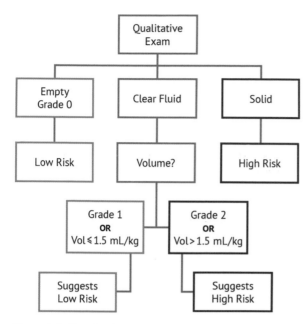

Figure 7.8 Algorithm for interpreting gastric contents and risk of aspiration. Reproduced from gastricultrasound.org. with permission.

Further Reading

Kristensen MS. (2011). Ultrasonography in the management of the airway. *Acta Anaesthesiologica Scandinavica*, **55**, 1155–1173.

Kristensen MS, Teoh WH. (2018). Front of neck: continued discovery of this anatomy essential for airway management. *British Journal of Anaesthesia*, **120**, 895–898.

Kristensen MS, Teoh WH, Graumann O, Laursen CB. (2014). Ultrasonography for clinical decision-making and intervention in airway management: from the mouth to the lungs and pleurae. *Insights into Imaging*, **5**, 253–279.

Kristensen MS, Teoh WH, Rudolph SS. (2016). Ultrasonographic identification of the cricothyroid membrane: best evidence, techniques, and clinical impact. *British Journal of Anaesthesia*, **117**(Suppl 1), i39–i48.

Mallin M, Curtis K, Dawson M, Ockerse P, Ahern M. (2014). Accuracy of ultrasound-guided marking of the cricothyroid membrane before simulated failed intubation. *American Journal of Emergency Medicine*, **32**, 61–63.

Perlas A, Van de Putte P, Van Houwe P, Chan VW. (2016). I-AIM framework for point-of-care gastric ultrasound. British Journal of Anaesthesia,**116**, 7–11.

Teoh WH, Kristensen MS. (2014). Ultrasonographic identification of the cricothyroid membrane. *Anaesthesia*, **69**, 649–650.

Oxygenation: before, during and after Airway Management

Søren Steemann Rudolph and Anil Patel

Introduction

Hypoxia is one of the most serious risks facing patients during anaesthesia, with prolonged hypoxia leading to arrhythmia, haemodynamic decompensation, hypoxic brain injury and death. Preventing hypoxia throughout airway management is a major priority for all clinicians who manage the airway. Patients can experience hypoxia during induction, maintenance and recovery from general anaesthesia. To counter the risk of hypoxia during airway management pre-oxygenation, which is an essential component of airway management, is recommended in all patients before induction of general anaesthesia, management of the airway or extubation.

In this chapter, we will review pre-oxygenation and peri-intubation oxygenation techniques, which may reduce the risk of critical hypoxia during airway management.

Pre-oxygenation

Pre-oxygenation is the administration of oxygen prior to induction of general anaesthesia and airway management and is considered a minimum standard of care. The main goal of pre-oxygenation is to delay the onset of oxyhaemoglobin desaturation during apnoea, often referred to as the 'safe apnoea time'. The safe apnoea time can be defined as the period of time until critical arterial oxygen desaturation (S_aO_2 88–90%) occurs following cessation of breathing/ventilation. Arterial saturation at 88–90% marks the upper inflection point on the oxygen–haemoglobin dissociation curve beyond which further decreases in P_aO_2 lead to a rapid decline in S_aO_2 ($\approx$30% every minute) (Figure 8.1).

During apnoea oxygen consumption is approximately 200–250 mL min^{-1} ($\approx$3 mL kg^{-1} min^{-1}). The physiological objective of pre-oxygenation is to increase the total body store of oxygen thereby increasing the time until depletion, and hypoxia, occurs. This

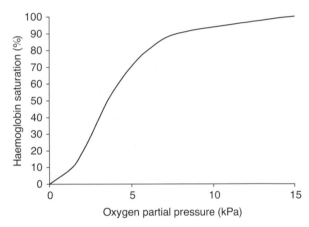

Figure 8.1 Oxygen–haemoglobin desaturation curve.

is achieved by increasing the oxygen stores in the lungs, blood, tissue fluids and in combination with myoglobin. The most significant increase takes place in the lungs where replacing nitrogen in the functional residual capacity (FRC) with oxygen (often referred to as 'denitrogenation') can increase oxygen stores from $\approx$450 mL breathing air to 3000 mL breathing 100% oxygen.

The FRC is the most important oxygen store in the body and in simple terms the greater the FRC, the longer the safe apnoea time. In a healthy pre-oxygenated patient the safe apnoea time is up to 8 minutes, compared to $\approx$1 minute breathing air. There are multiple conditions that will decrease safe apnoea time. These include

- conditions leading to reduced FRC (e.g. obesity, pregnancy, intra-abdominal pathology, ventilation/perfusion mismatching)
- airway occlusion
- increased oxygen consumption
- anaemia
- dyshaemoglobinaemia

- inadequate pre-oxygenation.

Many of these conditions frequently coexist in critically ill patients

Efficacy and Efficiency

The efficacy of pre-oxygenation relates to the ability to achieve end-tidal oxygen (ETO_2) > 90% and is dependent on the anaesthesia circuit used, oxygen flow rate, FRC and alveolar ventilation ($\dot{V}A$).

The efficiency of pre-oxygenation is defined by the rate of decline in arterial oxygen saturation and ultimately this is what is important in pre-oxygenation, i.e. the extension of the safe apnoea time. This is dependent on (i) the efficacy of pre-oxygenation (oxygen stored at the beginning of apnoea), (ii) the capacity for additional oxygen to be bound to haemoglobin during apnoea (e.g. by apnoeic oxygenation) and (iii) oxygen consumption (which is increased in many conditions including sepsis, pyrexia, pregnancy, obesity and in infants).

As an example, it is useful to consider the efficacy and efficiency of pre-oxygenation in a pregnant mother. She has *good efficacy* with her increased alveolar ventilation (rapidly filling her lung) and reduced FRC (less lung to fill), but *poor efficiency* with rapid oxygen desaturation due to reduced FRC (reduced oxygen store) and increased oxygen consumption.

ETO_2 monitoring is the gold standard in clinical practice for assessing denitrogenation of the lungs during pre-oxygenation and is a measure of efficacy. Optimal efficacy is achieved with ETO_2 > 90%, although this may not be achieved in some patients regardless of the method or duration of pre-oxygenation.

Methods

Methods of pre-oxygenation can be divided into slow and fast techniques. The rate of denitrogenation depends on the inspired fraction of oxygen, the inspired tidal volume relative to the FRC, and the respiratory rate.

Slow technique: *tidal-volume breathing technique.* Provide 100% oxygen via a tight-fitting face mask and ask the patient to breathe at normal tidal volumes for three or more minutes. If there are difficulties in achieving a good seal, a two-handed mask technique can be applied to create a better seal. Pre-oxygenation may be augmented by asking the patient to fully exhale before pre-oxygenation starts.

Fast technique: *deep breathing technique.* Provide 100% oxygen via a tight-fitting face mask and ask the patient to take eight deep vital capacity breaths in 60 seconds. The alveolar oxygen fraction increases rapidly, but total tissue oxygenation may not be as great as with the slow technique. An important limitation to this technique is that in many anaesthetic circuits the vital capacity (up to 5 L) may far exceed the volume of the circuit reservoir bag (usually 2 L), which will completely empty during inspiration and continuing inspiratory efforts will cause atelectasis, so counteracting the benefits of pre-oxygenation. Using an extra-large reservoir bag, increasing oxygen flow or by deploying the oxygen flush throughout this period may counteract this limitation.

Devices

Oxygen delivery devices may be divided into low flow and high flow systems. The principal difference being that low flow oxygen systems depend on inspiration of room air to meet the patient's inspiratory flow and volume demands, whereas high flow oxygen delivery systems are designed to provide the patient's entire inspiratory demands by providing either large oxygen reservoirs or flow rates. Low flow devices include standard nasal cannula, simple face masks, partial rebreather masks, non-rebreather mask and tracheostomy collars (Figure 8.2). The FiO_2 delivered by these systems depends on the degree of mixing of delivered oxygen with ambient air. This in turn depends on the patient's ventilatory pattern (tidal volume, peak inspiratory flow, respiratory rate and minute ventilation), the size of any device oxygen reservoir and the oxygen flow rate. These devices therefore deliver an unpredictable FiO_2 and are less suitable for optimal pre-oxygenation than high flow devices.

Low flow oxygen delivery systems may be used in combination (e.g. nasal cannula and non-rebreather mask) or at very high flow rates to provide efficient pre-oxygenation. Non-rebreather masks may thus provide an $FiO_2 \geq 0.9$ by increasing the oxygen flow rate to 30–60 L min^{-1} and provide a similar FiO_2 as bag-valve-mask (BVM) delivering 15 L min^{-1}. A BVM may be subjectively more difficult to breathe through and cause hypoventilation or rebreathing.

High flow oxygen delivery systems have flow rates and reservoirs large enough to provide the total inspired gases regardless of the patient's respiratory pattern. High flow devices include anaesthesia circuits, manual resuscitation bags with one-way valves on the expiratory port, aerosol masks and T-pieces

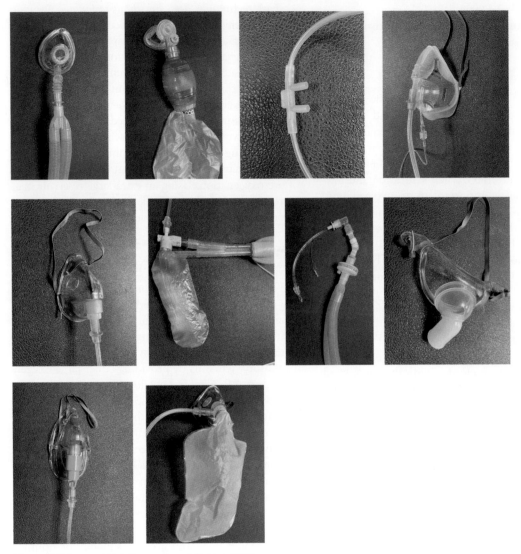

Figure 8.2 Low and high flow oxygen delivery systems.

that are powered by air-entrainment nebulisers or air-oxygen blenders and Venturi masks (Figure 8.2). These devices provide a fixed FiO_2 and most are capable of delivering an FiO_2 of 1.0. The primary limitations in regard to pre-oxygenation are cost, availability and bulkiness.

Positioning

Patients should be pre-oxygenated sitting up whenever possible.

In spontaneously breathing patients, a fully supine position will cause the diaphragm to move cephalad leading to compression atelectasis of the lower and dependent parts of the lung. The resulting reduction in FRC of 0.5–1.0 L will increase ventilation–perfusion mismatch (leading to hypoxia) and reduce pulmonary compliance. With increasing body mass index (BMI) and in pregnancy FRC and lung compliance are reduced with an exponential decrease in the oxygenation index (P_aO_2/P_AO_2).

Elevating the head of the bed reduces atelectasis and several studies have shown that the time to desaturation is increased by 20–30% in both normal-weight and obese patients by positioning the patient with the head of the bed elevated or in reverse Trendelenburg position.

An additional benefit of head elevation may be better laryngeal exposure during direct laryngoscopy, improved ease of intubation and reduced odds of intubation-related complications (see Chapter 14).

Increased Mean Airway Pressure

Pre-oxygenation with a high FiO_2 can lead to resorption atelectasis and while decreasing the FiO_2 to 0.8 prevents resorption atelectasis formation it reduces the duration of safe apnoea. Positioning and general anaesthesia, even in healthy patients, also increase atelectasis and intrapulmonary shunt, which further impair pulmonary gas exchange. The degree of atelectasis is greater in obese patients and pregnant patients. During pre-oxygenation, if patients have not achieved a saturation greater than 93% to 95% after 3 minutes of tidal-volume breathing with a high FiO_2 source, it is likely that they have a clinically significant physiological shunt; any further augmentation of FiO_2 is likely to be unhelpful. Physiological shunt can be partially overcome by augmenting mean airway pressure, thereby improving the effectiveness of pre-oxygenation and extending the safe apnoea time. Mean airway pressure may be increased during pre-oxygenation by continuous positive airway pressure (CPAP) masks. These may be connected to non-invasive ventilator machines or standard ventilators, or by using a positive end-expiratory pressure (PEEP) valve on a standard bag-mask. Both techniques will reduce atelectasis and improve safe apnoea time and are especially useful in the critically ill patient.

Evidence supports the use of increased mean airway pressure during pre-oxygenation in the operating theatre, emergency department and intensive care unit. Studies have consistently shown that CPAP improves oxygenation without negative cardiovascular effects or appreciable gastric insufflation.

Delayed Sequence Intubation: the 'Cannot Pre-oxygenate Patient'

In some patients altered mental status may prevent adequate pre-oxygenation and they can be categorised as 'cannot pre-oxygenate'. This may be due to agitated delirium from hypoxia, hypercapnia or the underlying medical condition. These patients are most often critically ill and induction of anaesthesia without adequate pre-oxygenation may lead to life-threatening adverse events. In these patients the technique of delayed sequence intubation (DSI) may be used as an alternative to traditional pre-oxygenation. The technique is particularly suitable for intubation out of hospital and in the emergency department (see Chapter 30).

DSI is procedural sedation, where the procedure is pre-oxygenation and it allows for a calm and controlled environment for optimised pre-oxygenation before airway management in an otherwise uncontrollable patient. Ketamine is the ideal agent for DSI as it preserves airway reflexes and respiratory drive.

Aliquots of ketamine are administered until the patient is dissociated, after which the patient can be positioned and pre-oxygenation can proceed using the techniques described above. Where necessary procedures such as gastric tube insertion can also be undertaken. When optimal pre-oxygenation is achieved a further dose of induction agent is administered if required, along with the muscle relaxant. Alternatively, if difficult laryngoscopy is expected the airway may be managed with preserved spontaneous ventilation.

DSI is only supported by limited observational data, but in these studies DSI was effective in improving oxygenation before intubation.

Apnoeic Oxygenation

During regular breathing approximately 250 mL min^{-1} of oxygen diffuse from the alveoli into the bloodstream and 200 mL min^{-1} of carbon dioxide return from the bloodstream to the alveoli. During apnoea oxygen continues to be used at a rate of 250 mL min^{-1}, while only 8–20 mL min^{-1} of carbon dioxide enter the alveoli from the bloodstream. The differential rates of oxygen removal and carbon dioxide diffusion into the lungs create a pressure gradient from the pharynx (atmospheric pressure) to the alveoli (subatmospheric pressure). This will in turn contribute to oxygen flow from the pharynx into the alveoli by a mass movement of gas if the upper airway is patent.

Apnoeic oxygenation has been known since the 1950s under various names, such as diffuse respiration, apnoeic diffusion oxygenation and aventilatory mass flow. Apnoeic oxygenation can be delivered via:

- nasal cannulae
- a buccal cannula
- a nasopharyngeal or oropharyngeal catheter with its distal tip lying above the vocal cords
- nasal or oral catheters with the distal tip lying beyond the vocal cords in the trachea
- bilateral endobronchial catheters in the right and left main-stem bronchi

- delivering oxygen through a side channel of a laryngoscope blade

Nasal cannulae are used most frequently and may be simple low flow devices (nasal specs) or more specialised high flow devices. High flow nasal cannulae are made by a number of manufacturers and can deliver humidified nasal oxygen over a broad range of FiO_2 and flows ($0-70$ L min^{-1}) and this technique is discussed further below.

Apnoeic oxygenation using standard nasal cannula typically uses nasal oxygen flow rates of $5-15$ L min^{-1}. Typically, pre-oxygenation uses both face mask and simple nasal cannula (the latter at oxygen flow rates of up to 5 L min^{-1}). Following induction of anaesthesia nasal oxygen is continued during intubation and the flow rate is increased to $10-15$ L min^{-1}.

Standard apnoeic oxygenation can only be applied for a limited amount of time as carbon dioxide levels rise, which can lead to severe respiratory acidosis. Usually laryngoscopy and tracheal intubation are achieved within minutes, in which case hypercarbia is of limited concern. Although no significant side effects of hypercapnia have been reported, prolonged apnoeic oxygenation should be used only in selected cases and avoided in patients with increased intracranial pressure, haemodynamic instability and cardiac arrhythmia.

Studies performed on elective surgical patients in the operating room have demonstrated that apnoeic oxygenation through various routes (nasal, buccal, nasopharyngeal, tracheal or endobronchial administration) prolongs safe apnoea time and reduces the incidence of oxygen desaturation without adverse effects.

High Flow Nasal Oxygenation

High flow nasal oxygen (HFNO) devices have been used for many years for management of the critically ill patient where the technique has been useful in preventing the need for intubation and for managing patients after weaning from mechanical ventilation.

More recently the technique has been introduced into anaesthetic practice and it has provided a number of new opportunities for safe airway management before and during surgery. HFNO requires the gas to be warmed and humidified to prevent damage to the nasal mucosa and for patient comfort. These are high flow oxygen delivery devices (as the oxygen flow

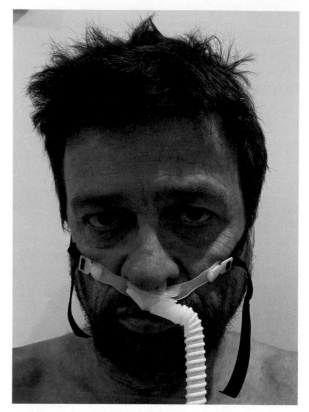

Figure 8.3 High flow (humidified) nasal oxygen.

is greater than peak inspiratory flow) and they are capable of delivering any desired FiO_2 up to 1.0 (Figure 8.3).

Advantages of HFNO with *spontaneous* breathing during pre-oxygenation at flow rates around 30 L min^{-1} include: (i) a reduction in the work of breathing, (ii) washout of pharyngeal dead space, (iii) PEEP, (iv) improved mucociliary clearance and (v) a constant FiO_2. Modern high flow nasal oxygen cannulae are soft and comfortable for patients to wear. Flow rates may be slowly increased to up to $70-80$ L min^{-1} and may provide PEEP at approximately 1 cmH$_2$O for every 10 L min^{-1} flow.

When HFNO is used during apnoea this has been termed transnasal humidified rapid-insufflation ventilatory exchange (THRIVE). This has been shown to have significant potential benefits during anaesthesia in some settings and some patient groups.

The rate of carbon dioxide rise during apnoea is generally considered to be ≈0.5 KPa min^{-1} but with HFNO this may be reduced to $0.15-0.2$ KPa

min^{-1}. The enhanced carbon dioxide clearance observed under apnoeic conditions with HFNO compared with classical apnoeic oxygenation is achieved by the combination of cardiopulmonary oscillations in the lower airway moving gases to the lower trachea where the turbulent gases from the HFNO are able to clear it to outside the patient's respiratory tract. This effect significantly slows the rise of P_aCO_2 and has the capacity to dramatically extend the safe duration of apnoeic oxygen making it a viable technique for surgery for some patients. HFNO has greater efficiency and efficacy than other methods of pre-oxygenation.

High Flow Nasal Oxygen Use in Anaesthesia

HFNO has been used for procedural sedation with spontaneous breathing to improve oxygenation and decrease the risk of desaturation during (i) awake tracheal intubation, (ii) bronchoscopy, (iii) transoesophageal echocardiography, (iv) gastrointestinal endoscopy and (v) awake tracheostomy. A recent survey of international experts with a track record of academic and clinical expertise in airway management showed the majority now use HFNO for awake tracheal intubation.

Two randomised controlled trials have compared pre-oxygenation between face mask and HFNO/THRIVE in adults undergoing rapid sequence induction (RSI) for emergency surgery. More accurately this could be termed *peroxygenation* – the period from the start of pre-oxygenation in an awake spontaneously breathing patient, induction of general anaesthesia, neuromuscular blockade, subsequent apnoea, laryngoscopy, confirmation of tube placement and finally lung ventilation. In the first study the P_aO_2 was similar in both groups immediately following intubation with the HFNO group having longer apnoea times and slower intubation. The second study showed 12.5% of patients in the control group desaturated below 93% compared to none in the HFNO group. These early studies offer the possibility of HFNO having benefit over traditional standard face mask pre-oxygenation but more evidence is required.

In the shared airway setting when surgical procedures are undertaken on the larynx or trachea the presence of a tracheal tube may make surgery more difficult (Chapter 26). An open airway with unimpeded surgical access can be provided in an apnoeic patient using apnoeic HFNO/THRIVE. To date 12 studies have described the use of apnoeic HFNO in shared airway microlaryngoscopy and pharyngolaryngoscopy procedures by otorhinolaryngologists including benign and malignant laryngeal lesions, head and neck pathology including hypopharyngeal obstruction and subglottic stenosis in adults.

As with any airway procedure shared decision making between anaesthetist and surgeon is essential. Apnoeic HFNO does not rescue total airway obstruction, does not replace good airway management or planning and requires an understanding of set-up, equipment, indications and contraindications. Apnoeic HFNO may fail to prolong the apnoea time as anticipated and a secondary plan for oxygenation should always be available. The efficacy of apnoeic HFNO varies between different groups and may be limited in paediatrics, increasing BMI (particularly super morbid obesity), severe shunt and restrictive lung disease.

The evidence supporting the use of HFNO outside the operating room, including the intensive care unit, emergency department and pre-hospital encounters, is less compelling but also less mature. While the current evidence shows that HFNO used for pre-oxygenation and continued throughout intubation may reduce hypoxaemic events in critically ill patients with normal or mild hypoxaemia, this has not been demonstrated in patients with significant hypoxaemia. It is important to understand that HFNO will support oxygen stores but it will not overcome airway obstruction or true shunt.

Risk Stratification

Not all patients have the same risk of hypoxia during airway management. Patients undergoing anaesthesia for elective surgical procedures, with no pulmonary pathology, adequate haemoglobin, low metabolic demand and pulse oximetry readings of 100% on room air, may be considered as low-risk patients. In contrast, patients undergoing anaesthesia for emergency surgical procedures, patients with physiological shunt, patients with increased oxygen consumption and those with hypoxia with pulse oximetry readings of ≤ 90% whilst breathing supplemental oxygen are

Table 8.1 A practical approach to oxygen therapy

Risk category	Patient factors	SpO$_2$	Pre-oxygenation	Onset of apnoea
Low	Normal weight Fasting Non-pregnant No cardio-pulmonary pathology Elective surgery	96–100% - on room air or 96–100% - emergency airway breathing supplemental O$_2$	Head of the bed elevated High flow system or augmented low flow system 3 minutes 8 vital capacity breaths EtO$_2$ 85–90%	Apnoeic oxygenation using simple nasal cannula or HFNO if prolonged laryngoscopy or emergency case
Intermediate	BMI > 40 kg m^{-2} Pregnant Cardio-pulmonary pathology Emergency	91–95% on supplemental O$_2$ or 91–95% after 3 minutes of pre-oxygenation	As above CPAP/PEEP Nasal O$_2$	As above Manual/mechanical ventilation
High	BMI ≥ 40 kg m^{-2} Critically ill Delirious/cannot pre-oxygenate	< 90% Hypoxic	As above Consider DSI approach	As above Consider awake intubation with spontaneous ventilation

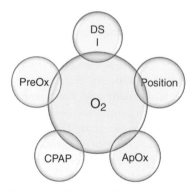

Figure 8.4 Techniques for providing or improving oxygenation throughout airway management. PreOx, pre-oxygenation; CPAP, continuous positive airway pressure; ApOx, apnoeic oxygenation; DSI, delayed sequence intubation.

high-risk patients. Patients with pulse oximetry readings of 93% or less are likely to continue to desaturate during the apnoeic period. Anaesthesia and airway management outside the operating room is a further risk factor for hypoxia. These patients are most often non-fasted, critically ill patients with decreased respiratory reserve and physiological shunt and will continue to be hypoxic despite pre-oxygenation. There is a higher risk of unexpected difficult intubation, a notably high rate of failure of primary intubation attempts and an associated high risk for numerous critical incidents and adverse

events (see Chapter 28). Some patients with features of each group can be categorised as of intermediate risk. The principles of management of low-, intermediate- and high-risk patients are summarised in Table 8.1 and of maintenance of oxygenation throughout anaesthesia and surgery in Figure 8.4.

Further Reading

Hermez LA, Spence CJ, Payton MJ, et al. (2019). A physiological study to determine the mechanism of carbon dioxide clearance during apnoea when using transnasal humidified rapid insufflation ventilatory exchange (THRIVE). *Anaesthesia*, **74**, 441–449.

Higgs A, McGrath BA, Goddard C, et al.; Difficult Airway Society; Intensive Care Society; Faculty of Intensive Care Medicine; Royal College of Anaesthetists. (2018). Guidelines for the management of tracheal intubation in critically ill adults. *British Journal of Anaesthesia*, **120**, 323–352.

Patel A, Nouraei SAR. (2015). Transnasal Humidified Rapid-Insufflation Ventilatory Exchange (THRIVE): a physiological method of increasing apnoea time in patients with difficult airways. *Anaesthesia*, **70**, 323–329.

Sakles JC, Chiu S, Mosier J, Walker C, Stolz U. (2013). The importance of first pass success when performing orotracheal intubation in the emergency department. *Academic Emergency Medicine*, **20**, 71–78

Simon M, Wachs C, Braune S, et al. (2016). High-flow nasal cannula versus bag-valve-mask for preoxygenation before intubation in subjects with hypoxemic respiratory failure. *Respiratory Care*, **61**, 1160–1167.

Weingart SD, Levitan RM. (2012). Preoxygenation and prevention of desaturation during emergency airway management. *Annals of Emergency Medicine*, **59**, 165–175.

Awake Tracheal Intubation

Charlotte Vallentin Rosenstock and Iljaz Hodzovic

Introduction

Awake tracheal intubation implies securing the airway in an awake spontaneously breathing patient with or without the use of sedation. Awake intubation is regarded as a gold-standard technique for difficult airway management. It will keep many options for airway management open when compared with those available after general anaesthesia and should be considered in any patient whose airway is predicted to be difficult to manage.

The ability of anaesthetists to predict airway management difficulty is uncertain due to a lack of reliable predictive tests. The decision-making process is further impeded by anaesthetists' apparent reluctance to perform awake intubation, even when clearly indicated, occasionally resulting in major airway complications or death. The potential for difficult airway management to cause harm cannot be emphasised enough and is supported by considerable evidence.

Awake intubation requires four vital elements for the anaesthetist to master: (i) continuous oxygenation, (ii) topicalisation, (iii) equipment handling skills and (iv) sedation. Laboratory and clinical training should provide opportunities for anaesthesiologists to practise equipment handling skills and awake intubation. In this chapter, we focus on the *awake* aspect of intubation. The details of intubation *techniques* are described in other chapters (see Chapters 16 and 17). Awake tracheostomy or cricothyroidotomy are discussed in Chapter 20.

Decision making

The decision to perform awake tracheal intubation should be guided by the most senior anaesthetist's skill and equipment availability and on thorough assessment of the patient's airway.

The authors use the following as broad guidance to decision making on whether to perform awake tracheal intubation or not. Predicted difficulty to oxygenate using a face mask or supraglottic airway (SGA) are clear indications for awake intubation. All patients with predicted difficult tracheal intubation should be considered for awake intubation: further information from imaging and nasendoscopy may be valuable. The need for awake tracheal intubation becomes clearer in patients with predicted difficult intubation when there is added aspiration risk, reduced apnoea tolerance (e.g. obesity) or a predicted difficult front of neck airway (FONA). Patients who have a previously documented difficult airway should also be considered for awake intubation.

Tip. Consider awake tracheal intubation if you think there is even a small chance that your patient may not be easy to oxygenate. This may include patients with obstructive sleep apnoea, morbid obesity, limited mouth opening or impending airway obstruction in patients with head and neck pathology.

Preparation for Awake Tracheal Intubation

Consent

The process of consent forms an important part of the awake tracheal intubation procedure. When the clinician judges it is desirable to perform awake tracheal intubation, the procedure should be clearly explained to the patient, to ensure informed consent. Before the procedure, it is good practice to document the patient's agreement to awake tracheal intubation and a summary of the discussion.

Complication. Consent refusal.

Solution. Patient refusal is a contraindication. However, by preparing your rationale for awake tracheal intubation prior to discussing with the patient and explaining the reasons it is a safer option, very few will disregard your claim. Explain to the patient that they will remain in control of the procedure as they can stop it at any time if they feel any discomfort and this will be dealt with before continuing.

Set-Up

Meticulous preparation before the start of the awake tracheal intubation procedure is likely to increase success. Decide the positioning of the operator, the patient, and the screen display from the device that you are using. They should be aligned so the operator, the patient and screen are in one line of sight requiring minimal head movement to refocus attention on each component (Figures 9.1 and 9.2). Two set-up positions are favoured by most anaesthetists:

- *Face-to-face*: this is the authors' preferred position for all awake flexible optical bronchoscope (FOB)-guided intubations (Figure 9.1). This set up enables the patient to be sitting upright (especially relevant in dyspnoeic patients) and encourages patient communication and visual monitoring of

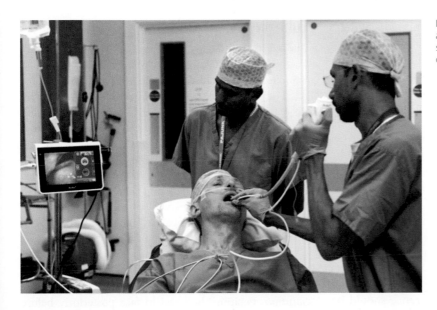

Figure 9.1 Face-to-face position for awake FOB-guided intubation. Degree of sitting up is adjusted according to patient condition and operator preference.

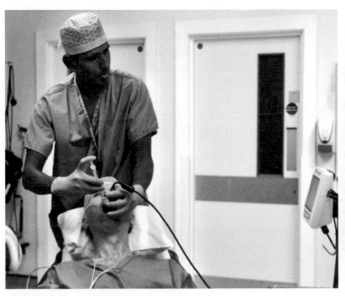

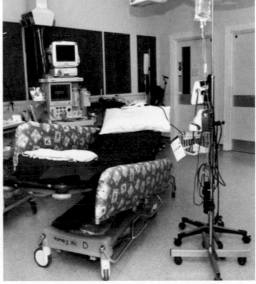

Figure 9.2 Head-end position for awake FOB- and videolaryngoscope-guided intubation using deckchair set-up.

the patient's level of sedation and comfort. It is also likely to be less intimidating for the patient.

- *Tip.* Face-to-face may be more difficult for the operator initially but after a few procedures the benefits are realised and few change back to head-end positioning.

- *Head-end*: some operators find it easier to stand at the head end of the patient due to the similarity of this set-up to direct laryngoscopy in an anaesthetised patient. This set-up, however, may reduce the flexibility of patient positioning (head-up position difficult to achieve) and reduces the ability to visually monitor and communicate with the patient. It may be the only option when performing awake videolaryngoscope-guided intubation. An acceptable compromise for awake videolaryngoscope-guided intubations may be a *deckchair position* with the patient sat up, but the trolley position adjusted so the head end is lowered to the desired level, aiming to keep both patient and operator comfortable (Figure 9.2).

The safest environment for performing awake tracheal intubation is in the operating theatre as this is large enough to accommodate extra equipment and additional anaesthetic and surgical personnel if needed.

When deciding about the route of intubation (nasal vs. oral) factors such as surgical access, presenting airway pathology, post-surgery airway management plan and the operator's preference should be considered. There is no evidence to support one route of intubation over the other.

Equipment

Laryngoscope

Awake tracheal intubation can be performed using any known method for intubation (see more options in Chapter 32) but in this chapter, we will focus on FOB- and videolaryngoscope-guided intubation. Current evidence suggests that awake videolaryngoscope-guided intubation is faster than FOB-guided intubation with equivalent success rate, safety profile and patient acceptance. Currently, there is no evidence to support the use of any individual videolaryngoscope design for awake intubation, but as there are few studies this may simply reflect a lack of evidence. A device with a blade that moves around the tissues rather than requires tissue displacement is logically preferable.

Tip. When learning to perform awake videolaryngoscope-guided intubation, prepare the patient and have both FOB and videolaryngoscope available. Try the videolaryngoscope first. If you or your patient becomes uncomfortable with the procedure, stop it and secure the airway with the FOB. Repeat this with different patients until you complete the intubation using a videolaryngoscope. Once acquired, you will find the skill of awake videolaryngoscope-guided intubation a very useful addition to your skill mix.

Tube Type

The size, type and bevel position of the tracheal tube have a significant impact on ease of awake tracheal intubation. Standard PVC tracheal tubes are not recommended for nasal or oral awake tracheal intubation as they are more likely to impinge on glottic structures and more difficult to railroad when compared to Parker-tip tubes (Bridgwater, CN, USA), intubating laryngeal mask airway tracheal tubes (LMA Fastrack TT, Teleflex, Beaconsfield, UK) and soft wire-reinforced tracheal tubes (Figure 9.3a). When advancing the tube over an FOB or over a bougie or stylet (when used to aid videolaryngoscope-guided intubation) the tracheal tube bevel should face posteriorly (Figure 9.3b).

Complication. Difficulty in railroading the tracheal tube.

Solution. Position the bevel to face posteriorly before entering the airway and keep that orientation throughout the railroading. This works better than 90° anticlockwise rotation during tube advancement for the tubes with bevels facing laterally. Trying to rotate the tube tip after advancing the tube over the scope may not work if the tube is constrained in the nose or impinging on the aryepiglottic folds. Try soft-tipped, tapered tracheal tubes such as ILMA or Parker tip (Figure 9.3a).

Oxygenation Technique

There is compelling evidence supporting the administration of oxygen during awake intubation. The incidence of desaturation ranges widely but may be up to 60% and is similar for both videolaryngoscope- and FOB-guided awake intubation. In many countries administration of oxygen is a required standard of care when administering sedation.

High flow (> 30 L min^{-1}) humidified nasal oxygen during awake tracheal intubation is gaining popularity and is the authors' preferred technique (Figure 9.4).

(a)

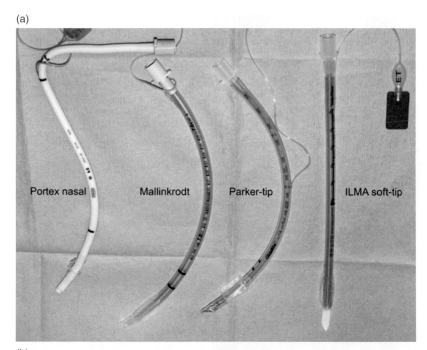

Portex nasal   Mallinkrodt   Parker-tip   ILMA soft-tip

Figure 9.3 (a) Tracheal tubes used for awake FOB-guided intubation. (b) Position of tracheal tube tips during tube advance. Note a large gap between the tip of the tube and FOB when the tube bevel is facing laterally.

(b)

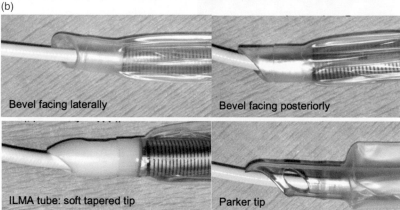

Bevel facing laterally   Bevel facing posteriorly

ILMA tube: soft tapered tip   Parker tip

Other techniques of oxygen administration during awake tracheal intubation, including nasal specs and nasal catheters, have also been reported.

Topicalisation and Nerve Blockade

Several techniques of local anaesthetic administration for awake tracheal intubation (topicalisation) have been described. These techniques include application of local anaesthetic using nebulisers, spray-as-you-go technique, transtracheal injection and glossopharyngeal and superior laryngeal nerve blocks. There is very little evidence supporting one technique of local anaesthetic application over another. Nerve blocks have been associated with lower patient comfort and

systemic toxicity and should not be undertaken by inexperienced operators.

Lidocaine is the most commonly used anaesthetic agent. Preparations of 2%, 4% and 10% lidocaine have been used for oral and nasal topicalisation. There is evidence of similar efficacy of 2% and 4% lidocaine when used in this setting. Although doses of 9.3 mg kg^{-1} lean body weight have been used without any manifestation of local anaesthetic toxicity, the British Thoracic Society recommends 8.2 mg kg^{-1} as a maximum dose of lidocaine administered topically for bronchoscopy. In general airway anaesthesia should be achievable with much more modest doses.

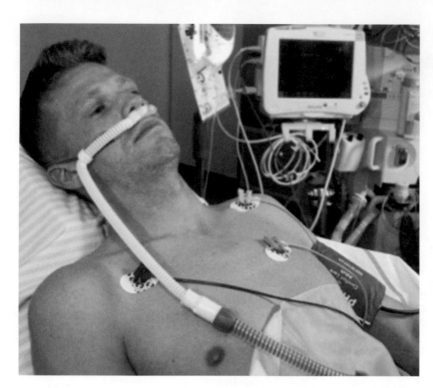

Figure 9.4 Oxygenation techniques during awake intubation: high flow humidified nasal oxygen (shown). Lower oxygen flow via nasal specs or nasal catheter is an alternative (not shown).

Cocaine, being a combined local anaesthetic and vasoconstrictor, was considered a suitable agent for nasal topicalisation but reports of myocardial infarction and coronary spasm associated with its use suggest it is best avoided.

Before nasal intubation a vasoconstrictor is recommended to reduce the incidence of bleeding and improve the view. Co-phenylcaine (5% lidocaine and 0.5% phenylephrine) has comparable anaesthetic and nasal vasoconstriction properties to cocaine without increasing risk of cardiovascular toxicity.

Administration of an anti-sialogogue, such as glyco-pyrrolate 0.1–0.2 mg, 40–60 minutes before the start of procedure may improve the view, but evidence that it provides benefit for awake tracheal intubation is limited.

Complications. Excessive secretions or blood in the airway. Inadequate topicalisation resulting in gagging and non-acceptance of the procedure. Non-acceptance of the videolaryngoscope blade during awake videolaryngoscope-guided intubation.

Solutions. Topicalise the airway sufficiently to enable you to remove most of the secretions using machine suction before continuing to topicalise for the actual procedure. Use a different local anaesthetic application technique to that you have used already (e.g.

gargling 4% or 10% lidocaine, swab application of lidocaine gel at the base of the tongue).

One of the authors uses atomised 10% lidocaine keeping the tip of the nozzle in the upper part of the oropharynx, applied liberally during first phase of inspiration. Successful application is marked with coughing during application. In case of awake video-laryngoscope-guided intubation try placing the blade after you are completely happy with topicalisation of the oropharynx. Be very meticulous and generous (dose adjusted) when applying your local anaesthetic.

With awake videolaryngoscope-guided intubation, larynx and trachea are anaesthetised once the blade is *in situ* using the display to guide your nozzle position.

Specific Nerve Blocks

These blocks are infrequently used. They require multiple bilateral injections, may fail and are more liable to complications than topical anaesthesia. However, in skilled hands they provide excellent airway anaesthesia.

The *sphenopalatine ganglion*, which lies in the posterior nose between the upper and middle turbinates, can be topicalised by administration transnasally of local anaesthetic with a soaked cotton wool tipped applicator or an atomiser spray. Onset is slow over several minutes.

The *glossopharyngeal nerve* lies deep to mucosa low down on the palatoglossal arch. It supplies sensation to much of the oropharynx, hypopharynx and the afferent arm of the gag reflex. With the tongue retracted medially it can be anaesthetised with several sprays of topical 10% lidocaine or injection of 1–2 mL lidocaine submucosally. Care is required as the carotid artery lies deep to the nerve.

The *internal branch of the superior laryngeal nerve* supplies sensation to the upper larynx. It runs over the hyoid bone just lateral to the greater cornu and then enters the thyrohyoid membrane. Walking a needle off the hyoid at the greater cornu and just penetrating this membrane enables nerve blockade with 2 mL of local anaesthetic.

A trans-cricothyroid membrane puncture and administration of 2–3 mL of 2–4% lidocaine will topicalise below the larynx and much of the trachea and due to the patient coughing also above the vocal cords. While not a specific block of the recurrent laryngeal nerve, it provides effective infra- and supra-laryngeal anaesthesia.

Sedation

In many cases, no sedation is required. A clinician's skill, gentleness and their reassurance of the patient may be all that is needed.

Patients scheduled for awake tracheal intubation may suffer from respiratory distress from either airway or respiratory pathology and may have pre-existing impairment of consciousness. These conditions need to be carefully evaluated prior to sedation of any kind. In these circumstances consider not using sedation at all. The administration of even minor amounts of sedation may result in complete loss of the airway thereby endangering the patient. Backup plans should be prepared and readily at hand.

When sedation is required, it is desirable to reach a situation where the patient is comfortable but remains able to cooperate during the procedure. The term *conscious sedation* is often used in this context. We recommend that the patient is monitored during the process by one person with the sole responsibility of administering and monitoring sedation necessary. The anaesthetist should aim for a patient who is cooperative, oriented and tranquil.

Requirements for drugs used for sedation are fast onset and effectiveness in reaching comfort, a minimum impact on airway tone and respiration and quick recovery following cessation. The combination of an anxiolytic and an analgesic would seem to be the rational choice for awake intubation. However, the requirements may vary from case to case. Most evidence supports the use of two drugs namely dexmedetomidine (bolus 0.7 to 1.0 µg kg^{-1} over 10 minutes followed by infusion rate 0.3 to 0.7 µg kg^{-1} h^{-1}) or remifentanil (bolus 0.75 µg kg^{-1} followed by infusion rate 0.0075 µg kg^{-1} min^{-1}). The anaesthetist must reach experience in using monotherapy or combining drugs as well as titrating doses to the desired effect.

Complications. Lack of patient compliance despite meticulous instructions, topicalisation and sedation necessitating general anaesthesia. Respiratory depression, hypoxaemia and loss of airway due to oversedation. Aspiration. Hypotension and bradycardia.

Solution. Avoid using sedation as a compensation for inadequate topicalisation. Time and patience in reaching a cooperative, oriented and tranquil state. Avoidance of the single sedationist-operator. Backup plans for failure with personnel and instruments prepared and ready for use.

Performing Awake Intubation

Prior to performing the intubation, topicalisation can be tested simply by asking the patient if he or she feels anaesthetised in the mouth and throat. This can be evaluated by touching the base of the tongue, uvula, bilateral pharyngopalatine fauces and posterior pharyngeal wall with a wooden spatula. The posterior nares can be stimulated with a suction catheter. Testing topicalisation with a suction catheter enables clearance of secretions at the same time just before undertaking the intubation procedure.

Videolaryngoscope-Guided

Awake videolaryngoscope-guided intubation is a valuable alternative to awake FOB-guided intubation. A major advantage is that the videolaryngoscope is used far more frequently than the FOB in routine daily clinical practice. Videolaryngoscope-guided intubation provides a wider view of the glottis aiding in recognition of anatomical landmarks and the tracheal tube may be seen during the whole intubation process, which may reduce airway trauma. The direct line of sight during laryngoscopy also improves clearing of secretions and blood. However, awake videolaryngoscope-guided intubation is impossible in patients with very restricted mouth opening or a space-occupying lesion within the mouth and in some patients with restricted access to the mouth (high body mass index, fixed flexed neck deformity in ankylosing spondylitis, obese term pregnancy). Videolaryngoscopes differ in blade design and methods of use and evidence is lacking on the most appropriate device for awake intubation. Most studied are the GlideScope, the Airway scope, the C-MAC Mac blade and the McGrath series V. In this context, different types of videolaryngoscopes may be relevant for different types of difficult airways.

FOB-Guided

The anatomical landmarks to follow naturally differ according to the approach. The type of surgery may determine whether the nasal or oral route should be used. If, however, left to the decision of the anaesthetist, the inexperienced operator may favour the nasal approach since the route to the trachea is more straightforward. Nasal railroading of the tube may be difficult; tube type, size and length as well as appropriate space for passage is crucial for success. For the oral approach, an oral conduit such as a Berman (see Chapter 16) or Ovassapian airway is generally used (placing this is a good test of topicalisation). The operator should look for the anatomical landmarks once the FOB has left the intubation conduit. If landmarks are not visible, repositioning of the conduit as well as tongue and jaw protrusion by the patient may improve visibility. Occasionally jaw thrust or gentle pulling on the tongue with a gauze swab by the assistant may be needed. Anatomical landmarks can be distorted or missing due to prior surgery, radiation therapy, oedema, a malignant or infectious process in the pharynx/larynx. Looking for air bubbles may direct the intubator to the tracheal inlet in case of distorted anatomy. After the identification of tracheal rings and the carina the tracheal tube is railroaded. As the FOB is removed it is useful to confirm the tip of the tracheal tube is an appropriate distance above the carina. The tracheal tube is then connected to the anaesthetic circuit and the cuff inflated. Provided topicalisation is of good quality the inflated cuff is well tolerated. Only after a capnography curve confirms positioning of the tube in the trachea and the cuff is inflated should general anaesthesia be induced. The suggested checks of tube position prior to induction of general anaesthesia apply to both FOB- and videolaryngoscope-guided awake intubation.

Complications. Blood or secretions in the upper airway obtunding or blurring the view of the glottic structures. Loss of the airway. Airway trauma.

Solutions. Thorough training and instruction of assistants reduces procedural complications. In the event of failure due to secretions or blood in the airway, placement of an SGA may keep the glottic structures clear of secretions and FOB-guided intubation can be continued through the SGA while preserving continuous oxygenation. It is important to confirm compatibility (length and diameter) of the SGA tube and the tracheal tube before changing to this technique (see also Chapter 13).

Extubation

In any patient with a difficult airway extubation requires the same level of planning and care as intubation. Delayed extubation, use of specialised airway adjuncts or techniques or a tracheostomy may each be appropriate. This is no different after awake tracheal intubation. This topic is discussed in Chapter 21.

Further Reading

Ahmad I, El-Boghdadly K, Bhagrath R, et al. (2020). Difficult Airway Society guidelines for awake tracheal intubation (ATI) in adults. *Anaesthesia*, **75**(4), 509–528.

Alhomary M, Ramadan E, Curran E, Walsh SR. (2018). Videolaryngoscopy vs. fibreoptic bronchoscopy for awake tracheal intubation: a systematic review and meta-analysis. *Anaesthesia*, **73**, 1151–1161.

Cook TM, Woodall NM, Frerk CM; Fourth National Audit Project. (2011). Major complications of airway management in the UK: results of the Fourth National Audit Project of the Royal College of Anaesthetists and the Difficult Airway Society. Part 1: anaesthesia. *British Journal of Anaesthesia*, **106**, 617–631.

Frerk C, Mitchell VS, McNarry AF, et al. (2015). Difficult Airway Society 2015 guidelines for management of unanticipated difficult intubation in adults. *British Journal of Anaesthesia*, **115**, 827–848.

Hinkelbein J, Lamperti M, Akeson J, et al. (2018). European Society of Anaesthesiology and European Board of Anaesthesiology guidelines for procedural sedation and analgesia in adults. *European Journal of Anaesthesiology*, **35**(1), 6–24.

Joseph TT, Gal JS, DeMaria SJ, et al. (2016). A retrospective study of success, failure, and time needed to perform awake intubation. *Anesthesiology*, **125**, 105–114.

Meghjee SPL, Marshall M, Redfern EJ, McGivern DV. (2001). Influence of patient posture on oxygen saturation during fibre-optic bronchoscopy. *Respiratory Medicine*, **95**, 5–8.

Roth D, Pace NL, Lee A, et al. (2018). Airway physical examination tests for detection of difficult airway management in apparently normal adult patients. *Cochrane Database of Systematic Reviews*, **5**, CD008874.

Chapter 10

Drugs for Airway Management

Lars S. Rasmussen

Difficulties in airway management can be related to anatomical factors, airway pathology and poor positioning but we should not forget the importance of the anaesthetist. Experience and manual skills are essential and the anaesthesia provider can have an important impact on the ability to manage the airway by administering drugs, which in turn can significantly increase the chance of securing the airway on first attempt. The optimal choice, timing and dosage of anaesthetic drugs for airway management will be described in this chapter.

The first step is always to have an airway management strategy, including alternatives if the primary plan fails. Anaesthetic drugs are used to optimise conditions according to that strategy. The results of the airway assessment and the anaesthetist's experience will guide decision whether to manage the airway with general anaesthesia or with local anaesthesia with or without sedation.

General anaesthesia can be managed with the intention to maintain spontaneous ventilation or with controlled ventilation. Airway tone will be reduced by most anaesthetics and this facilitates insertion of devices by jaw relaxation and depression of reflexes. Tracheal intubation is facilitated when the vocal cords are fully abducted and there is no vocal cord movement or coughing. This likely creates less laryngeal morbidity, including hoarseness and sore throat. The possible drawback is that it may not be possible to maintain spontaneous ventilation or an open airway.

Local anaesthesia for airway management may be combined with sedation. Sedation is used to ameliorate anxiety and discomfort in order to facilitate the airway management, but it carries the risk of overdosing with a transition to general anaesthesia. Sedation is a drug-induced alteration of consciousness during which patients should be able to respond purposefully to verbal commands. Variation in patient response to sedative agents and delayed onset of action may make titration of sedative drugs to obtain a desired level of sedation challenging.

Rapid reversal (to restore spontaneous ventilation and airway tone) is sometimes possible, particularly for opioids and benzodiazepines, for which there are direct antagonists. That is not the case for propofol or barbiturates. For some neuromuscular blocking drugs (NMBDs), sugammadex may also provide rapid reversal of effect.

Where No Airway Management Difficulty Is Anticipated

Hypnotics and Opioids

The most important aspect in this situation is to optimise conditions by giving enough drug with optimal timing in an attempt to secure the airway on first attempt. Subsequent attempts will have lower success rates and the risk of complications increases dramatically, including hypoxaemia, aspiration, dental injury and oesophageal intubation. All anaesthetics depress the level of consciousness and most impair spontaneous ventilation, but they have differential effects on airway reflexes and airway muscle tone. The anaesthetist must carefully assess whether bag-mask ventilation will be possible or not and also what the secondary plan is in case of an inability to ventilate after induction of general anaesthesia.

Bag-mask ventilation, laryngoscopy and insertion of airway devices are all procedures that require decreased muscle tone and the anaesthetist should not attempt any of these without being confident that the desired depth of anaesthesia has been achieved. Inadequate depth of anaesthesia is a common reason for the inexperienced anaesthetist to encounter difficult airway management. This is especially common in patients who consume large doses of opioids or alcohol and in children. Large doses of propofol are effective in depressing reflexes and reducing muscle tone, especially if combined with a rapid-onset opioid such as remifentanil. Other hypnotics (e.g. barbiturates, etomidate and benzodiazepines)

Table 10.1 Neuromuscular blocking drugs

Drug	Intubation dose (mg kg^{-1})	Onset time (min)	Approximate duration of action (min)
Suxamethonium	1	1	8*
Rocuronium	0.6	1.5	40
Vecuronium	0.1	2.5	40
Cisatracurium	0.15	4	50
Mivacurium	0.2	2.5	20*

* Elimination prolonged if plasma cholinesterase is not normal.

are less potent in reducing muscle tone, and an NMBD may be necessary to facilitate airway management. Spontaneous ventilation may be maintained with ketamine and upper airway obstruction is also less common with this hypnotic although secretions can be a problem. An NMBD can create optimal conditions but the anaesthetist must be familiar with the onset time and appropriate dose (Table 10.1).

Use of NMBDs and Reversal

If an NMBD is used a quick onset is often preferable. For suxamethonium onset time is approximately 45 seconds. For rocuronium, increasing the dose to 1 mg kg^{-1} will reduce the onset time to around 60 seconds. This enables it to be used for rapid sequence induction instead of suxamethonium. One drawback, however, of rocuronium is the pronounced variability in the duration of action. Suxamethonium should be used with caution because of the risk of serious side effects, including hyperkalemia, arrhythmias and malignant hyperthermia.

Neuromuscular monitoring is strongly recommended if an NMBD is used to guide the anaesthetist when the drug is working and also to guide offset and need for reversal. Onset time depends on the type of drug and the dose but may also be impacted by distribution related to cardiac output. Duration of action is quite unpredictable, especially in the elderly and those with an impairment of elimination, including renal or hepatic dysfunction and abnormal cholinesterase (for mivacurium and suxamethonium). Neuromuscular recovery is faster for the laryngeal muscles, the diaphragm, orbicularis oculi and slower for upper airway muscles and the adductor pollicis. For this reason, neuromuscular monitoring using the adductor pollicis muscle is preferable to using facial muscles.

Historically it was taught that no NMBD should be administered before it has been established that bag-mask ventilation is possible. Recent evidence indicates that it is easier to ventilate the patients who are paralysed and this includes patients in whom there is some difficulty initially.

Reversal of neuromuscular blockade – whether by neostigmine (routinely 50 µg kg^{-1}, accompanied by an antimuscarinic agent) or by sugammadex (for rocuronium or vecuronium) – should be guided by *quantitative* neuromuscular monitoring and complete before allowing emergence from general anaesthesia. Reversal should be judged inadequate until a T1:T4 ratio of > 0.9 is achieved. Manual assessment of T1:T4 ratios is insensitive between ratios of 0.4–0.7 and risks inadequate reversal and consequent airway and respiratory complications.

Tracheal Intubation

Optimal conditions facilitate prompt and uncomplicated intubation. Pharmacological muscle relaxation with an NMBD facilitates tracheal intubation and is used routinely. Alternatively, this can be achieved by a combination of large doses of a hypnotic and an opioid but NMBDs improve conditions for intubation and lessen side effects both of the procedure and of hypnotic overdose. A combination of propofol and remifentanil may be used to achieve tracheal intubation without neuromuscular block, but large doses are needed, typically 2 mg kg^{-1} propofol and 4 µg kg^{-1} remifentanil in young healthy individuals. In the elderly, lower doses (propofol to 1 mg kg^{-1} and remifentanil to 1.5 µg kg^{-1}) are suitable.

Supraglottic Airway Insertion

Inserting a supraglottic airway can be achieved routinely without an NMBD if an adequate dose of propofol has been administered. Other induction agents are less useful. Opioids, nitrous oxide and IV lidocaine each independently facilitate supraglottic airway insertion. NMBDs may be used where there is insertion difficulty or first-attempt success is essential.

Re-establishing Spontaneous Ventilation during Unanticipated Airway Difficulty

It is a great challenge to restore airway tone and spontaneous ventilation soon after induction of general anaesthesia with or without neuromuscular blockade. Even the shortest-acting drugs profoundly depress ventilation for so long that an inability to ventilate is a true emergency with a risk of life-threatening hypoxaemia. Spontaneous ventilation can be re-established following $1–1.5$ mg kg^{-1} suxamethonium after 8 to 10 minutes, though duration may be much longer in patients with low pseudocholinesterase levels (e.g. elderly, pregnant, septic, malnourished). Rocuronium may be reversed with sugammadex (16 mg kg^{-1}) within a few minutes after injection but it takes time to find the drug, fill the syringe and inject the drug. When trying to wake a patient because of airway difficulty soon after induction of anaesthesia the airway will require active management during the time it takes for offset and reversal of drugs.

When Airway Management Difficulty Is Anticipated

Maintaining Spontaneous Ventilation

One key question here is whether spontaneous ventilation should be maintained during airway management, such as tracheal intubation. This is possible with inhalational anaesthesia, but also with propofol or ketamine using small boluses or by incremental infusion. Either technique requires familiarity with the drug chosen and considerable patience (Table 10.2) Reflexes will be depressed and airway tone diminished to some extent but it is difficult to titrate the dosage to reach an anaesthetic level allowing intubation. It may therefore be advantageous to combine these techniques with local anaesthesia. Any spontaneous breathing technique is challenging as vigorous coughing, laryngospasm or vomiting may result if the patient is not adequately anaesthetised and airway obstruction or apnoea may occur if the patient is too deeply anaesthetised.

Table 10.2 Typical doses of intravenous drugs for sedation during airway management. Patient response is variable, requiring skilled titration, and doses may need to be dramatically reduced in the elderly, in unwell patients and in those at risk of airway obstruction

Drug	Bolus dose (mg kg^{-1})	Infusion rate (mg kg^{-1} h^{-1})
Propofol	0.5–1	0.5–3
Midazolam	0.01–0.05	0.02–0.1
Remifentanil	NR	0.005–0.01
Ketamine	0.15–0.5	0.5–2

NR, not recommended.

Inhalational Anaesthesia

Sevoflurane is the recommended drug as it does not cause airway irritation and is well tolerated. The concentration should gradually be increased up to 8% and the mask must fit well to maximise uptake and to ensure reliable monitoring of end-tidal volatile concentration. End-tidal concentration of around two minimal alveolar concentrations (around 5% in young individuals) is usually sufficient to enable airway management and this takes typically 5 minutes to achieve but is much longer in patients with respiratory insufficiency. Thus, inhalational induction takes time and requires patient cooperation. The gradual reduction in airway tone sometimes requires insertion of a nasopharyngeal or oral airway to relieve obstruction. Local anaesthesia is valuable but should not be administered during light anaesthesia as laryngeal spasm may occur. Addition of nitrous oxide to the inhalation gases hastens anaesthesia, but risks hypoxia in patients with significant respiratory compromise.

Local Anaesthesia

Local anaesthesia can be extremely useful in situations where spontaneous ventilation should be maintained, for example because of airway pathology with limited mouth opening or tumours where it is unlikely that bag-mask ventilation will be adequate.

Lidocaine 1% or 2% is a good choice and it can be used for inhalation, spray, atomisation, bilateral blocks of the glossopharyngeal and superior laryngeal nerve, or for injection through the cricothyroid membrane. Lidocaine 4% and 10% may also be used during topicalisation. Topical amethocaine is an effective alternative.

Inhalation of aerosolised local anaesthetic is a simple technique where a nebuliser is attached to a mouthpiece or a face mask. After inhalation for 15–30 minutes, topical anaesthesia covering the oropharynx and trachea is achieved.

It is also possible to spray or apply local anaesthetic directly onto the mucosa of the mouth, pharynx, tongue and nose. Topicalisation with lidocaine-soaked cotton swabs takes 5–15 minutes.

The glossopharyngeal nerve can be blocked using an injection either at the base of the anterior tonsillar pillar or near the base of the posterior tonsillar pillar. The injection at the base of the anterior tonsillar pillar is done while the tongue is swept to the opposite side and the needle is inserted 0.5 cm with injection of 2 mL of lidocaine 2% on each side. The injection near the base of the posterior tonsillar pillar requires more mouth opening and the tongue is pressed down. An injection of 5 mL of lidocaine 2% in the submucosa is recommended.

The superior laryngeal nerve can be blocked near the greater cornu of the hyoid bone which should be displaced towards the site of injection After contacting the bone, the needle is then moved in a caudal direction until it slips off the hyoid. The nerve can be blocked with 2 mL of lidocaine 2%.

Injection of 2–3 mL of lidocaine 2–4% through the cricothyroid membrane is highly effective in anaesthetising the larynx and trachea.

Whenever lidocaine is used the lowest dose should be used. During injections this should not exceed 3 mg kg^{-1} without adrenaline and 7 mg kg^{-1} with adrenaline. When used topically doses up to 8 mg kg^{-1} have been used safely but are rarely necessary.

Further Reading

Bouvet L, Stoian A, Rimmelé T, et al. (2009). Optimal remifentanil dosage for providing excellent intubating conditions when co-administered with a single standard dose of propofol. *Anaesthesia*, **64**, 719–726.

Mencke T, Echternach M, Kleinschmidt S, et al. (2003). Laryngeal morbidity and quality of tracheal intubation: a randomized controlled trial. *Anesthesiology*, **98**, 1049–1056.

Wang H, Gao X, Wei W, et al. (2017). The optimum sevoflurane concentration for supraglottic airway device Blockbuster™ insertion with spontaneous breathing in obese patients: a prospective observational study. *BMC Anesthesiology*, **17**, 156

Chapter 11

How to Avoid Morbidity from Aspiration of Gastric Content to the Lungs

Richard Vanner and Takashi Asai

The Problem

Pulmonary aspiration of gastric contents during general anaesthesia can be fatal. If acidic liquid or bile is inhaled it can cause pneumonitis with bronchospasm and pulmonary oedema and, less often, if particulate matter is inhaled it can cause airway obstruction or massive atelectasis. Conversely, if no symptoms, signs or hypoxaemia occur within 2 hours of aspiration, respiratory complications are unlikely. In one report, of those patients who aspirated, 64% developed no respiratory sequelae, 20% required ventilation on an intensive care unit (ICU) for > 6 hours and 5% died.

Since a 1956 report identified pulmonary aspiration as the commonest cause of death during general anaesthesia, major efforts have been made to reduce its incidence. The UK Confidential Enquiries into Maternal Deaths (CEMD) was an important triennial national audit that correlated airway management with death from aspiration (Figure 11.1). In the 1950s, during emergency caesarean sections, most aspirations occurred during spontaneous breathing through a face mask. In 1963 CEMD recommended tracheal intubation to protect the lungs. However, in the following 6 years, deaths from aspiration increased 50%, despite intubation being planned in all but one case. Aspiration occurred after induction with thiopentone and suxamethonium during face mask ventilation, before tracheal intubation: cricoid force (cricoid pressure), although first described in 1961, was not used. During the 1970s and 1980s various methods were introduced almost simultaneously: pre-oxygenation, rapid sequence induction and intubation (RSI), cricoid force, antacid therapy, fasting policies and regional anaesthesia. Maternal mortality from aspiration fell with this package of care, but deaths from hypoxaemia with other airway problems increased.

Landmark studies of the 1980s and 1990s reported that the incidence of pulmonary aspiration was 1:4000 during elective general anaesthesia and 1:900 for emergency anaesthesia, with a mortality rate of 1:70,000 for general anaesthetics. In 2011 the 4th National Audit

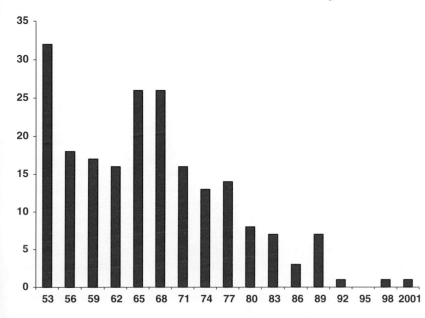

Figure 11.1 Maternal mortality from aspiration from each Confidential Enquiry into Maternal Deaths in England and Wales report. Middle year of each triennial report on the *x* axis, cases on *y* axis.

Project (NAP4) (see Chapter 3) reported that pulmonary aspiration remains the commonest cause of death or brain damage from anaesthetic airway complications. Aspiration was responsible for 50% of such deaths and 52% of cases of death or permanent brain damage.

The most frequent cause of aspiration during anaesthesia has changed over the last few decades. In the 1980s and early 1990s before the use of supraglottic airways (SGAs), the trachea was intubated routinely with the aid of neuromuscular blocking drugs. Pulmonary aspiration mainly occurred in emergency cases during induction of anaesthesia, before tracheal intubation or after extubation. Two more recent national audits (NAP4 included 23 cases and the Australian Anaesthesia Incident Monitoring Study (AIMS) in the 1990s included 133 cases of aspiration in the first 5000 incidents) have both shown that the combination of obesity and the use of a first generation SGA, in fasted elective patients, is now the most frequent cause of aspiration.

Avoiding Morbidity from Aspiration

Preoperative Assessment

The NAP4 report pointed out that 'Poor judgement was the likely root cause in many cases which included elements of poor assessment of risk (patient and operation) and failure to use airway devices or techniques that would offer increased protection against aspiration.' AIMS suggested universal use of a simple guideline would have prevented 60% of reported aspiration cases. Therefore, when planning airway management during anaesthesia, the anaesthetist should routinely assess both the risks of pulmonary aspiration and airway difficulty.

The risk of pulmonary aspiration should be predicted based on (at least) patient, operation, anaesthesia factors and airway device (Table 11.1). If the operation is an emergency, time from the last ingestion should be confirmed. Factors associated with aspiration in AIMS are shown in Table 11.2. Aspiration risk is in practice a continuous spectrum, which the anaesthetist should then match with an appropriate airway technique.

Aspiration Risk and Choice of Airway Device

Ninety-three per cent of aspiration cases in NAP4 and 75% in AIMS had at least one risk factor for aspiration. In particular, almost all patients who aspirated during the use of an SGA were at increased risk. Therefore, the risk assessment should influence the anaesthetic technique.

Routine airway management with an SGA should not be used where there is a contraindication, though it is notable that tracheal intubation and neuromuscular blockade have their own risks.

Although the mean gastric volume after fasting is 26–30 mL, it can be 180 mL. Use of ultrasound to assess the volume of gastric contents is a validated, clinically relevant and increasingly important tool. It is discussed in further detail in Chapter 7. In one study of 200 fasted elective patients, 7% had a gastric volume > 100 mL, including one patient (150 mL preoperatively) without other risk factors who regurgitated after extubation. Therefore, when an SGA is chosen for airway management, even with a low risk of aspiration, it is perhaps prudent to use a second generation device (see Chapter 13).

Preoperative Plans

For elective cases, patients should be fasted preoperatively so that the stomach is almost empty. Fasting of clear liquid is generally limited to 2 hours, though some in paediatric practice are reducing this to 1 hour. Prolonged starvation increases the volume of acid in the stomach. Small and medium-sized meals of low fat content are emptied from the stomach within 6 hours.

There is little evidence to support the universal use of gastric acid reducing therapy or prokinetic drugs such as metoclopramide, but the former is used routinely in obstetrics and in patients with symptoms of gastro-oesophageal reflux.

When the patient is at increased risk of aspiration, and difficult tracheal intubation is also predicted, avoiding general anaesthesia by use of regional anaesthesia is sensible, but is not always feasible. For example, in a patient with small bowel obstruction undergoing emergency laparotomy, regional anaesthesia would not be effective or safe, as this risks massive regurgitation and aspiration during surgery, while awake in the supine position. If general anaesthesia is planned, securing the airway while awake should be considered, but if topical anaesthesia is used this technique also has a risk of aspiration (see Chapter 9).

When the patient is at increased risk of aspiration and no difficulty in tracheal intubation is predicted, RSI should be planned. Cricoid force is routinely used with RSI in the UK, but its value is unproven and some anaesthetists avoid it because of concerns that it may increase airway difficulty. NAP4 identified several cases where the omission of RSI, despite strong indications for its use, was followed by patient harm, or death from

Table 11.1 Risk factors for aspiration

Patient factors

(a) Full stomach
- Emergency surgery
- Inadequate fasting time
- Gastrointestinal obstruction

(b) Delayed gastric emptying
- Systemic diseases, including diabetes
- Recent trauma
- Opioids preoperatively
- Raised intracranial pressure
- Previous gastrointestinal surgery including bariatric surgery
- Pregnancy, in active labour and for 48 hours after

(c) Incompetent lower oesophageal sphincter
- Hiatus hernia
- Recurrent regurgitation
- Dyspepsia
- Previous upper gastrointestinal surgery
- Pregnancy, after 20 weeks

(d) Oesophageal disease
(e) Morbid obesity
(f) Sedation or unconscious

Surgical factors
- Upper gastrointestinal surgery
- Lithotomy or head-down position
- Laparoscopy

Anaesthetic factors
- Light anaesthesia
- Positive pressure ventilation
- Length of surgery > 2 hours
- Difficult airway

Device factors
- First generation supraglottic airway devices

Table 11.2 Risk factors in 133 cases of aspiration

Aspiration (n.133)	
1 Emergency surgery	21
2 Light anaesthesia	18
3 Abdominal pathology, acute and chronic	17
4 Obesity	15
5 Opioid medication preoperatively	13
6 Neurological deficit and sedation	10
7 Lithotomy position	8
8 Difficult intubation/airway	8
9 Reflux symptoms	7
10 Hiatus hernia	6

From Kluger MT, Short TG. Aspiration during anaesthesia: a review of 133 cases from the Australian Anaesthetic Incident Monitoring Study (AIMS). *Anaesthesia* 2002; 54: 19–26. Reproduced with permission from Wiley.

aspiration. The NAP4 report states 'much more trouble resulted from failure to protect an airway by intubation than was caused by the process of intubation and the same applied to RSI. There were no cases where cricoid force was reported to lead to major complications.' Within a whole year's data, there was only one case report of aspiration during RSI with cricoid force applied. This was a case of small bowel obstruction where a nasogastric tube (NGT) had not been inserted before induction of anaesthesia. The report also stated, 'Rapid sequence induction with cricoid force does not provide 100% protection against regurgitation and aspiration of gastric contents but remains the standard for those patients at risk. On balance, rapid sequence induction and intubation should continue to be taught as a standard technique for protection of the airway.'

Birenbaum's recent large randomised controlled trial from France compared real or sham cricoid force as part of RSI and failed to show any benefit or harm. They studied 3472 patients requiring RSI, each having at least one risk factor for aspiration, including elective and fasted patients with reflux or high body mass index (BMI). It is likely the cricoid force applied was closer to 15 than 30 N. There was no statistically significant difference in the incidence of aspiration (0.56% vs. 0.52% respectively) or difficult intubation (4% vs. 3%) between the two groups. This important study would seem to indicate that cricoid force is an unnecessary part of RSI in those patients at lower risk (such as those fasted with a history of reflux or a high BMI) and should be reserved for those with a high risk of aspiration.

Conduct of RSI in High-Risk Cases

Patients with small bowel or gastric outflow obstruction are at highest risk of pulmonary aspiration. In an international survey of 10,000 anaesthetists in 2019, 60% would use an NGT, 70% head-up tilt and 71% cricoid force in cases of intestinal obstruction. A large NGT is passed before induction of anaesthesia and stomach contents removed by suction. A double-lumen NGT (Salem sump tube) is more effective at emptying the stomach than a single-lumen NGT as a single-lumen tube may simply suck up mucosa and block the end of the tube. An RSI is then performed in the head-up position. This involves pre-oxygenation, an intravenous induction (with or without opioid)

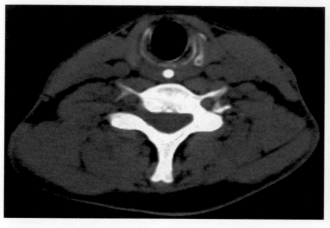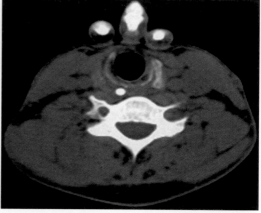

Figure 11.2 CT scans of the neck in transverse section at the level of the cricoid cartilage in a subject with a 14FG NGT filled with contrast medium. The first without, and the second with, firmly applied cricoid force. (Permission from Wiley, Vanner RG, Pryle BJ. Nasogastric tubes and cricoid pressure. *Anaesthesia* 1993; 48: 1112–1113.)

followed by a large dose of a fast-acting neuromuscular blocking drug (suxamethonium or rocuronium), cricoid force and then tracheal intubation with a cuffed tracheal tube. As the NGT is not compressed by cricoid force (Figure 11.2), leaving it open to atmospheric pressure during induction, by connecting it to a bag, enables it to vent liquid or gas. The NGT reduces the pressure of gastric contents and the head-up tilt reduces the pressure of any oesophageal contents, thereby increasing the effectiveness of cricoid force.

Excessive cricoid force increases airway difficulty. A force of > 30 N may cause difficult mask ventilation, difficult laryngoscopy, laryngeal distortion and an increased chance of failed intubation. Cricoid force of > 10 N while the patient is awake is uncomfortable, can cause retching and itself lead to pulmonary aspiration (or very rarely, if cricoid force is not released, oesophageal rupture). Cricoid force should be applied at < 10 N (< 1 kg) while the patient is awake, increasing to 20–30 N (2–3 kg) after loss of consciousness (Figure 11.3). These forces can be practised beforehand on weighing scales or using the more easily available 'syringe compression' technique: using a 50 mL syringe, compressing 50 mL of air to 33 mL needs 30 N. It is important to practise with correct volumes as lower volumes may result in an inadequate force being applied (cf. Birenbaum, 2019). Although UK guidelines by both the Difficult Airway Society (DAS) and the Obstetric Anaesthetists' Association in 2015 each advise that cricoid force should be used during RSI, both recommend its release if there

is intubation difficulty. In this way cricoid force protects against aspiration in the majority of patients with an easy airway and, as its effects on the airway are completely reversible, does no harm in those with a difficult airway.

Mask ventilation during RSI has traditionally been avoided to minimise gastric inflation and the associated increased risk of regurgitation. However, cricoid force prevents gas from passing into the stomach. Since 2015, DAS guidelines have recommended low-pressure mask ventilation to help maintain oxygenation during the apnoeic period.

Repeated attempts at tracheal intubation should be avoided, to prevent worsening mask ventilation and increased risk of aspiration. Videolaryngoscopy may reduce attempts at intubation, enables monitoring of correct placement of cricoid force and its impact on the airway and facilitates adjusting manoeuvres if necessary.

Release of cricoid force, after confirming tracheal intubation using capnography, can be followed by copious regurgitation. Micro-aspiration can occur even if the tracheal tube cuff has been adequately inflated, so any regurgitated material should be immediately removed by suction.

What Part of the Gullet Is Cricoid Force Occluding?

Anatomically cricoid force does not occlude the oesophagus, because this starts at the caudal border of the cricoid cartilage. It is the post-cricoid part of the hypopharynx that is compressed, lying within the cricopharyngeus muscle. Cricopharyngeus, which is the upper oesophageal sphincter, is attached to each side of the cricoid cartilage like a sling, and therefore always lies behind the cricoid even when the larynx is moved laterally. The lumen here is crescent shaped and wider than the lumen of the oesophagus. Figure 11.2 shows the structures behind the cricoid cartilage and that when two convex structures, the cricoid cartilage and the cervical vertebral body, are pressed together with cricoid force, only part of the pharyngeal lumen is compressed between them and the NGT is squeezed sideways. There is also lateral movement of the cricoid cartilage, and the rest of the pharynx is compressed against the muscle in front of the transverse process on that side of the spine. Figure 11.2 clearly shows the compression of these muscles with cricoid force.

Application of left-sided paratracheal direct oesophageal force has recently been proposed as an alternative to cricoid force but requires more evaluation before it can be widely recommended.

Lower-Risk Cases

In patients with risk factors but who are regarded as at lower risk of pulmonary aspiration (such as those that are fasted with a history of reflux or a high BMI), an RSI with tracheal intubation but without cricoid force could be used. If tracheal intubation is indicated for surgical reasons in patients at low risk of aspiration, for example open abdominal surgery, RSI is unnecessary. A face mask or an SGA is suitable when tracheal intubation is unnecessary. As the SGA is less stimulating it

may be possible to maintain a lighter depth of anaesthesia, but this also risks aspiration if the patient coughs or strains during too light anaesthesia. The contraction of the crus of the diaphragm normally augments the lower oesophageal sphincter pressure during straining, but this effect is lost during general anaesthesia.

Treatment of Aspiration

Table 11.3 describes the steps needed to treat the patient if regurgitation with possible aspiration occurs during anaesthesia.

Table 11.3 Treatment of regurgitation with possible aspiration – several elements may be performed concurrently depending on urgency of clinical situation

- Suction the drainage port of the SGA
- Suction the oropharynx
- Remove SGA if vomitus in the airway tube*
- Head-down position to limit pulmonary aspiration
- Left lateral position, if feasible
- Give 100% oxygen
- Apply cricoid force if ventilating by face mask or SGA removed
- RSI and tracheal intubation when supine
- Tracheal suction catheter
- Bronchoscopy to look for and remove food particles
- Treatment of bronchospasm
- Insert a gastric tube and remove stomach contents
- Chest X-ray if there are symptoms or signs
- Transfer to ICU if there is significant aspiration or if hypoxaemia develops

* If small volumes of fluid consider inserting suction catheter and flexible optical bronchoscopic inspection via SGA. Proceeding to intubation if indicated either via SGA or without SGA.

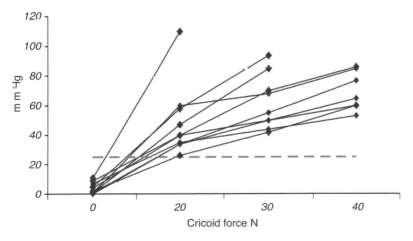

Figure 11.3 Regurgitation in cadavers. Pressure of oesophageal saline was increased until regurgitation occurred (y axis) in 10 cadavers at each increment of cricoid force (x axis) applied with a 'cricoid yoke' with force transducer. The dashed yellow line represents the maximum likely gastric pressure. (Permission from Wiley, Vanner RG, Pryle BJ. Regurgitation and oesophageal rupture with cricoid pressure: a cadaver study. *Anaesthesia* 1992; 47: 732–735).

Extubation and Post-operative Care

Pulmonary aspiration may occur during or after airway removal. During caesarean section, mortality from aspiration is now more frequent after tracheal extubation than during induction of anaesthesia.

According to AIMS many cases of aspiration occurred in the sitting or supine position during extubation, emergence or in the recovery room. AIMS therefore recommended that tracheal extubation in the emergency patient should be with the patient awake and on their side. While this practice used to be routine, a recent survey noted increases in extubation in the head-up or sitting position, even in emergency cases. There are issues turning obese patients and it may be that this is changing practice for all patients. Modern trolleys with a small headpiece may also hamper management in the lateral position.

The risk factors for post-operative pulmonary aspiration include a full stomach, ileus, ageing and obesity. Incomplete recovery from neuromuscular blockade, which is common after general anaesthesia, is an important cause of aspiration-induced pneumonia and complete reversal of neuromuscular blockade should be assured. Risk is increased further by residual anaesthetic agents, depressed conscious level and opioids. Risk is also higher after tracheal intubation than use of an SGA during anaesthesia, as laryngeal reflexes are inhibited beyond extubation and laryngeal competence does not return after tracheal extubation for at least 1 hour.

Further Reading

Asai T. (2016). Videolaryngoscopes: do they have role during rapid-sequence induction of anaesthesia? *British Journal of Anaesthesia*, **116**, 317–319.

Birenbaum A, Hajage D, Roche S, et al. (2019). Effect of cricoid pressure compared with a sham procedure in the rapid sequence induction of anesthesia The IRIS Randomized Clinical Trial. *JAMA Surgery*, **154**, 9–17.

Kluger MT, Short TG. (2002). Aspiration during anaesthesia: a review of 133 cases from the Australian Anaesthetic Incident Monitoring Study (AIMS). *Anaesthesia*, **54**, 19–26.

Salem MR, Khorasani A, Zeidan A, Crystal GJ. (2017). Cricoid pressure controversies. *Anesthesiology*, **126**, 738–52.

Vanner RG, Asai T. (1999). Safe use of cricoid pressure. *Anaesthesia*, **53**, 1–3.

Warner MA, Warner ME, Weber JG. (1993). Clinical significance of pulmonary aspiration during the perioperative period. *Anesthesiology*, **78**, 56–62.

Face Mask Ventilation

Adrian Matioc

Basic Face Mask Ventilation Technique

Adult face mask ventilation (FMV) is an airway management technique used by healthcare providers with variable levels of training, inside and outside the operating room for the oxygenation and ventilation of the unconscious patient.

FMV devices are the face mask, the oropharyngeal and nasopharyngeal airway, a suction device and a positive pressure gas-delivery system. The latter may be driven by the rescuer's expiratory effort (mouth-to-mask ventilation), hand (the bag of an anaesthesia circuit or a self-inflating resuscitator bag) or a machine (any mechanical ventilator). The face mask is the oldest airway management device specifically designed for inhalational anaesthesia. John Snow's (1847) had all the characteristics of a modern face mask: a symmetrical dome, a soft edge to provide a tight gas seal and increase the patient's comfort and a connector to the breathing circuit. (Figure 12.1)

Proper handling of the face mask is critical, as the grip generates both the airtight seal and an optimal airway manoeuvre. The generic left-hand 'E-C' technique is performed with the thumb and index finger resting on the dome (the 'C'), the third and fourth on the mandible and the fifth at the mandibular angle (the 'E'). It has never been validated for positive pressure ventilation (Figure 12.2) and has been carried over from an era when anaesthesia was a single-agent inhalational technique administered to a spontaneously breathing patient.

Airway Manoeuvres

Airway manoeuvres are blind techniques used to provide upper airway patency by manipulating solid anatomical structures – the mandible, cervical spine and hyoid bone – to stretch soft pharyngeal tissues connected to them – the soft palate, tongue, epiglottis and lateral pharyngeal wall. The stronger the solid–soft tissue connection, the more effective a correct airway manoeuvre (e.g. base-of-tongue and epiglottis obstruction). The weaker the connection, the less effective the manoeuvre (e.g. soft palate obstruction during inspiration and expiration in obstructive sleep apnoea patients). Nasal cavity obstruction is not affected by

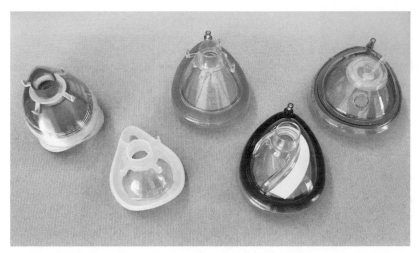

Figure 12.1 Face masks (from left to right): early transparent mask (circa 1960), face mask with anatomical shape for soft seal, generic modern face mask, ergonomic asymmetrical face mask, specialty endoscopy face mask. (Picture taken by the author, at the Wood Library-Museum of Anesthesiology, Schaumburg, Illinois, with their kind support.)

airway manoeuvres and requires an oropharyngeal or a nasopharyngeal airway for correction.

Airway manoeuvres have been validated only as two-hand techniques for mouth-to-mouth ventilation. With hands on the chin and forehead/occiput the torque generated in the sagittal plane corresponds to and maximises craniocervical extension. Jaw thrust is applied in the transverse plane with hands on the mandibular angles for maximal subluxation of the temporomandibular joints. Both techniques generate chin elevation, positioning the mandibular teeth in front of the maxillary, and increase the distance between chin and sternum, resulting in upper airway stretching. Additionally, it increases the distance between chin and cervical spine, resulting in upper airway enlargement (Figure 12.3). Combining both techniques with an open mouth (with or without an oropharyngeal airway) generates the most effective technique: the *triple airway manoeuvre*. Turning the

extended head to the side may also prove effective. Airway manoeuvres are used in both partial and complete upper airway obstruction.

A maximal airway manoeuvre is limited by anatomy (maximal mobility permitted by normal tissues) or pathology (e.g. trauma or degenerative changes of bony structures and joints). Maximal head extension in patients with normal cervical spines is approximately 45°. This can be estimated by the angle between a horizontal (longitudinal axis of the operating table) and the longitudinal axis of the face mask at the cushion level. Maximal mandibular advancement measured on normal anaesthetised volunteers at the mandibular-maxillary incisors level is 16.2 ± 3.2 mm. These measurements can be used as technical objective markers for an FMV attempt. Inability to generate a measurable airway manoeuvre may signal the need for an airway adjunct before the ventilation attempt.

Adjuncts

The modern oropharyngeal airway was described in 1933. The bite block opens the mouth and encourages oral ventilation by bypassing nasal and velopharyngeal obstruction. The curved portion supports the tongue. Insertion of the wrong size oropharyngeal airway or in light planes of anaesthesia may lead to iatrogenic airway obstruction, laryngospasm or regurgitation. A correctly sized and positioned nasopharyngeal airway has the benefit of clearing nasal obstruction and bypassing soft palate and base-of-tongue obstruction. Potential complications are nasal bleeding, trauma and airway obstruction.

Measuring Adequacy of Face Mask Ventilation

Unreliable, subjective ventilation outcome markers, such as cyclical condensation on the mask dome or bag compliance, are routinely used inside and outside

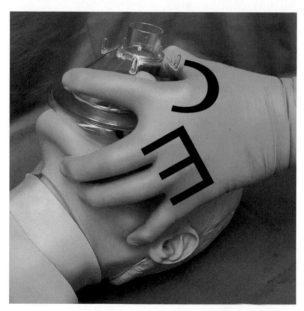

Figure 12.2 The one-hand 'E-C' grip face mask technique.

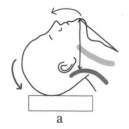 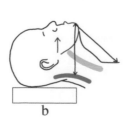 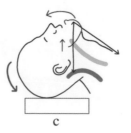

Figure 12.3 Airway manoeuvres generate chin elevation positioning the mandibular teeth in front of the maxillary and increase the chin–sternum and chin–cervical spine distance (a – head extension, b – jaw thrust, c – mouth opening added to the two previous mentioned manoeuvres: = 'triple airway manoeuvre').

the hospital. The use of a stiff, self-inflating resuscitation bag gives limited feedback about the effectiveness of the technique during inspiration and expiration. Chest expansion and bilateral breathing sounds are difficult to observe in trauma and obese patients. Oxygen desaturation is a late marker of ventilation failure.

Objective ventilation outcome markers are tidal volume, airway pressure and the capnogram. Effective ventilation is represented by a capnogram with plateau, acceptable airway pressure (< 20–$25\ cmH_2O$ to minimise gastric inflation) and satisfactory tidal volume (4–5 mL kg^{-1}, sufficient to maintain oxygenation for a prolonged time). Spirometry tracing, when available, can accelerate the diagnosis of expiratory flow limitation.

A Technique for Routine One-Hand Face Mask Ventilation

An optimal FMV attempt should generate an effective seal and the best possible airway manoeuvre (active upper airway enlargement) and should be evaluated with objective technical and outcome markers. A first step is positioning the patient's head in the *sniffing position*, with lower cervical flexion and upper cervical extension (Figure 12.3), or the *ramp position* in obese patients (passive upper airway enlargement). Administration of muscle relaxants may help the FMV attempt.

The 'E-C' grip applies an asymmetrical seal on a symmetrical face mask with suboptimal results when applied with a large mask, large patient or by a practitioner with small hands. The generic E-C grip generates both an imperfect seal as the C does not control the whole dome and a suboptimal airway manoeuvre as the E cannot generate and maintain maximal extension of the cervical spine or subluxation of the temporomandibular joints. An imperfect seal forces the practitioner to push the mask on the chin or to use head straps, flexing the neck, compromising the airway manoeuvre and inducing iatrogenic airway obstruction.

The *chin lift grip* is a power grip with the web space between the thumb and index finger against the connector. It is implemented with a new asymmetrical face mask or a symmetrical generic mask with the hook ring removed. The grip controls the whole dome, fingers three, four and five reach for the chin generating and optimised torque for head extension in the sagittal plane (Figure 12.4).

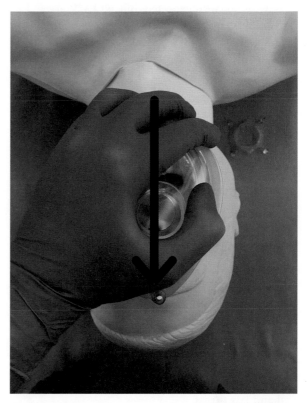

Figure 12.4 The one-hand 'chin lift' grip is applied in sagittal plane for an optimised head extension.

Difficult Face Mask Ventilation

Prediction

Difficult FMV, occurs in 5–9% of the general population. Many predictors of FMV difficulty are revealed by inspection of the patient.

- *Predictors of excessive airway obstruction* stem from excessive soft tissue collapsibility as seen with male patients, increased weight or neck circumference, snoring, obstructive sleep apnoea, increased age, lack of teeth, Mallampati class III–IV or tumour.
- *Predictors of technical difficulty* are related to airway manoeuvres and seal and are associated with a limited mandibular protrusion test, acute or chronic cervical spine pathology, presence of a beard, short thyromental distance, lack of teeth, thick neck or previous radiation therapy.
- *Other predictors* may be operator-specific, such as small hands or poor technique or due to inadequate devices or difficult access to the patient.

99

- *Categories* with expected difficult FMV are obstetric, morbidly obese, full stomach, fixed cervical spine and pre-hospital patients.

Management

When FMV is difficult an oropharyngeal or nasopharyngeal airway should be used. The best technique for ventilation is the two-hand *E-V technique*, with thumbs and thenar eminences placed longitudinally along both sides of the mask to create a symmetrical seal and fingers two, three, four and five along the mandible for head extension, jaw thrust and mouth opening: the triple airway manoeuvre (Figure 12.5). The first and second fingers create a 'V' and the third, fourth and fifth fingers an 'E'. The symmetrical hand-device and hand-jaw interaction optimises the FMV attempt. A second practitioner controls the bag, or ventilation can be provided by a ventilator. Practitioners with small hands should routinely use the two-hand approach.

The two-hand approach can be augmented with a two-person four-hand approach where the assistant positioned at the side of the patient is facing the primary rescuer positioned at the patient's head. The assistant's hands reinforce the primary's two-handed seal and jaw thrust.

When FMV difficulty is diagnosed preinduction or the FMV attempt fails in an anaesthetised or unconscious patient, early recourse to a supraglottic airway or intubation may resolve the situation.

The traditional difficult FMV scale used in literature was described by Han (2004). It has four grades of difficulty: (1) one-hand ventilation, (2) one hand with airway adjuvants, (3) 'inadequate, unstable or requiring two providers' with airway adjuncts and (4) impossible ventilation. This subjective scale reflects a trial and error time-consuming difficult FMV tactic, escalating from simple to complex techniques as attempts fail. It also ignores the difficult FMV predictors (to acknowledge

and address an expected difficult attempt) and objective ventilation outcome markers (to quickly diagnose and address an unexpected difficult or failed FMV). Undiagnosed difficult FMV prolongs apnoea, consuming the buffer provided by pre-oxygenation and precipitating subsequent advanced airway management attempts.

Lim and Nielsen proposed an objective scale for FMV difficulty based on the best capnography tracing achieved: (A) plateau present, (B) no plateau, $ETCO_2 \geq$ 10 mmHg, (C) no plateau, $ETCO_2 < 10$ mmHg, (D) no $ETCO_2$. They represent in order effective, adequate, inadequate and failed ventilation (Figure 12.6). Both

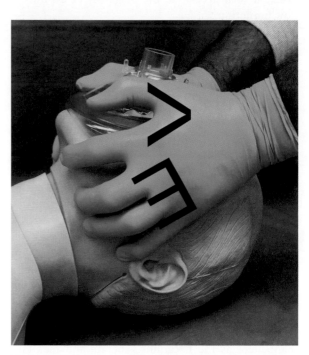

Figure 12.5 The two-hand 'E-V' grip is applied symmetrically on the mask and jaws for an optimised triple airway manoeuvre.

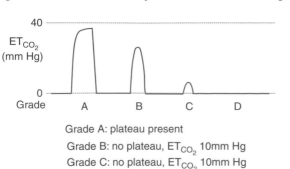

Grade A: plateau present
Grade B: no plateau, ET_{CO_2} 10mm Hg
Grade C: no plateau, ET_{CO_2} 10mm Hg
Grade D: no ET_{CO_2}

☐ 1 hand for mask
☐ 2 hands for mask
☐ Guedel airway
☐ Nasopharyngeal airway

Figure 12.6 Lim's objective face mask ventilation grading using capnography (A – effective, B – adequate, C – inadequate, D – failed).

ventilation and oxygenation status can be predicted by capnography.

Conclusions

Assessment of basic (FMV), advanced (supraglottic, glottic) and invasive (subglottic) airway management difficulty should be concurrent. The results should be integrated into an airway management strategy that optimises upper airway instrumentation and administration of medications (sedatives, induction agents, muscle relaxants). The misperception of FMV as a simple technique, the lack of rigorous validation of the one-hand technique, and the lack of routine use of objective technical and outcome ventilation markers can lead in many cases to a suboptimal approach. An optimal first FMV attempt should be tailored to patient predictors, operator limitations and clinical context.

FMV difficulty should be defined objectively as with any other airway management technique. An effective attempt, as shown by a tidal volume of 4–5 mL kg^{-1}, achieved at acceptable airway pressures of < 20–25 cmH$_2$O, and with a capnogram plateau, means that FMV can support life by oxygenation for a prolonged time without complications. An ineffective attempt (low tidal volume, high airway pressure and capnogram with rapid upswing without plateau) or a failed attempt (lack of measurements) should trigger an appropriate response. Using these principles, a clinician can challenge their routine, redefine FMV difficulty and develop specific FMV strategies.

Further Reading

Fei M, Blair JL, Rice MJ, et al. (2017). Comparison of effectiveness of two commonly used two-hand mask ventilation techniques on unconscious apnoeic obese adults. *British Journal of Anaesthesia*, **118**, 618–624.

Kuna ST, Woodson LC, Solanki DR, et al. (2008). Effect of progressive mandibular advancement on pharyngeal airway size in anesthetized adults. *Anesthesiology*, **109**, 605–612.

Langeron O, Masso E, Huraux C, et al. (2000). Prediction of difficult mask ventilation. *Anesthesiology*, **92**, 1229–1236.

Lim KS, Nielsen JR. (2016). Objective description of mask ventilation. *British Journal of Anaesthesia*, **117**, 828–829.

Matioc A. (2019). An anesthesiologist's perspective on the history of basic airway management. The 'modern' era, 1960 to present. *Anesthesiology*, **130**, 686–711.

Paal P, Goedecke V, Brugger H, et al. (2007). Head position for opening the upper airway. *Anaesthesia*, **62**, 227–230.

Chapter 13

Supraglottic Airways

Tim Cook

The term supraglottic airway device (SGA) describes a group of airway devices designed to establish and maintain a clear airway during anaesthesia. SGAs' wider roles include use during airway rescue in or out of hospital, during cardiopulmonary resuscitation and as a conduit to assist (difficult) tracheal intubation. For this reason, a full understanding of the currently available devices and techniques is fundamental to modern anaesthetic practice. SGAs' roles are described in many other chapters in this book: this chapter aims to fill the gap of information not provided elsewhere, including areas of controversy.

Prior to 1998 almost all general anaesthesia was conducted with face mask or tracheal tube. The classic laryngeal mask airway (cLMA) was introduced in 1988 and rapidly transformed the way in which anaesthesia was practised through much of the world. In many countries, SGAs are used to maintain the airway in the majority of anaesthetics, but usage varies considerably by country. There has subsequently been an explosion of new SGAs designed to compete with the cLMA. These devices vary considerably in the degree to which they have been evaluated before and since marketing. Several devices have been modified multiple times since introduction so interpretation of literature on device performance must be made with great care to ensure the device reported on is the device currently produced. There are currently too few comparative trials between devices to determine the clinical role (if any) of some devices. The ProSeal LMA (PLMA), i-gel and laryngeal tube (LT) are the most extensively investigated of the newer SGAs. The LMA Supreme and LMA Protector are also supported by an increasing body of evidence.

The majority of SGAs are designed to lie with their tip at the origin of the oesophagus, effectively 'plugging' the oesophagus. A seal around the larynx is then achieved by a more proximal cuff, which acts to elevate the base of the tongue, lift the epiglottis and seal the oropharynx. Some cuffs encircle the laryngeal inlet while others simply lie above it. All conventional SGAs are inserted beyond the epiglottis and may lead to downfolding of the epiglottis and airway obstruction. One of the design challenges of these devices is to enable placement of the distal portion of the device behind the cricoid cartilage without displacing the epiglottis during insertion.

Efficacy, Safety and New SGAs

As described above, SGAs may have a number of roles, and different designs and performance characteristics may be required for each role. In anaesthesia the cLMA was originally used almost exclusively for brief, peripheral operations, performed in slim patients, usually breathing spontaneously.

SGAs may be used for most operations. Contraindications include:

- Major oral or pharyngolaryngeal pathology
- Increased risk of full stomach and pulmonary aspiration
- Reduced lung compliance such that airway pressures above the pharyngeal seal pressure are required
- SGA would interfere with access to the surgical site
- Surgery prevents access to the SGA during surgery

All are relative contraindications and require judgement and interpretation. Thresholds for use will therefore vary with device, clinician experience and individual opinion.

SGAs have become increasingly used for longer, more complex operations and in obese patients, during laparoscopic (and even open) abdominal surgery, during controlled ventilation and even in the prone position by some practitioners.

All these expansions of use offer potential benefit to patients but also raise questions of efficacy and safety. In low-risk patients the cLMA provides

Table 13.1 (cont.)

	First generation SGAs
CobraPLA and Tulip	The Cobra perilaryngeal airway (CobraPLA) is a single-use soft plastic SGA designed for use during anaesthesia. It has a wide tubed design with a proximal (pharyngeal) balloon and distally a soft plastic head (shaped a little like a cobra head) designed to seat in and seal the hypopharynx. The head's anterior surface should abut the larynx and has a grille of soft bars, which are easily displaced for airway instrumentation.
	The Tulip airway is a single-use SGA comprising a tube which lies in the upper airway and a circumferential cuff that seals within the oropharynx. The airway does not extend into the hypopharynx or oesophagus. In this regard it strongly resembles the COPA (cuffed oropharyngeal airway) which was available in the early 1980s but superseded by the cLMA. It is marketed for airway management during resuscitation, including by bystanders, rather than anaesthesia.
	A concern with both the CobraPLA and Tulip airway is that they seal the oro/ hypopharynx but do not seal below the larynx. There is therefore a concern that, especially during controlled ventilation, their use may lead to gastric inflation. If regurgitation occurs there is no route of egress and the designs might be judged to increase the risk of pulmonary aspiration (0 generation SGA).
	SGAs designed for intubation
Intubating LMA	Described in the text. Single-use and reusable versions. Includes specific tracheal tube and stabilising device to assist removal of SGA after removal.
LMA classic excel	Based on the cLMA but with a wider stem, easily detachable connector and with the grilles replaced by an epiglottic elevator. Available in North America only.
Ambu Aura-i	A first generation LM designed for routine use and for tracheal intubation.
Ambu AuraGain	A second generation LM designed for routine use and for tracheal intubation.
iLTS-D	An LT designed specifically for intubation. The only second generation intubating SGA.

FOB, flexible optical bronchoscope; ILMA, intubating LMA; SLIPA, streamlined liner of the pharynx airway.

(a)

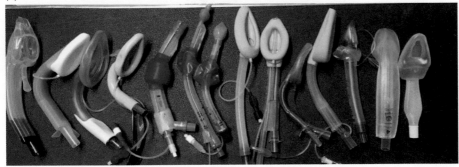

(b)

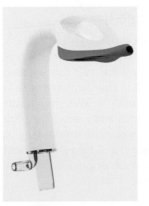

Figure 13.1 (a) A number of SGAs are illustrated here. From left to right: Baska mask, LMA protector, Ambu Aura-i, intubating LMA, Gastro-LT, laryngeal tube suction II, laryngeal tube, classic LMA, ProSeal LMA, LMA Supreme, Guardian CPV, Cobra perilaryngeal airway, i-gel, Streamlined liner of the pharynx airway (SLIPA). (b) The Eclipse.

Table 13.2 Characteristics of cLMAs

Size	Patient group	Weight range (kg)	Maximum cuff volume (mL)	Length of airway tube (mm)	Maximum size of tracheal tube that will pass
1	Neonate	< 5	4	108	3.5
1.5	Infant	5–10	7	135	4.5
2	Child	10–20	10	140	5.0
2.5	Child	20–30	14	170	6.0
3	Child/small adult	30–50	20	200	6.5
4	Adult	50–70	30	205	6.5
5	Adult	70–100	40	230	7.0
6	Large adult	> 100	50	–	–

Length of airway tube: from connector to grille.

Maximum size of tracheal tube: based on an uncuffed, well lubricated, Portex blue line tracheal tube, without forcing.

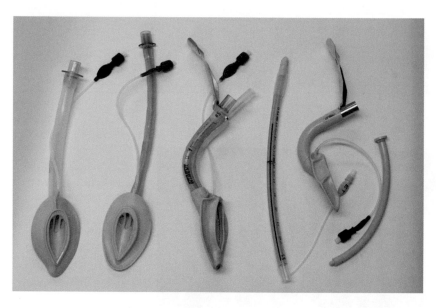

Figure 13.2 LMA family. From left to right: classic LMA, flexible LMA, ProSeal LMA with introducer attached, ILMA tracheal tube, ILMA and ILMA stabilising rod.

The lateral cuff lies against the pyriform fossa and the proximal cuff the base of the tongue. The mask is held in a stable position by the hypopharyngeal constrictor muscles laterally and cricopharyngeus inferiorly. Inflation of the mask cuff produces a low-pressure seal around the larynx.

The cLMA is designed for use up to 40 times. Standard masks are not MRI compatible due to metal in the pilot tube valve. MRI compatible masks are available with a metal-free valve and are colour coded with yellow pilot balloons.

Practicalities and Routine Use

There are eight sizes of cLMA available (1, 1½, 2, 2½, 3, 4, 5, 6) for use from neonates to large adults. Features of each size mask are described in Table 13.2. Size selection is according to patient weight in children (up to size 3) and in adults, as a 'rule of thumb' in Western patients a size 4 is used for adult women and a size 5 for adult men. In smaller Asian patients one size smaller may be appropriate. Using a larger size cLMA for a given patient is likely to result in an improved airway seal, but may increase minor airway trauma.

The cLMA is designed to be used during spontaneous or controlled ventilation. It is an alternative both to anaesthesia with face mask or tracheal tube. Its introduction transformed the routine practice of anaesthesia and face mask anaesthesia is now rarely practised. Good case selection is the first key to successful, safe use, with good insertion technique being the second.

Importantly, like all SGAs, the cLMA does not reliably protect against aspiration of regurgitated gastric contents and is contraindicated for patients who are not starved or who may have a full stomach. The cLMA seals with the pharynx to a pressure of 18–22 cmH$_2$O and the oesophagus to a pressure of 30–50 cmH$_2$O but has no drain tube. The cLMA does provide good protection from pharyngeal secretions above the cuff entering the larynx.

The depth of anaesthesia required for cLMA insertion is greater than that needed for insertion of a Guedel airway, but less than for several other SGAs or for tracheal intubation. Prior to insertion there should be no eyelash reflex and no response to purposeful jaw thrust. Propofol is the ideal anaesthetic induction agent for insertion as it profoundly reduces airway reflexes (in contrast to thiopentone). Addition of a rapidly acting opioid, intravenous lidocaine (up to 1.5 mg kg^{-1}) and nitrous oxide each improve insertion conditions. Neuromuscular blocking drugs are not needed. The cLMA may also be inserted with topical anaesthesia of the airway or bilateral supraglottic nerve blocks. Insertion causes minimal haemodynamic response.

Insertion is best performed with the patient in the 'sniffing position' (flextension). The cLMA should be visually inspected, free from foreign bodies and the mask completely deflated. Failure of a cLMA to maintain complete deflation indicates a cuff leak.

The smaller the leading edge of the device is, the less likely it is to catch on the tongue or epiglottis during insertion, both of which may impair placement. Full deflation enables the cLMA to slide behind the cricoid cartilage. The posterior of the mask should be well lubricated. During insertion the non-intubating hand holds the head to prevent flexion of the head. The airway is held like a pen, with the index finger placed at the anterior junction of the airway tube and mask. The mouth is opened, the mask inserted and its posterior aspect pressed onto the hard palate. The index finger is then advanced towards the occiput, which causes the cLMA to pass along the roof of the mouth and then the posterior pharynx (Figure 13.3).

The device is advanced in a single smooth movement until it is felt to stop, on reaching the cricopharyngeus muscle. Chin lift or jaw thrust applied by an assistant aids insertion. Once fully inserted the tube should be held while the intubating finger is withdrawn.

The cuff should be inflated before attaching the anaesthetic circuit. When correctly inserted the black line on the posterior of the cLMA tube will remain in the midline and during cuff inflation the device rises out of the mouth some 1–2 cm as the anterior neck fills. The manufacturer indicates volumes of air that may be inserted into the mask (Table 13.2). These are *maximum* volumes and half this maximum is often sufficient. During or after cuff inflation the intracuff pressure should be measured and maintained at 60–70 cmH$_2$O. Most of the airway seal is achieved with the first 10 mL of air inserted into the cuff and is achieved with cuff pressure of below 30 cmH$_2$O. High intracuff pressure maintained for a long period may cause pharyngeal and laryngeal mucosal or nerve damage. Inflation to manufacturer's maximum volumes routinely leads to intracuff pressure > 120 cmH$_2$O. If nitrous oxide is used during anaesthesia this will diffuse into the cuff and lead to increases in volume and pressure particularly in the first 30 minutes of anaesthesia. Injuries to the lingual (particularly when large masks are used), hypoglossal and recurrent laryngeal nerves have been infrequently reported. These injuries, and post-operative sore throat and hoarseness, are likely to be minimised by meticulous insertion, positioning and maintaining intracuff pressure below 70 cmH$_2$O.

Once the cLMA is inserted ease of manual ventilation should be assessed. Adequate ventilation should be achieved with no audible gas leak at a pressure below 20 cmH$_2$O. If this cannot be achieved consider use of an alternative size of cLMA or a different airway. Airway noise, poor filling of the reservoir bag (impaired expiration) or a 'scalloped' expiratory trace on flow:volume spirometry are all signs of expiratory airway obstruction, likely due to poor placement, and should lead to further investigation or repositioning of the airway.

The cLMA should be secured by tape or tie to reduce the likelihood of extrusion or displacement. Use of a bite block (rolled gauze placed between the molar teeth) is recommended until removal. This is particularly important during emergence.

Misplacement may occur due to rotation, the tip of the device bending backwards, folding of the

(a)

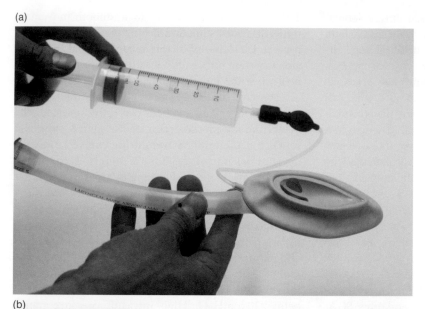

(b)

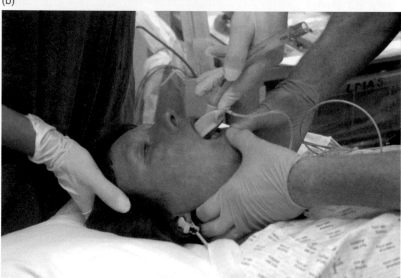

Figure 13.3 (a and b) cLMA insertion technique. (a) Preparation by full deflation and inspection and (b) insertion maintaining the head and neck in position with one hand and pushing the cLMA posteriorly and caudally with the other.

epiglottis or insertion of the tip of the device into the glottis. Careful technique reduces all these misplacements. Insertion of the tip of the device into the glottis may mimic laryngospasm with high airway pressures, slow expiration and wheeze. The presence of the cLMA tip behind the larynx may occasionally shorten the vocal cords leading to partial extrathoracic airway obstruction during spontaneous ventilation and paradoxical cord movement during controlled ventilation. If the origin of the oesophagus lies within the bowl of the cLMA the use of controlled ventilation may lead to gastric distension. This misplacement may occur in up to 15% of cases and may not be clinically apparent.

At the end of surgery, where controlled ventilation has been used, the transition to spontaneous ventilation is usually seamless. The cLMA is tolerated until very light planes of anaesthesia. The cLMA can be left in place during transfer to the recovery unit with the patient remaining supine. Oxygen is administered by T-piece, Venturi or T-bag. Of these the T-bag is preferred. The T-Bag (LMA-T-Bag Oxygen Enhancement Device) is an inflatable plastic bag that serves as an oxygen reservoir, is economical, provides a high oxygen concentration with as little as 2 L min^{-1} gas flow and provides an auditory and visual indicator of breathing as well as enabling controlled ventilation if required.

Though not all studies support this the consensus and recommendations are that removal of the bite block and cLMA should not be attempted until the patient regains consciousness and airway reflexes return. It is recommended to deflate the cuff at the time of removal; however, removal without cuff deflation is usually well tolerated and without complications. Airway suction is not necessary or desirable unless secretions are excessive as pharyngeal secretions are removed with the airway. The cLMA may be removed with the patient supine or on their side. The evidence on timing of removal of the cLMA in children is conflicting and confusing: some clinicians prefer to remove the cLMA in infants and small children before emergence. Removal of any SGA during partial emergence (e.g. coughing, moving or swallowing but unresponsive) is most likely to cause complications, including breath-holding, laryngospasm, regurgitation and hypoxia.

After use the cLMA should be promptly and thoroughly cleaned before being sterilised by autoclave (up to 137 °C for 3 minutes with the cuff fully deflated) and stored in sterile packaging thereafter (see Chapter 37).

Predictors of difficult laryngoscopy/tracheal intubation do not correlate with ease or difficulty with cLMA placement, though markedly reduced mouth opening will also impede cLMA placement. In patients who are edentulous with loss of alveolar bone, it may prove difficult to achieve a stable airway with the cLMA.

During use of the cLMA airway resistance (tube plus laryngeal resistance) is similar to that of a conventional tracheal tube (size 4 cLMA vs. 7.0–8.0 mm ID tracheal tube). Correct positioning of the cLMA is important for reduced resistance and a downfolded epiglottis, rotation of the cLMA or mechanical shortening of the vocal cords may increase laryngeal and therefore overall resistance.

Movement of head and neck does little to alter cLMA position over the larynx. However, head and neck flexion or rotation both lead to an increase in intracuff pressure and airway seal. Head and neck extension has the opposite effects.

Since its introduction there has been a gradual but inexorable widening of the applications and reduction in the contraindications to cLMA use. Whether the more laissez-faire approach to use of the device is appropriate is not known, but the effect that the cLMA has had on routine anaesthesia care is remarkable, as is its safety record. A large 1993 study showed 30% of all surgical cases were performed with a cLMA and one in 2002 reported its use in 65% of cases, half with controlled ventilation.

The incidence of airway-related critical incidents has been reported as 0.16% during spontaneous ventilation and 0.14% during controlled ventilation. The incidence of aspiration in carefully selected elective patients is variously estimated as 1 in 5000–11,000. The accuracy of these figures is unclear but is of a similar order to reported incidences of aspiration during tracheal tube anaesthesia (1 in 2000–4000).

Meta-analysis has been used to compare cLMA anaesthesia with tracheal tube or face mask anaesthesia. Advantages over the face mask include improved oxygenation and lesser hand fatigue. Advantages over tracheal intubation include improved haemodynamic stability, reduced anaesthetic requirements during maintenance, improved emergence (better oxygenation and less cough) and reduced sore throats in adults. The cLMA lessens laryngeal morbidity compared with tracheal intubation with reduced mechanical and neurological vocal cord dysfunction.

The use of the cLMA for controlled ventilation remains controversial. The main concern is the possibility of gastric distension during controlled ventilation and the reliability of airway protection from regurgitated gastric contents. Detractors point to several factors; while the cLMA has been shown to modestly reduce lower oesophageal sphincter pressure, much more importantly as peak airway pressure increases the risk and extent of gastro-oesophageal insufflation increases. However, when oropharyngeal leak occurs during controlled ventilation with the cLMA the leak is into (and out of) the mouth in approximately 95% of cases. Cadaver work shows the cLMA does provide some protection from oesophageal fluid when compared with the unprotected airway. Large series have reported use of controlled ventilation in 44–95% of cases with no increase in aspiration or airway-related critical incidents. Proven aspiration with the cLMA remains infrequent and there are few reports of long-term sequelae after aspiration during cLMA use. When the cLMA is used for controlled ventilation case selection and correct positioning are both critical. Imperfect position should not be accepted. Airway pressures should be kept to a minimum and pressures above 20 cmH$_2$O should be avoided altogether. Several second generation SGAs – with higher airway seal and a drain tube – are more suitable for controlled ventilation than the cLMA.

Use of the cLMA for laparoscopic surgery is also controversial. The use of controlled ventilation, raised intra-abdominal pressure and the lithotomy position all theoretically increase aspiration risk. Several small trials support the use of the cLMA for gynaecological laparoscopy and suggest controlled ventilation with muscle relaxation or spontaneous ventilation are both acceptable. Proof of safety is absent but series of up to 1500 cases with no cases of aspiration are reported.

Despite these reassuring data, in NAP4 the commonest cause of events and of airway-related death was pulmonary aspiration: half of these cases involved use of an SGA and in most cases a first generation device. Poor case selection and acceptance of a poor airway were common themes.

Another useful role for the cLMA is to maintain the airway after tracheal extubation. Tracheal extubation can be associated with undesirable haemodynamic and respiratory complications and in particular coughing and oxygen desaturation and these are reduced by use of a cLMA (this technique is described in Chapter 21).

The breadth of cases that the cLMA has been used for is enormous. There are reports of the use of the cLMA for elective laparotomy, abdominal aortic aneurysm surgery, caesarean section, neurosurgery and cardiac surgery. In intensive care medicine the cLMA has been used for brief periods of controlled ventilation in selected cases, as a bridge to extubation, as an aid for weaning from mechanical ventilation and during percutaneous dilational tracheostomy. However, successful use does not indicate safety or even efficacy. 'Can do' does not equate to 'should do'! In many of these advanced settings a second generation SGA may be more suitable.

Use in Difficult Airway Management

The cLMA has multiple uses in difficult airway management – some are described below. However, it is notable that second generation SGAs have likely superseded the cLMA in difficult airway management in most circumstances.

Use during Cardiopulmonary Resuscitation and Neonatal Resuscitation

During the 1990s and 2000s the cLMA developed an important role during cardiopulmonary resuscitation and neonatal resuscitation. Again, the best of the second generation SGAs have generally superseded the cLMA for this role (see Chapter 31).

Second Generation SGAs

The most important include

- ProSeal LMA
- i-gel
- LMA Supreme
- LMA Protector
- Laryngeal tube suction II (reusable and disposable versions)
- Gastro-LT and LMA Gastro airway
- Streamlined liner of the pharynx airway

Other second generation devices include the Baska, Eclipse, Combitube and Easytube: key features are listed in Table 13.1 and some devices shown in Figure 13.1.

ProSeal Laryngeal Mask Airway (PLMA)

The PLMA, introduced to the UK in January 2001, was designed by Dr Archie Brain based on the cLMA with modifications intended to improve controlled ventilation, improve safety and enable diagnosis of misplacement.

Compared to the cLMA the PLMA has a softer, larger bowl, a posterior extension of the cuff, a drainage tube running parallel to the airway tube and an integral bite block (Figure 13.4). The modifications improve the airway seal, enable leaking gas to vent via the drain tube and facilitate passage of an orogastric tube (OGT). The drain tube enables early diagnosis of PLMA misplacement, which is not possible with the cLMA (Box 13.1).

Figure 13.4 ProSeal LMA.

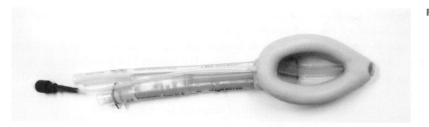

Box 13.1 Algorithm for checking ProSeal LMA (PLMA) positioning

Note any resistance or hold up during insertion. This suggests folding over of the mask tip.

Inflate cuff to 60–70 cmH$_2$O.

Assess depth of insertion. More than 50% of the bite block should usually be beyond the incisors.

Start controlled ventilation while assessing for unobstructed inspiratory and expiratory flow, observing capnometry and spirometry. Poor compliance or reduced expiratory flow may indicate mechanical obstruction of the vocal cords.

Place gel (or a film of soapy liquid) over the drain tube. (i) If this blows (or inflates) immediately with ventilation (or oscillations of the film are seen in time with the pulse) the PLMA may be sited in the glottic opening. Pressure on the chest leading to displacement of the gel confirms this. (ii) Blowing of the gel with applied airway circuit pressure of < 20 cmH$_2$O suggests the PLMA needs advancing further. The airway may be advanced to resolve a leak, otherwise it should be removed and reinserted.

Unexpectedly high inflation pressures may also indicate folding over of the tip.

If hold up was noted during insertion further tests to exclude tip folding should be used even if ventilation is successful. Press briefly on the suprasternal notch. This raises the pressure in the oesophagus and if this pressure rise is not transmitted to the drain tube the tip of the mask may be folded over. Inability to freely pass an OGT 30 cm to the tip of the drain tube may be used to confirm this. If the tip is folded over the PLMA should be reinserted.

(a) (b)

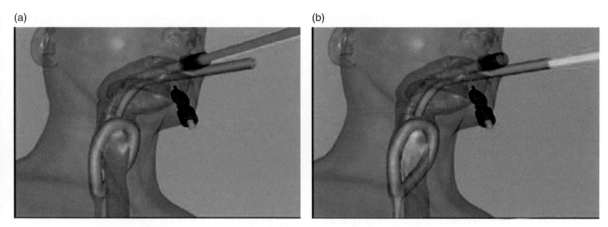

Figure 13.5 (a and b) ProSeal LMA showing the (a) airway tube lying over the glottis and (b) drain tube and access to the oesophagus.

Correctly placed, the PLMA lies with the drain tube in continuity with the oesophagus and the airway tube in continuity with the trachea (Figure 13.5). As the airway and oesophageal seals are both increased this creates functional separation of the alimentary and respiratory tracts. The drain tube vents gas leaking from the mask into the oesophagus and prevents gastric distension. It also may vent regurgitated liquid stomach contents.

Sizes 1–5 are available and size selection is as for other LMA devices: the smallest sizes lack the posterior cuff.

The PLMA may be inserted with or without an introducer that is supplied with it (Figure 13.2). Without the introducer the technique is the same as that for the cLMA (see above) and with the introducer is as for the ILMA (see below). There is no convincing evidence that one method is preferable. An important alternative method involves prior placement of a bougie, straight tip first (or a gastric tube), into the oesophagus, over which the PLMA drain tube is then railroaded. After insertion the cuff is inflated. While maximum volumes are published by the manufacturers, inflation to an intracuff pressure of 60–70 cmH$_2$O is preferred.

Table 13.3 Tests of PLMA positioning

Position	Bite block position	Pressure on chest	Suprasternal notch pressure	Airway seal	Other
Correct position	< 50% (often < 25%) visible at mouth	–	Gel blows off drain tube	Median 32 cmH$_2$O	Able to pass OGT with ease
Tip in glottis	–	Gel blows off drain tube	–		Obstructed airway
Mask folded over	> 50% may be visible	–	–	May be high or low	Resistance on insertion Airway may be obstructed Unable to pass OGT
Tip in pharynx	> 50% visible	–	–	Low (< 20 cmH$_2$O)	

A lubricated OGT can be passed through the drain tube when indicated.

When correctly positioned the tip of the PLMA (corresponding to the distal end of the drain tube) lies behind the cricoid cartilage. There are three important misplacements possible with the PLMA:

- If placed too proximally, ventilated air is vented via the drain tube
- If the tip enters the glottis airway obstruction is likely; a forced exhalation (pressure on the chest wall) leads to gel displacement from the drain tube
- If the tip folds over during insertion the functionality of the drain tube is lost. This misplacement is readily diagnosed by inability to pass an OGT to the tip of the PLMA.

A small amount of gel placed over the drain tube enables diagnosis of misplacements (Table 13.3). This enables early correction of position and optimal function.

Successful insertion and ventilation rates of approximately 99% can be achieved. First time insertion rates are somewhat lower (85%) than for the cLMA (92%) and time taken for insertion a few seconds longer. However, use of a bougie-guided technique leads to almost 100% first-attempt success rates, without an increase in trauma or sequelae. This insertion technique is specifically recommended when other techniques fail or for rescue after failed tracheal intubation.

Median airway seal pressure with the PLMA is approximately 32 cmH$_2$O, almost twice that of the cLMA, and exceeds 40 cmH$_2$O in 20% of cases. Results are similar with or without muscle relaxation.

The improved seal enables successful ventilation in many cases where this would not be achieved with the cLMA. The PLMA exerts lesser mucosal pressure than the cLMA for any given cuff pressure or airway seal.

OGT passage is successful in nearly 100% of correctly placed PLMAs: ease of passage correlates with positioning of the PLMA over the larynx. Where there is doubt over correct PLMA positioning, pass an OGT and if this fails reposition the PLMA.

The PLMA is designed to decrease risks of regurgitation and of aspiration if regurgitation occurs. There is extensive robust evidence from bench work, cadaver and clinical studies to support these claims, but it is unproven and probably unprovable. Cadaver studies show an oesophageal seal of 70–80 cmH$_2$O and efficacy of the drain tube in venting regurgitated fluid.

Considering all the available evidence the PLMA lessens the risk of aspiration compared with the cLMA and there is an argument for its routine use. However, no SGA should be used for cases of significant aspiration risk, except as a temporary rescue device.

Complications associated with the PLMA include minor airway obstruction and difficult placement. It is unclear whether these occur more frequently with the PLMA than the cLMA. Complications when using controlled ventilation are less frequent when the PLMA is used.

There are several studies comparing PLMA performance with other SGAs. In all of these to date the PLMA performs as well as or better than other SGAs, making it the benchmark for a high quality second generation SGA.

Based on the available evidence the PLMA is an appropriate SGA for use in several 'extended roles' *in selected patients*. These roles include use in moderately obese patients, for laparoscopic surgery, selected open abdominal surgery, as an adjunct for difficult intubation and a rescue device after failed intubation. Use in such cases mandates careful assessment of risk and benefit, a good understanding of the device and its limitations, experience in lower-risk cases and excellent technique.

Other advanced uses reported include use in the super-obese as a bridge to intubation, and for prone and emergency surgery.

The recommended product life is for 40 sterilisations. Cost is very similar to the cLMA.

i-gel

The i-gel is a cuffless, single-use SGA made of a medical grade elastomer gel. Features (and potential benefits) include a short wide-bore airway tube with no grilles (low resistance to gas flow and good access to the airway as a conduit), an elliptical stem (stability) and 'anatomically' shaped bowl (improved pharyngeal seal), an integral bite block (prevention of obstruction) and a drain tube (safety against regurgitation). A full range of paediatric sizes are available but are considerably less well evaluated than adult devices.

Insertion is performed in the sniffing position and requires that the i-gel is lubricated *on all surfaces* before insertion. Due to its bulk, good mouth opening and jaw thrust assist insertion. Standard insertion mimics cLMA insertion with the passage of the i-gel following the roof of the mouth and posterior pharynx until stopped by cricopharyngeus muscles. A rotatory insertion technique is also described in which the device is inserted laterally and when resistance is felt it is rotated and advanced into place.

Evidence confirms that the i-gel is remarkably easy to insert, both by experienced and novice users. This is because of a combination of remarkably low frictional properties and the fact there is no cuff to inflate. The pharyngeal seal is approximately 24–28 cmH$_2$O in most cases but in 2–5% it is considerably lower, and ventilation is not possible: choosing another size may help. Its tip is shorter than many SGAs and it therefore does not penetrate so far into the post-cricoid area. This has two consequences; first it has a low oesophageal seal (13–21 cmH$_2$O) and relies on the drain tube to reduce risk of aspiration; second its use is associated with less dysphagia and dysphonia than other SGAs.

Gastric access is as reliable as for the PLMA, though the drain tube is smaller. The myth that the 'thermoplastic' nature of the elastomer leads to an increase in seal pressure over time as the device warms has been disproved. It is likely the seal of all SGAs improves in the first 10–15 minutes of use and may occur as the pharynx adapts to the shape of the device.

The i-gel offers the potential for improved ease of use, improved ventilation and increased safety compared with the cLMA, in a disposable SGA. Its performance characteristics and design have made it a popular alternative to the cLMA. It is widely used for airway management during CPR and during out-of-hospital airway management (see Chapters 30 and 31). It is suitable for airway rescue and its short wide stem makes it especially suited as a conduit for direct (accepting a 7.0 mm ID tracheal tube) or flexible optical bronchoscope (FOB)-guided intubation. Even though direct intubation is relatively successful compared with many other SGAs an FOB should be used for this procedure, when available.

Complications reported with the i-gel are few. Laryngopharyngeal trauma and pain after use appear very infrequent indeed. Transient nerve injuries and lingual congestion have been reported but their frequency appears low.

LMA Supreme and LMA Protector

The LMA Supreme and LMA Protector are single-use SGAs made of PVC and silicone, respectively. They are designed to combine the most useful elements of the PLMA (improved airway seal, drain tube, integral bite block) with those of the ILMA (rigid anatomical stem enabling reliable insertion without needing to place hands in the patient's mouth) and the LMA Unique (single use). The LMA Supreme is available in a full range of sizes and the LMA Protector only in adult sizes at present. The manufacturers recommend their use for the same indications as the PLMA.

Ease of insertion may be improved compared with the PLMA but other benefits are unproven. The LMA Supreme is somewhat rigid and this, combined with its PVC construction, may lead to increased rates of minor airway trauma. The silicone LMA Protector may solve this problem. Once inserted, correct depth of insertion (and sizing) is indicated by a tab on the upper surface of the device: this should sit 0.5–2.0 cm from the upper lip. The tab is also designed for fixation of the device using adhesive tape. The LMA Supreme achieves an airway seal of 24–28 cmH$_2$O while early

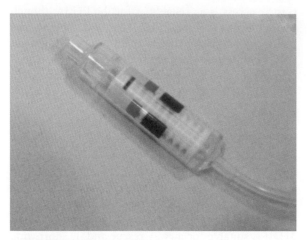

Figure 13.6 The cuff pilot technology on the LMA Protector, which provides a visual indication of the safety of the intracuff pressure.

studies suggest that for the LMA Protector may be higher. The airway sits over the larynx as frequently as the cLMA or PLMA. An OGT can usually be passed via the drain tube. Both have good sized drain tubes.

A limitation of the LMA Supreme is that the drain tube is central in the stem with two narrow (5 mm) airway channels running either side. This has been addressed in the LMA Protector and the airway lumen is large (facilitating use as a conduit for intubation) and central. Both devices are suitable for many of the same roles as the PLMA but as yet there is no evidence of any benefit of using these devices instead of the PLMA and their per case costs are notably higher than for reusable SGAs.

The LMA Protector has a 'cuff pilot' which replaces the pilot balloon. The pilot gives a visual representation of whether the intracuff pressure is correct, using a traffic light system (Figure 13.6).

Laryngeal Tube Suction II

In 2002 a new version of the laryngeal tube (LT) (see below) was introduced, the LT-suction (LTS), with a drain tube running posterior to the airway tube to enable OGT placement and prevent gastric inflation during ventilation. While the design aimed to increase device safety (a similar step to that from cLMA to PLMA) the change in design led to a much bulkier device that was harder to insert and potentially traumatic: thereby losing two of the LT's major advantages. In 2005 the LTS was further modified (LTS-II) with the addition of a slim profile tip and asymmetric oesophageal balloon. Like the LT the LTS-II is

reusable after sterilisation up to 50 times. Size selection and insertion technique for the LTS-II is identical to the LT. A single-use device (LTS-D) is also available.

The LTS device is easily inserted and achieves relatively high airway and oesophageal seals. It may be suitable both for elective anaesthesia, for use out of hospital and during CPR. It is somewhat prone to axial rotation and its relatively small airway orifice may not sit over the glottis. This and its narrow airway orifice make it rather unsuited as a conduit for intubation whether directly or with an Aintree intubation catheter (see below).

Recently a version designed to facilitate intubation – the intubating laryngeal tube with drain tube (iLTS-D) – has been released.

Gastro-LT and LMA Gastro Airway

Both the LT series and LMA series include SGAs designed for use in upper gastrointestinal endoscopy. The drain tube has been expanded to a size that will accept a gastrointestinal endoscope and the airway tube reduced to minimal calibre. Small case series attest to their efficacy and greater speed than performing procedures with tracheal intubation, but there are no substantial studies confirming safety.

Streamlined Liner of the Pharynx Airway (SLIPA)

The streamlined liner of the pharynx airway (SLIPA) is a single-use, cuffless, 'boot-shaped', second generation SGA of novel design: a soft plastic blow-moulded airway with the shape mimicking a 'pressurised pharynx'. It is designed to sit with the toe of the boot in the hypopharynx. Lateral prominences in the device midportion are designed to sit in the pyriform fossae displacing the tongue base anteriorly, so improving airway seal, reducing airway obstruction by the epiglottis and stabilising the device's position.

The SLIPA is included in the second generation SGAs on the basis of design only. It lacks a drain tube but the inventor describes the hollow interior as a protective reservoir (sump) with the capacity to accommodate 50–70 mL of fluid in the event of regurgitation.

There are six sizes and while size selection is based on height the aim is to match the maximum diameter of the SLIPA with the maximum diameter of the larynx (measured as the maximum width of the thyroid cartilage in millimetres).

Early cohort and comparative trials by the inventor showed satisfactory insertion performance (90% first-attempt insertion success and a pharyngeal seal comparable or above the cLMA). A few small independent trials have been performed showing adequate insertion success and airway seal. One trial suggested increased gastric inflation. Trauma, bleeding and the ability to protect the airway are potential concerns.

Other Second Generation SGAs

The Baska mask, Eclipse, Combitube and Easytube are described in Table 13.1. Second generation SGAs of use for intubation are shown in Figure 13.7.

First Generation SGAs

Key features of several first generation SGAs are listed in Table 13.1. Several are also described below.

The Flexible (Reinforced) LMA (fLMA)

The flexible or reinforced LMA is identical to the cLMA except for the airway tube, which is made of soft silicone with spiral wire reinforcement. This means that the airway tube is more flexible and is less prone to kink when bent. Unlike the cLMA, the fLMA airway tube can be moved as necessary to improve surgical access without displacing the mask and this is especially useful when surgery is close to the face. It is available in single-use and reusable versions in sizes 2–6.

The fLMA stem is long and narrow such that the overall airway resistance with an fLMA is somewhat higher than for a tracheal tube. The increased work of breathing during spontaneous ventilation is rarely clinically important. The long narrow stem also makes the fLMA poorly suited as a conduit for tracheal intubation. The wire in the airway tube makes it unsuitable for use in the MRI scanner.

Insertion technique is identical to the cLMA but requires considerably greater attention to detail to prevent axial rotation. Poor technique may lead to a 'backwards facing' device, with a substandard airway and the potential for reduced airway protection. Device performance is as per the cLMA. A modified version, the LMA Flexyplus, has a more rigid curved distal stem, designed to ease insertion and positioning, while preserving the flexibility of the proximal stem. Its performance is largely unevaluated.

The fLMA is particularly suitable for head, neck and especially intra-oral surgery. During ophthalmological

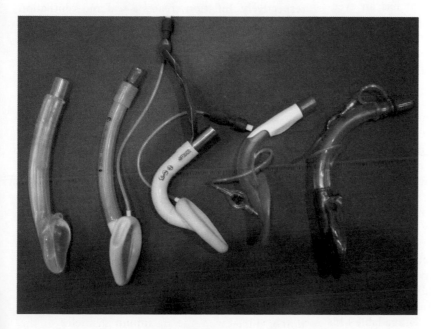

Figure 13.7 SGAs suitable or designed for intubation. From left to right, i-gel, LMA Classic Excel, Intubating LMA, Ambu Aura-I, AirQ. The Ambu AuraGain is not pictured.

surgery, compared with a tracheal tube, it causes less rise in intraocular pressure and less coughing and airway complications during emergence. Its use during maxillofacial and ENT surgery is described in Chapters 25 and 26.

Laryngeal Masks (LMs): Single-Use and Reusable

Since 2003, when many cLMA patents lapsed, many manufacturers have produced competitors to the cLMA and fLMA both in single-use and reusable form. As the term laryngeal mask airway (LMA) is registered the newer devices are referred to as laryngeal masks (LMs). The manufacturers propose the main driving force for the introduction of single-use devices has been concerns over sterility of cleaned reusable devices. This has been a particular issue in the United Kingdom since 2001 with concerns over elimination of proteinaceous material and the risk of transmission of prion disease (variant Creutzfeldt–Jakob Disease, vCJD – see Chapter 37); the relevance of this is now diminished as vCJD has been eliminated from the food chain for more than a decade. The scientific rationale for a change in practice to single-use LMs on the basis of infection risk is, at best, questionable and the environmental impact of the rush to single-use plastic equipment has an ever-increasing importance. The financial opportunities of the cLMA market are another obvious reason for the proliferation of such devices.

For patent reasons all LMs differ from LMAs and there is also much variation between LMs. All LMs do not have the grille at the distal end of the airway tube. Some have angulated stems and some enlarged masks. Particularly with the larger sizes there is a possibility of tongue entrapment or epiglottic downfolding during insertion. Many single-use LMs are made of PVC, which increases the rigidity of the mask and may increase trauma. Silicone devices, both single use and reusable, are now also available. Nitrous oxide does not diffuse into PVC cuffs.

Generally, there is little robust evidence to advise whether the currently available single-use LM devices perform similarly to equivalent LMAs nor to advise which LM performs best. What the limited evidence does show is that all LMs and LMAs are not equivalent. A systematic review of 27 available LMs reported that only two had substantial publications to compare efficacy with the cLMA; for one device the body of evidence strongly suggests poorer performance than the cLMA while for the Ambu Aura LM evidence from about 400 patients suggested equivalence. For the other 25 devices there appeared to be a vacuum of published evidence. A publication from the National Health Service centre for evidence-based purchasing illustrates the difficulty in determining the relative merits and demerits of these competitors to the cLMA: the document listed more than 25 alternative standard LMs and reported a total of 18 comparative trials between devices. Some of these studies were of poor quality. This contrasts to the > 2500 publications on the cLMA alone.

The Laryngeal Tube

The laryngeal tube (LT) consists of a slim airway tube with a small balloon cuff attached at the tip (distal cuff) and a larger asymmetric cuff encircling the middle part of the tube (proximal cuff) (Figure 13.1). Both cuffs are inflated through a single pilot tube and balloon, through which the cuff pressure can be monitored. When the device is inserted, it lies along the length of the tongue. Proximal and distal cuffs sit in the oropharynx and oesophageal inlet, respectively. Inflation creates a seal and ventilation occurs through relatively small orifices between the cuffs.

It is designed for use during spontaneous breathing, controlled ventilation and airway rescue and has been used for all of these roles. Its narrow profile design makes insertion easy but this and the lack of a mask increase the risk of axial rotation: the airway orifice then misaligns with the glottis. This impacts spontaneous ventilation (causing airway obstruction) more than controlled ventilation. No advantages of the LT over the cLMA and PLMA during controlled ventilation have been demonstrated. It is not widely used during anaesthesia but easy insertion by relative novices gives it a potential role during CPR (see Chapter 31).

A family of devices exist, with the range matching that of the LMA family. The apparently considerable evidence base for the LT family is hampered by multiple iterations of device(s) compromising interpretation of studies.

LMA Unique, CobraPLA and Tulip

The LMA Unique, CobraPLA and Tulip airway are described in Table 13.1.

SGAs in Paediatric Practice

There is a general consensus that use of SGAs in children below 10 kg and especially 5 kg weight is of higher risk and is a specialised technique. Database evidence has recently confirmed this.

There is a considerably smaller evidence base to choose the best SGA in children compared with adults. A number of RCTs, in all age ranges, demonstrate improved performance by the PLMA compared with the cLMA. A network meta-analysis compared airway seal, first-attempt insertion failure, overall failure and risk of blood staining across a range of SGAs. The PLMA, i-gel and CobraPLA had the best airway seals. The i-gel was the only device with significantly reduced blood staining risk, but it was amongst a small number of devices with an increased risk of failure (6%). The authors concluded the PLMA was the 'best SGA for children'.

Clinician Choice of SGA

Several surveys have shown that the majority of anaesthetists pay little regard to what SGA they use – both in adult and paediatric practice: lowest cost of devices ranks as the highest priority and evidence base lowest. 'I use whatever I am handed' was a common response in one survey. This academic 'blind spot' regarding SGAs is unsatisfactory as there is evidence of differential performance, failure rates and likely safety of different devices. These adverse outcomes are evermore likely when SGAs are used for advanced indications. SGAs are also important rescue devices during difficult airway management and the optimal device should be deployed.

Understanding performance characteristics of SGAs and using those with the best characteristics is likely to improve efficacy, efficiency and safety of routine and difficult airway management.

SGAs and Difficult Airway Management

SGAs may be used to rescue an airway or as a conduit to manage tracheal intubation electively or after failed intubation.

Airway Rescue

SGAs are reliable after failed mask ventilation or failed tracheal intubation and are likely to 'rescue the airway' in more than 90% of such cases. Airway difficulty is more likely in the obese and during emergencies when patients may not be starved, both circumstances when a first generation SGA is not the device of choice. Airway rescue should generally be with a second generation SGA and this requires that they are available and that airway managers are skilled in their routine use. This is specifically recommended in some airway guidelines, including the UK DAS 2015 guidelines.

If an SGA is used to rescue the airway during rapid sequence induction it is important to understand how cricoid force impedes placement and function. For example, the tip of the cLMA seats behind the cricoid cartilage so placement is not possible in the presence of cricoid force. If cricoid force is being applied it should be removed to enable cLMA placement. Once the cLMA is placed cricoid force may be reapplied but it may interfere with effective ventilation. Conversely, although cricoid force needs to be removed to place the PLMA, once placed it still enables ventilation if cricoid force is reapplied.

Intubation via an SGA

When an SGA is correctly placed the glottis is visible with an FOB in at least 90% of cases, though rates vary between devices. Several SGAs are specifically designed to work as a conduit for tracheal intubation (ILMA, LMA Classic Excel, Ambu Aura-i, iLTS-D), others are well suited to use for intubation (i-gel, PLMA, LMA Protector, AirQ device) while some others because of a narrow stem or airway orifice are not (LMA Supreme, all other laryngeal tubes). SGAs with a very large stem may enable direct placement of a tracheal tube (e.g. i-gel, AirQ). For those with a narrower stem a two-stage technique using the Aintree intubating catheter (AIC) is suitable and this technique is included in several airway rescue algorithms. Intubation via the ILMA and with an AIC are described here.

Direct Intubation via an SGA

Blind intubation via an SGA with bougie or tube is unreliable (success 10–20%) and risks airway and oesophageal trauma. It is not recommended.

Intubation via selected SGAs with an FOB has a high success rate of at least 90%. This is described in Chapter 16.

The Intubating LMA (ILMA) (Fastrach)

The intubating LMA (ILMA) (Figure 13.2) was introduced into practice in the late 1990s. It was designed by Dr Archie Brain to provide a dedicated airway and enable tracheal intubation with a moderate-size tracheal tube through it, in both easy and difficult airways. The stem is short, rigid and anatomically curved. This enables easy mask insertion, even by novices. A plastic single-use version is available but is less well evaluated than the metal and silicone reusable device.

Intubation via the ILMA is facilitated by the anatomical shape of the stem, use of the dedicated ILMA tracheal tube (Figure 13.2) and optimal technique including ensuring the ILMA is optimally placed over the glottis before attempting intubation. Intubation via the ILMA can be performed blind or guided by an FOB, with first-attempt success rates by trained operators for each technique of approximately 75% and 97%, respectively. The most difficult part of the intubation technique is removal of the ILMA after intubation – failure to follow the correct technique will lead to avulsion of the pilot tube from the tracheal tube meaning it cannot be easily inflated. The ILMA has become less popular in the last decade but success rates for intubation are at least as high as for other SGAs and notably higher than others for blind intubation. Reports of harm during intubation generally relate to use of techniques not recommended by the manufacturer. Concerns about the ILMA include relatively high cost and the potential for mucosal trauma from the rigid tube pressing against the oral mucosa have limited its routine use, but it is highly successful if used correctly.

Technique is described in Box 13.2.

Intubation via an SGA Using an Aintree Intubation Catheter (AIC)

The AIC is a narrow 56 cm long tube of external diameter of approximately 6.5 mm and internal diameter of 4.5 mm. It is designed to facilitate FOB-guided exchange of an SGA to a tracheal tube. The technique is described in Box 13.3 and Figure 13.8.

Box 13.2 Intubation via an intubating LMA (ILMA)

- After anaesthesia is established, the ILMA is inserted and 100% oxygen is administered. As per routine LMA insertion the tip of the mask is placed against the hard palate and the airway advanced along the hard palate, soft palate and posterior pharyngeal wall, until the tip lies at the top of the oesophagus. The ILMA is best inserted by holding the handle and rotating it inwards.
- The ILMA position is optimised. This may be tested by manual or mechanical ventilation and assessing whether it is optimal by 'feel' or by examination of spirometry. Optimal ventilation is essential as this correlates with the ILMA orifice lying directly over the glottis.
- If ventilation is not optimal the ILMA may be repositioned by gently moving it inwards and outwards. If this does not produce easy ventilation a downfolded epiglottis may be corrected by withdrawing the ILMA 6–8 cm and reinserting.
- Once optimal ventilation is achieved the ILMA should be held by its handle and gently lifted to hold the mask against the glottis. The anaesthetic circuit is now disconnected ready for intubation.
- The ILMA tracheal tube is inserted. A 6.0 mm ID tube is recommended unless there is a reason to use a larger one. The tracheal tube connector should be partially inserted so that it is easy to remove after intubation.
- *Blind technique*. The ILMA tracheal tube is inserted, with the longitudinal line facing cephalad, until the horizontal black line on the tube enters the ILMA stem – at this point the tracheal tube tip exits the ILMA tube, pushing up the epiglottic elevator. The tracheal tube is advanced approximately 6–8 cm further. There should be no resistance as the tracheal tube enters the trachea. If there is resistance the tracheal tube should be removed and the process of ILMA position optimisation should be restarted.
- We recommend that a flexible bronchoscope is always used for intubation via the ILMA when available.

Box 13.2 (cont.)

- *Flexible optical bronchoscope-guided technique.* There are two techniques. In the 'tube first technique' after optimising the ILMA position the ILMA tracheal tube is inserted 2–3 cm beyond the horizontal black line, to lift the epiglottic elevator. The FOB is then inserted via the tracheal tube, into the trachea to the carina and then the tracheal tube railroaded over the FOB. In the 'scope first technique' the FOB (with the tracheal tube loaded) is inserted first and is negotiated around the epiglottic elevator and into the trachea before the tracheal tube is railroaded over it. The former technique may be quicker for 'easy' airways where the glottis is likely to lie behind the epiglottic elevator, while the latter may be more successful in more complex airways and where there is displacement of the glottis or trachea.
- After tracheal tube insertion the tube cuff is inflated until there is no leak during ventilation. Note the reusable ILMA tracheal tube (pink tip and pilot balloon) has a low-volume high-pressure cuff and the single-use version (white tip and pilot cuff) has an intermediate size and pressure cuff.
- Ventilation is re-established, correct positioning is confirmed with capnography and auscultation of the lungs and there is a further period of oxygenation.
- *ILMA removal.* The ILMA is not designed to be left in place beyond a few hours and should be removed in most cases. This is the most high-risk part of the process, but only because technique is often poor. The depth of insertion of the tracheal tube is noted. The tracheal tube connector is removed and kept for later use. The ILMA stabilising rod is placed into the tracheal tube – note it is not a 'pusher' – and stabilises the ILMA tracheal tube position while the ILMA (with its cuff deflated) is removed. The tracheal tube is not advanced. As the ILMA mask starts to exit the mouth the stabiliser is removed. The operator can then hold onto the tracheal tube in the mouth as the ILMA is completely removed.
- It is essential to remove the stabiliser before completely removing the ILMA as if this is not done the pilot cuff of the ILMA tracheal tube will be caught and avulsed between the stabiliser and the ILMA stem, and the tube cuff will deflate.
- Once the ILMA is fully removed the tracheal tube connector and anaesthetic circuit are reattached and ventilation re-established.
- Note – if the ILMA tracheal tube pilot tube is avulsed a small blunt needle or cannula (e.g. 18G) can be inserted into the pilot tube and used to re-inflate the cuff before clamping the pilot tube. The tracheal tube should then be replaced.

Box 13.3 Intubation via an SGA with an Aintree intubation catheter

- The Aintree intubation catheter (AIC) is placed over a flexible optical bronchoscope (FOB) of suitable size (< 4.5 mm).
- An angle piece with a rubber diaphragm through which the FOB can be inserted is attached between the SGA and the catheter mount. Ventilation of the patient should continue throughout, an increased FiO_2 is advised. Care during insertion of the SGA and optimising ease of ventilation (to increase the likelihood of the SGA lying over the glottis) is also important.
- The FOB and AIC combination, both slightly lubricated externally, are inserted through the diaphragm and into the SGA stem and advanced through the SGA stem to the mask portion. If the glottis is easily visible the FOB/AIC are passed through and advanced to just above the carina. If the glottis is not easily accessible the procedure should be stopped, the FOB/AIC removed, the SGA repositioned and then the procedure restarted.
- The FOB is then removed without removing the AIC and while maintaining the AIC at the same depth of insertion.
- The SGA is also removed, again without displacing the AIC.
- A suitable tracheal tube is railroaded over the AIC, and once this is in position the AIC is removed. Correct placement of the tracheal tube is confirmed by capnography and auscultation.
- The type of tracheal tube should be one suitable for FOB-guided intubation (see Chapter 16). For most tracheal tubes a size 7.0 mm ID tube is suitable. A 6.5 mm ID ILMA tracheal tube is also suitable.

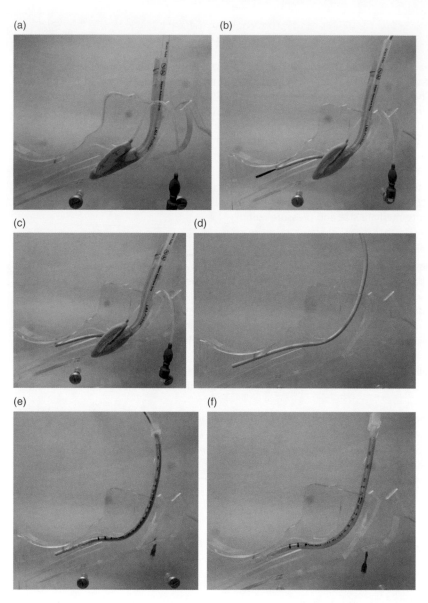

(a)   (b)   (c)   (d)   (e)   (f)

Figure 13.8 (a–f) Exchange of an SGA to a tracheal tube using the Aintree Intubating catheter (AIC). The technique is described in Box 13.3.

Further Reading

Asai T, Shingu K. (2005). The laryngeal tube. *British Journal of Anaesthesia*, **95**, 729–736.

Caponas G. (2002). Intubating laryngeal mask airway. A review. *Anaesthesia and Intensive Care*, **30**, 551–569.

Cook TM, Lee G, Nolan JP. (2005). The ProSeal™ laryngeal mask airway: a review of the literature. *Canadian Journal of Anaesthesia*, **52**, 739–760.

Keller C, Brimacombe J, Bittersohl P, Lirk P, von Goedecke A. (2004). Aspiration and the laryngeal mask airway: three cases and a review of the literature. *British Journal of Anaesthesia*, **93**, 579–582.

Mihara T, Asakura A, Owada G, et al. (2017). A network meta-analysis of the clinical properties of various types of supraglottic airway device in children. *Anaesthesia*, **72**, 1251–1264.

NHS Purchasing and Supply Agency, Centre for Evidence-based Purchasing. (2008). *Buyers' guide: Laryngeal masks*.

Schmidbauer W, Bercker S, Volk T, et al. (2009). Oesophageal seal of the novel supralaryngeal airway device I-Gel in comparison with the laryngeal mask airways Classic and ProSeal using a cadaver model. *British Journal of Anaesthesia*, **102**, 135–139.

Theiler L, Gutzmann M, Kleine-Brueggeney M, et al. (2012). i-gel™ supraglottic airway in clinical practice: a prospective observational multicentre study. *British Journal of Anaesthesia*, **109**, 990–995.

Verghese C, Brimacombe J. (1996). Survey of laryngeal mask airway usage in 11,910 patients: safety and efficacy for conventional and non-conventional usage. *Anesthesia & Analgesia*, **82**, 129–133.

Tracheal Intubation: Direct Laryngoscopy

Keith Greenland and Richard Levitan

'If you know the enemy and know yourself, you need not fear the result of a hundred battles...'
Sun Tzu, The Art of War (5th century BC)

Successful direct laryngoscopy and tracheal intubation is based on a clear understanding of upper airway anatomy and how it can be manipulated to achieve successful airway management and patient safety. Understanding the mechanisms of normal and difficult direct laryngoscopy can be illustrated by two concepts: the two curve theory and three column model. This enables the difficult airway to be managed predictively rather than reactively.

Airway assessment and preparation before performing airway manoeuvres have been highlighted in a number of airway management audits, including NAP4. These topics are covered in detail in Chapters 5–7. The reader should be familiar with these subjects before reading this chapter.

The Key Elements of Successful Direct Laryngoscopy

These are
1. Correct positioning of the head and neck
2. Correct insertion and manipulation of the laryngoscope blade within the upper airway

The two curve theory is an alternative to the three axes alignment theory and allows an understanding of airway configuration in different head and neck positions (Figure 14.1). This theory divides the airway passage into two curves:
1. Primary or oropharyngeal curve
2. Secondary or laryngotracheal curve

How to Flatten the Primary Curve through Patient Positioning

When the adult is in the neutral position (i.e. no pillow and the patient has a vertical gaze with no head extension, such as the position commonly found during manual in-line neck stabilisation) each curve has a small radius of curvature making airway manoeuvres difficult.

The optimal airway position is that which enables easy airway management. This occurs when the external auditory meatus and the sternal notch lie on the same horizontal plane. This occurs in a small child with a small head-ring under the head, in a large child and adult with a single pillow and in the obese patient with 'ramping' using several pillows or wedges under the upper torso and head (Figure 14.2).

In the 'sniffing position' there is a combination of lower cervical flexion and upper cervical extension. This flattens both curves (Figure 14.1B) and makes airway manipulation easier, thereby improving the chance of successful direct laryngoscopy.

An alternative to the sniffing position is to tilt the upper body 25° 'head-up'. This rotates the oroglotto-tracheal curve and aligns it with the operator's viewing angle during direct laryngoscopy. This position may be of use for emergency airway management when ramping the patient is logistically difficult (e.g. an unconscious obese patient).

The Function of a Standard Macintosh Laryngoscope Blade

The laryngoscope blade displaces the tongue to the left and completes the flattening of the primary curve by elevating the mandible and compressing the tissues in the submandibular space. The operator pushes the laryngoscope blade anterodistally (not levering on maxillary teeth) to (i) lift the epiglottis anteriorly by pressure on the hyoepiglottic ligament, (ii) displace the submandibular tissues anteriorly and (iii) push the tongue laterally. The result is to provide sufficient space for the operator to view the vocal cords and insert the tracheal tube into the trachea.

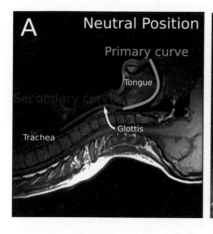
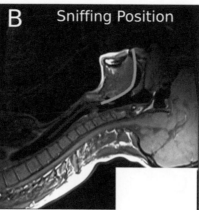

Figure 14.1 Airway passage (solid curved line) superimposed over MRI scan showing primary (solid green line) and secondary (solid red line) curves. (A) 'Neutral position' (no pillow): small radii of curvature of both curves. (B) 'Sniffing position': head lift (flexion of lower cervical spine) and head extension (extension of upper cervical spine) causes flattening of both curves.

Correct Technique When Using a Macintosh Laryngoscope Blade

The blade is optimally placed along the floor of the mouth to the right of the tongue and used to displace the tongue to the left (Figure 14.3A). This contrasts to placing the blade over the tongue (Figure 14.3B) where greater force is required as it is necessary to try to compress both the tongue and submandibular tissues.

An alternative technique is the retromolar approach when the patient's head is turned to the left and the blade is inserted over or behind the right molar teeth. This approach reduces the volume of submandibular tissue to be displaced and has been recommended for patients with a large tongue or at-risk upper teeth.

Anatomical Causes of Difficult Direct Laryngoscopy

An understanding of difficult direct laryngoscopy may be based on (i) why the two curves cannot be flattened and (ii) factors preventing correct insertion and manipulation of the laryngoscopy blade. These factors may be summarised in the three column model of difficult airways.

The Three Column Model of the Airway

In this model the airway is divided into three columns (Figure 14.4):

- Anterior column – formed by the mandible and submandibular tissues
- Middle column – formed by the airspace
- Posterior column – formed by the cervical spine

Factors Affecting the Anterior Column

Common factors that affect the ability to displace the anterior column with a laryngoscope blade include:

1. reduced volume (e.g. short mandible or short thyromental distance) that limits the space into which tissues can be compressed
2. reduced compliance of soft tissues (e.g. haematoma, infection, mass or previous radiotherapy to submandibular tissues) making compression more difficult

Factors Affecting the Middle Column

These problems generally lead to narrowing and/or distortion of the upper airway. They include:

1. laryngeal tumours
2. lingual tonsillar hypertrophy

Factors Affecting the Posterior Column

These occur when cervical spine mobility is reduced and impact the ability or not to achieve the 'sniffing position'. Problems include:

1. ankylosing spondylitis
2. manual in-line neck stabilisation
3. obesity, especially patients with enlarged dorsocervical fat pads ('buffalo humps') which prevent the head extending backwards

Use of Alternative Laryngoscope Blades to Resolve Difficulties

Different laryngoscope blades may be used logically by understanding the two curve and three column models.

123

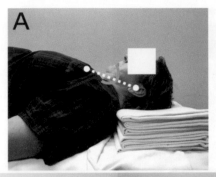

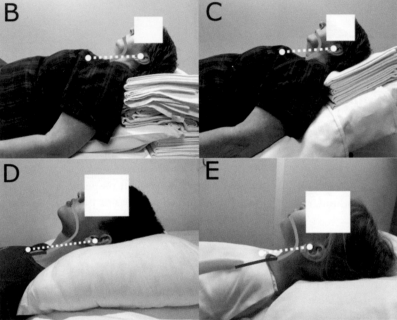

Figure 14.2 Head and neck positioning during airway management. (A) Obese patient with standard head lift: external auditory meatus and sternal notch are not in the same horizontal plane (white dotted line) leading to poor flattening of secondary curve (solid red line) and difficult direct laryngoscopy. (B) Obese patient in ramped position with head elevation and shoulder support: external auditory meatus and sternal notch are in the same horizontal plane (white dotted line) leading to flattening of secondary curve (solid red line) and easy direct laryngoscopy. (C) Obese patient with head-up positioning: similar effect to ramped position with external auditory meatus and sternal notch in the same horizontal plane (white dotted line) leading to flattening of secondary curve (solid red line) and easy direct laryngoscopy. (D) Non-obese patient with standard pillow: external auditory meatus and sternal notch are in the same horizontal plane (white dotted line) leading to flattening of secondary curve (solid red line). (E) Child with small pillow (i.e. relatively large head in relation to small antero-posterior diameter of chest): external auditory meatus and sternal notch are in the same horizontal plane (white dotted line) leading to flattening of secondary curve (solid red line).

The McCoy levering laryngoscope blade, in its flexed position, applies pressure at the base of the tongue lifting the epiglottis anteriorly and is therefore appropriate when there is a posterior column problem (e.g. manual in-line stabilisation of head and neck) where the mandible and submandibular tissues are normal. In contrast when there is an anterior column problem (a mismatch of submandibular space and tissue compressibility) the Miller straight blade may succeed as its low profile produces a higher pressure on the submandibular tissues with the same force (pressure = force/area) and it can be used to lift the epiglottis directly.

Use of Airway Adjuncts

If the primary curve is only partially flattened (e.g. Cormack and Lehane Grade 3 laryngoscopy), a curve-tipped device such as the bougie, stylet or an optical stylet may be used as an intubation adjunct to negotiate the distal part of the curve.

External laryngeal pressure will depress the glottic region and flatten the distal part of the primary curve helping to bring the larynx into the direct line of sight.

A Suggested Technique for Direct Laryngoscopy and Tracheal Intubation

Indications:

- Maintenance of oxygenation
- Maintenance of ventilation (controlling PCO_2)
- Maintenance of airway patency
- Prevention of pulmonary aspiration of gastric contents, blood etc.

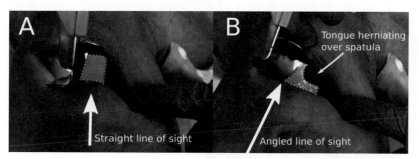

Figure 14.3 (A) Laryngoscope blade in paraglossal position causing lateral displacement of tongue and lifting submandibular tissues, providing wide field of view (yellow shaded area); straight line of sight over patient's head. (B) Laryngoscope blade placed over the tongue reducing field of view due to: (1) less displacement as the tongue is anterior to the blade and (2) tongue bulging over spatula into field of view; angled line of sight to view around bulging tongue.

- Access to the lower airway for tracheal toileting/suctioning

Preparation:

- Close communication with staff regarding the airway management strategy
- Appropriate monitoring
- Reliable intravenous access
- Testing tracheal tube cuff integrity
- Backup laryngoscope light source, selection of blades and different tracheal tube sizes
- Suction device available

Positioning of patient:

- If possible, the patient is placed in the sniffing position before induction of anaesthesia.

Pre-oxygenation with an anaesthesia circuit or other device capable of delivering > 90% FiO_2 with a tight-fitting mask should be performed for 3–5 minutes or until expired oxygen concentration (FeO_2) is > 90%. If there is insufficient time, the patient can take five to eight vital capacity breaths of 100% oxygen. In patients at risk of hypoxaemia during intubation, continuous positive airway pressure ventilation before induction and supplementary oxygen during the procedure is valuable.

Oxygenation during laryngoscopy may be achieved via simple nasal cannulae (2–4 L min^{-1} before induction, increased to 15 L min^{-1} after induction) or delivery of humidified high flow nasal oxygen (HFNO at up to 70 L min^{-1}). These techniques are discussed further in Chapters 8 and 28. Importantly, apnoeic oxygenation is only beneficial while the airway is patent and an assistant should ensure airway patency by jaw thrust. Returning to bag-mask ventilation between attempts at intubation when laryngoscopy is difficult should be routine practice.

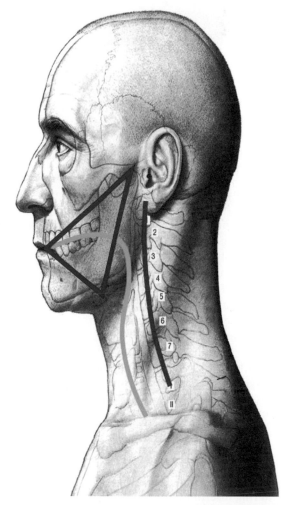

Figure 14.4 Three Columns: Anterior Column – mandible and submandibular tissues (blue triangle), Middle Column – airway passage (green line) and Posterior Column – cervical spine (red line). (Reappraisal of Adult Airway Management, K.B. Greenland *Australasian Anaesthesia* 2011 Publisher: Australian and New Zealand College of Anaesthetists 630 St Kilda Road Melbourne VIC 3004 ISBN 978–0-9775174–7-3 ISSN 1032–2515.)

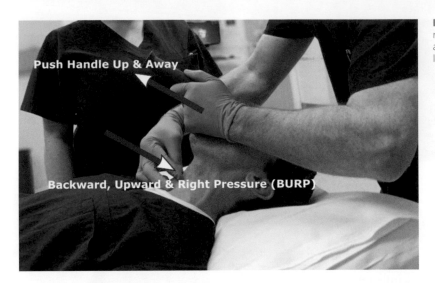

Push Handle Up & Away

Backward, Upward & Right Pressure (BURP)

Figure 14.5 Backwards, upwards and rightwards pressure to reverse the forces applied during laryngoscopy and improve laryngeal view.

Drugs for induction of anaesthesia and paralysis are discussed in Chapter 10.

Performing Direct Laryngoscopy

- Hold the laryngoscope handle in the left hand close to the hinge of the blade using a light ('two-finger') grip at the base of handle and blade. A common error of novice operators is forceful gripping of the handle and engaging the tongue with too much force. This can prevent optimal insertion of the blade tip into the vallecula and displacement of the tongue. It is important to slow the blade insertion from uvula to epiglottis to avoid over-insertion of the blade past the glottis.
- An assistant may open the mouth and apply jaw thrust. If operating alone, open the patient's mouth with the right hand pushing the front maxillary teeth cephalad with the third finger and mandibular teeth caudal with the index finger.
- Insert the blade tip to the right of the tongue, along the floor of mouth and into vallecula anterior to the epiglottis while using the blade to sweep the tongue to the left.
- Identify the tongue base, epiglottis and vallecula during insertion.
- Do not allow the tongue to herniate over the flange of the blade as it will obstruct the view.
- Place the blade tip into the base of the vallecula in the midline and lift the laryngoscope anterodistally. This lifts the blade away from

front maxillary teeth and the blade tip lifts the hyoid and epiglottis. With the blade tip placed well into the vallecula and strictly in the midline it will tighten the hyoepiglottic ligament, which will cause the epiglottis to pivot anteriorly revealing the larynx.

When using a Miller blade the tip is placed posterior to the epiglottis and used to lift it directly.

The tube tip is inserted from the right-hand side keeping the operator's hand out of the line of vision. Once the operator sees the tip of the tube pass through the glottis, the tube is inserted until the intubation marks are level with the glottic opening.

If the view is poor, check that the blade position is optimal and adjust if necessary.

The view may also be improved by backwards, upwards, rightwards pressure (BURP) applied to the thyroid cartilage. This counteracts the forces applied by the operator during laryngoscopy (Figure 14.5). This can be applied by the operator (variously referred to as 'bimanual laryngoscopy' or 'optimal external laryngeal manipulation') or by the assistant when it is referred to by its acronym: BURP.

If laryngoscopy remains difficult and oxygenation remains good, the tracheal tube tip may be guided around the epiglottis and into the trachea with either a stylet or a bougie.

- A stylet is inserted into the tracheal tube and should be straight (to mirror the straight line of sight) with a 35° bend angled at the proximal limit of the cuff (to mirror the bend required to negotiate the epiglottis). There is a risk of airway trauma including tracheal perforation when using a stylet and it should never enter the trachea. The stylet tip should not reach the tracheal tube tip and during intubation, as the tube tip reaches the glottis, the stylet should be progressively withdrawn so the tracheal tube, but not the stylet, enters the glottis and trachea.

- A bougie may be inserted into the trachea and the tracheal tube is then 'railroaded' over it into the trachea. A bougie may be inserted alone followed by railroading or may be inserted with the tube already mounted. Bougies may also cause airway trauma and should not be inserted beyond 25 cm from the teeth – so the tip remains above the carina. The tube may need to be rotated 90° anticlockwise over the bougie so that the tube tip enters the laryngeal inlet and does not catch on the arytenoid cartilages.

The tip of a bougie or styletted tube should pass over the interarytenoid notch (i.e. dividing line between larynx above and oesophagus below). The tube or bougie should always approach the glottis from below, enabling the operator to see it pass over the notch, rather than being inserted directly down the line of sight as this will obstruct the glottic view.

Significant Problems with Tracheal Tube Misplacement

Oesophageal Intubation

There are several techniques for detecting oesopha-geal tracheal tube placement. However, none has been shown to be 100% reliable. Several commonly used techniques include:

Clinical observation

- Seeing the tracheal tube passing through the glottis. Weaknesses: (i) operator needs to see at least part of the vocal cords, which may be obscured during intubation and (ii) does not provide assessment of ongoing tracheal tube placement.
- Condensation within the tracheal tube. Weaknesses: highly variable and inconsistent.
- Chest auscultation (five-point auscultation – lung apices, axillae and epigastric auscultation). Weakness: 'breath sounds' may be misdiagnosed in up to 15% of oesophageal intubations.

- Chest movement. Weaknesses: (i) decreased or absent chest excursion with obesity and lung diseases, (ii) oesophageal intubation does produce some degree of chest movement.
- Reservoir bag compliance. Weaknesses: highly variable and inconsistent.

Monitors

- Exhaled carbon dioxide (capnograph – digital or wave form, colorimetric carbon dioxide detector) after six lung ventilations is highly reliable for distinguishing tracheal and oesophageal intubation. Colorimetric capnometry requires approximately 2 kPa (15 mmHg) exhaled carbon dioxide to be positive, whereas capnography detects much lower levels. A capnography waveform is very useful for continuous monitoring of tube position. There are few weaknesses but in cardiac arrest an attenuated (not flat) trace is observed.
- Oesophageal detector device. A compressed bulb or syringe is attached to the tube. The suction in the device will collapse if the tube is in the trachea, whereas if it is in oesophagus the bulb or syringe will not re-expand. Weaknesses: (i) may create false readings in status asthmaticus, copious tracheal secretions and tracheal collapse, (ii) false readings in oesophageal intubation with air in stomach and (iii) not useful for continuous monitoring of tube position.
- An ultrasound probe placed transversely over the jugular notch with both trachea and oesophagus in view will reveal the 'double trachea sign' if the tube enters oesophagus. Strength: unlike capnography oesophageal intubation can be detected before initiation of ventilation. Weakness: demands a second operator (see Chapter 7).

Investigations

- Chest radiograph. Important to note that a radiograph taken in only one plane (e.g. AP chest X-ray) cannot rule out oesophageal tube intubation.
- Flexible optical bronchoscopic inspection to identify tracheal rings and carina.

In summary, clinical observation is not uniformly reliable. While it is useful for the intubator to directly observe the tube entering the glottis, capnography is the most reliable method for confirming correct pla-cement of the tracheal tube and for monitoring its

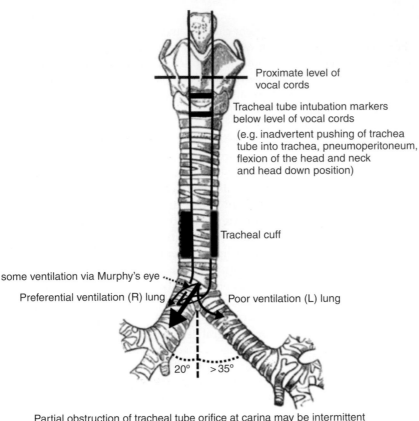

Proximate level of vocal cords

Tracheal tube intubation markers below level of vocal cords

(e.g. inadvertent pushing of trachea tube into trachea, pneumoperitoneum, flexion of the head and neck and head down position)

Tracheal cuff

some ventilation via Murphy's eye ....

Preferential ventilation (R) lung

Poor ventilation (L) lung

20° | >35°

Partial obstruction of tracheal tube orifice at carina may be intermittent and vary in degree with mediastinal movement caused from diaphragmatic and/or cardiac movements.
Obstruction replicates lower airway obstruction (e.g. asthma) on capnography

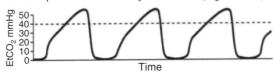

Note: Normal capnography does not exclude endobronchial intubation

Figure 14.6 Endobronchial intubation with preferential ventilation of right lung, especially during low volume/pressure ventilation. (Capnography trace © Farish SE, Garcia PS (2013) Capnography primer for oral and maxillofacial surgery: review and technical considerations. *Journal of Anesthesia & Clinical Research* 4: 295. doi: 10.4172/2155-6148.1000295.)

correct position thereafter. If there is no exhaled capnograph trace after intubation the tube should be assumed to be in the wrong place until proven otherwise ('no trace = wrong place').

Endobronchial Intubation

When using chest auscultation alone, clinicians may frequently miss endobronchial intubation because unilateral breath sounds are only detected when the tracheal tip is 2 cm beyond the carina. Steps to avoid endobronchial intubation are based on an understanding of normal tracheal anatomy along with how the tracheal tube tip moves in different clinical scenarios.

The tracheal tube tip may become endobronchial with Trendelenburg position, flexion of the neck and pneumoperitoneum. As an example, the tracheal tube tip may move up to 6.4 cm when moving the head from full extension to full flexion. In these situations, the tracheal cuff may be above the carina but the tip within the right main bronchus. Chest auscultation detects bilateral airway entry, especially if large-volume/high-pressure ventilation is used with hand ventilation. When subsequently using mechanical ventilation with lower volumes and pressures, preferential filling of the right lung along with inadequate filling of the left occurs. The latter leads to partial left lung collapse, ventilation/perfusion mismatching and hypoxia. Some degree of wheezing may occur leading to a misdiagnosis of acute asthma secondary to tracheal intubation (Figure 14.6).

A simple measure for reducing the risk of endobronchial intubation is to only insert the tube 20 cm from the teeth in woman and 22 cm from the teeth in men. While this will not universally eliminate bronchial intubation, it is rarely necessary to insert the tube further.

Ultrasonography can help in diagnosing if both lungs are being ventilated (see Chapter 7).

Endobronchial intubation should be considered if there is poor oxygenation, high airway pressures and a low or up-sloping capnography trace (noting that a normal capnography trace does not exclude endobronchial intubation).

To eliminate endobronchial intubation as a cause of hypoxia, the steps shown in Figure 14.7 are recommended.

Should endobronchial intubation be confirmed, the airway should be suctioned and re-recruitment of the collapsed lung should occur with large tidal volumes.

Summary

Understanding of the two curve theory and the three column model helps explain normal and difficult direct laryngoscopy. To optimise the airway for laryngoscopy the sternal notch and external meatus should be at the same horizontal level. In most adults the sniffing position achieves this. The direct laryngoscope blade should be advanced along the floor of mouth while displacing the tongue laterally. Waveform capnography is the modality to exclude oesophageal intubation. Endobronchial intubation may be missed when chest auscultation is the only method used to detect it.

- Stop stimulation and surgery
- Stop administration of suspected drugs & colloids
- FiO_2 changed to 1.0
- Hand-ventilated to assess:
  - ✓ the adequacy of ventilation
  - ✓ functionality of the equipment
- Ensure SaO_2 reading is accurate
- Check TT position in trachea by either:
  - ➤ Check TT intubation marks next to or just above the vocal cords
    - ✓ If C&L grade 1 or 2: direct laryngoscopy
    - ✓ If C&L grade 3 or 4: videolaryngoscopy alternatively
  - ➤ Check location of the tracheal tube tip by either fibreoptic bronchoscopy or chest X-ray
- Trial cuff deflation: either remove any cuff herniation that blocks the tube tip and/or remove any unequal cuff inflation that causes the tip to abut the tracheal mucosa
- Tracheal catheter inserted down TT to ensure patency

Figure 14.7 Steps for diagnosing endobronchial intubation.

Further Reading

Greenland KB (2008). A proposed model for direct laryngoscopy and tracheal intubation. *Anaesthesia*, **63**, 156–161.

Greenland KB (2010). Airway assessment based on a three column model of direct laryngoscopy. *Anaesthesia and Intensive Care*, **38**, 14–19.

Greenland KB. (2012). Reappraisal of adult airway management. In: Riley R (Ed.), *Australasian Anaesthesia 2011*. Melbourne: Australian and New Zealand College of Anaesthetists. pp. 57–65

Levitan RM, Heitz JW, Sweeney M, Cooper RM. (2011). The complexities of tracheal intubation with direct laryngoscopy and alternative intubation devices. *Annals of Emergency Medicine*, **57**, 240–247.

Chapter 15

Tracheal Tube Introducers (Bougies), Stylets and Airway Exchange Catheters

Massimiliano Sorbello and Iljaz Hodzovic

Tracheal tube introducers (commonly referred to as 'bougies'), stylets and airway exchange catheters (AECs) are widely used airway adjuncts for facilitating airway management in difficult circumstances. They are easy to use, relatively inexpensive and have success rates of ≥ 90% in most settings.

Bougies are 60–80 cm long narrow tubes of 4–5 mm external diameter designed to assist during tracheal intubation. They are inserted into the trachea during laryngoscopy and then used as a guide over which to pass a tracheal tube (called 'railroading the tracheal tube'). They often have a curved or angled ('coudé') tip (Figure 15.1). They are also used to aid supraglottic airway (SGA) insertion, videolaryngoscope (VL)-guided intubation and as adjuncts to emergency front of neck airway (eFONA) procedures.

Stylets are rigid or semi-rigid airway adjuncts, 30–50 cm long, that are inserted into the tracheal tube before intubation. They maintain the tracheal tube in a particular shape and may therefore assist during intubation (Figure 15.1).

AECs are semi-rigid hollow tubes of 80–110 cm designed to aid airway device (SGA, and single- or double-lumen tracheal tube) exchange or to manage 'at-risk' extubation (Figure 15.1).

The risk of serious airway trauma associated with the use of bougies, stylets and AECs, and the risk of barotrauma with the latter, invites cautious and educated use of these devices.

The usefulness of bougies and AECs is probably underestimated and, as a consequence, under-taught, perhaps due to the assumption that the basic techniques are easy and not worthy of the meticulous disciplined approach they deserve.

Tracheal Tube Introducers (Bougies)

Aid to Direct Laryngoscope-Guided Intubation

History

- 1949: Macintosh used a gum elastic urinary dilator (bougie) to facilitate tracheal tube placement in a patient with limited laryngeal view at laryngoscopy with a straight blade.
- 1973: Venn introduced the '*Eschmann endotracheal tube introducer*', with a *coudé* tip and just the right balance between stiffness and flexibility.
- 1996: Frova designed the first hollow single-use introducer using stiffer material.
- Current: there are numerous types of bougies described all differing somewhat (Table 15.1).

Bougies are highly effective aids to direct laryngoscope-guided intubation. Reported success rate is around 90% on first attempt rising to 94–100% with two attempts. During unexpected difficulty success rate is 80–90%.

Bougies are most effective when the view at direct laryngoscopy is limited to the epiglottis only but this can be lifted (Cook's modified Cormack and Lehane Grade 3a) or there is a better view but tube advancement is difficult. The use of a bougie in Grades 3b (epiglottis resting on the posterior pharyngeal wall over the glottic opening) and 4 (only the base of the tongue visible) is unlikely to be successful and may lead to airway trauma due to blind attempts at tracheal placement (Figure 15.2).

Bougies with a deflectable or steerable tip have been introduced relatively recently. These have the

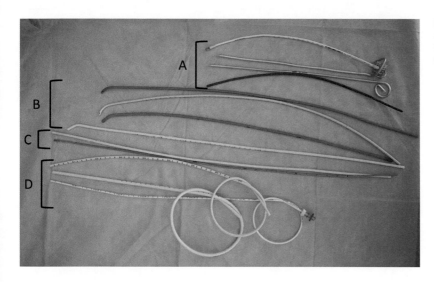

Figure 15.1 Airway catheters overview. A: malleable stylets; B: tracheal introducers (bougies); C. tracheal tube guides; D: airway exchange catheters.

potential to improve success rates of bougie-guided direct and VL intubation. However, they are likely to require practice to master and to be relative rigid. It is therefore possible they will slow down during routine intubations and have increased risk of trauma. Their place in airway management practice is yet to be established.

Tips on Optimal Use

- Hold the bougie 25–30 cm from the tip as this improves control when manoeuvring the bougie.
- Curve the distal 20 cm of the bougie so the curvature imitates the curvature of the airway. This is particularly relevant with Grades 2b (only posterior laryngeal structures visible) and 3a (only epiglottis visible). Different curves might be needed according to the bougie used, depending on the materials used and its shape memory.
- A bougie can be used in Grade 1 -2a (cords visible) views to minimise laryngoscopic traction, in order to reduce potential airway trauma.
- Advance the bougie into the trachea no more than 20–24 cm mark at the incisor level (in adults). This ensures the position of the bougie tip is above the carina and is likely to significantly reduce the risk of airway trauma.
- Load the tracheal tube over the bougie with the tube bevel facing posteriorly in relation to the patient. Advance it in this position. A 90°

anticlockwise rotation during tube advancement may achieve the same effect but tube impingement on the laryngeal aryepiglottic folds is more likely during rotation.

A multicoloured bougie has been described (traffic light bougie) which uses colours to highlight when the safe limit of insertion depth has nearly (orange) or has (red) been reached. This decreases over-insertion but is not yet commercially available.

Preloading a curved bougie prior to intubation is advocated by some users to be faster and may be especially useful to airway managers working without assistance. It may help awkward intubations but in truly difficult intubations the presence of the tracheal tube may hamper bougie manipulation.

Single-Use or Reusable Bougie?

The original Eschmann 'gum elastic' bougie has been in use for more than 50 years with very few reports of airway trauma. Some hospitals use this reusable bougie as a single-use device because of cross-infection concerns.

Some single-use bougies have been introduced into clinical practice with little or no clinical evidence of comparative performance or safety. Success rates are generally lower than with the Eschmann reusable bougie, with the Frova bougie approaching equivalence. Single-use bougies are variably stiffer and have greater airway trauma potential, with reports of severe airway trauma. The potential for airway trauma is increased if

Table 15.1 Tracheal introducers – bougies

Device	Material	Colour	Length (cm)	OD/ID Fr (mm)	Hollow/ports	Tip	Notes
Eschmann (Venn) GEB (Smiths Portex)	Woven polyester (inside) fibreglass (outside)	Golden brown	60	15 Fr (5)	NO	Coudé (35) 38°	For TT 6.0 mm ID Memory. Reusable.
ET Introducer (Smiths Portex)	PVC	Yellow (1997) Azure (2006)	60 70	15 Fr (5)	< 1 mm	Coudé	Hollow lumen < 1 mm
Frova (Cook Medical)	Intermediate density PET	Light blue	70	14 Fr (4.7) / 3	Yes (3 mm)/2	Curved 2 × 2 cm	For TT 5.5 mm ID Optional stiffening metal cannula. Pre-curved packaging available
Frova (Pediatric)	Polyurethane	Yellow	35	8 Fr (2.7) / 2	Yes/2	Curved 1 × 1 cm	For TT 3.0 mm ID Stiffening metal cannula
VBM (Coudé)	Stiff PET	Orange	65	15 Fr (5)	Yes/2	Coudé	For TT 6.0 mm ID
METTS (VBM)	PVC – metal core	Light green	40/65	8/12/14 Fr	NO	Flexible-coudé	Malleable For TT 6.0 mm ID
METTI (VBM)	PVC – plastic core	Dark green	80	12/14 Fr	NO	Flexible-coudé	For TI and TI with TT ID 4.5/5.5 and larger
Pocket Introducer (VBM)	Stiff PET	Blue	20→65	15 Fr	NO	Coudé	Folded, to be extended
S-Guide (VBM)	PVC – partially metal reinforced	White, orange tip	65	15 Fr (5)	Yes/3	Coudé 35°	Soft tip+ flexible + malleable segment ('airway dance')
ET introducer ET malleable (SunMed)	Low density PET	Light blue Violet	70	10/15 Fr	NO	Coudé/straight	
Bougie To Go (SunMed)	Low density PET	Light blue	60	15 Fr	NO	Coudé	Rolled-up-packed
Introes Pocket Bougie	Special blend PTFE (Teflon)	White	60	14 Fr (4.7)	NO	Flexible	Double-ended use, precurved
Interguide (Intersurgical)	NA	Green	53/70	6/10/15 Fr (2/3.3/5)	NO	Coudé	
Universal Stylet Bougie (Intersurgical)	Low density PET + metal inserts	White green dots	65	15 Fr	NO	Coudé	Hexagonal section – stylet & bougie function

Name	Material	Colour	Length	Size	Vented/ports	Tip	Features
DEAS (DEAS)	Stiff PET	Light blue	53.5/70/83	2/3.3/5	Yes/2	Coudé	
Vented Introducer (P3)	NA	Blue/yellow	47/60/75/80	5/10/14/15 Ch	Yes/2	Straight/angle/coudé	
Flexible Tip (P3)	Nylon + silicon tip	White-yellow	66	15 Fr/5	NO		Flexible/steerable tip; phosphorus coated (UV)
Boussignac (Vygon)	PVC	Transparent-green/orange	50/60/70	NA	Yes (double)	Coudé 40°	
CoPilot bougie (Occam design)	PET	Orange	60	15 Fr	NO	Coudé	
Cobralet bougie (Occam design)	PVC	Orange	60	15 Fr	Yes/3	Coudé/angled	Preshaped/shape-holding
COBRA bougie (Occam design)	PVC – wired	Orange	60→73	15 Fr	NO	Adjustable	Wire-in-bougie to change shape/length
Pro-Breathe (PROACT Medical)	PVC	Yellow	47/60/80	5/10/15 Fr	NO	Coudé	Barium tip
Probreathe vented (PROACT Medical)	PVC	Blue	75	14 Fr	Yes/2	Curved	
AviAir (Armstrong Medical)	NA	Orange	75/80	10/14/15 Fr	Yes (14 & 15 Ch)	Coudé luminescent	Luminescent tip; markers on left; memory & flexibility
Tracheal introducer (SUMI)	PVC	Blue or green	60/70/100	3.3/5	NO	Coudé	

Fr, French; ID, inner diameter; NA, information not available; OD, outer diameter; PET, polyethylene; PTFE, polytetrafluoroethylene; PVC, polyvinyl chloride; TI, tracheal intubation; TT, tracheal tube; UV, ultraviolet.

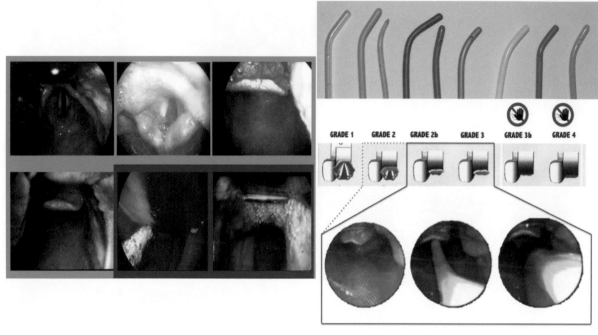

Figure 15.2 Indications for use of tracheal introducers (bougies): note that use of bougies in Grades 3b and 4 (Cook's modification of the Cormack and Lehane grading) – i.e. when the epiglottis either cannot be lifted from the pharyngeal wall or is not seen at all – is unlikely to be effective and is strongly discouraged. The top right figure illustrates the variation in shape and material of the bougies (Some images courtesy of Giulio Frova).

the 'hold-up' sign is elicited during placement (see below).

Single-use bougies with undocumented success rate and airway trauma potential should be avoided.

Confirming Tracheal Placement

Traditional techniques of confirming tracheal bougie placement, when not able to see its passage into the trachea, are 'clicks' (felt as the bougie tip runs against tracheal rings) and distal 'hold up' (when the tip of the bougie is wedged into the smaller bronchi). 'Clicks' occur in 90% and hold up in 100% of cases, making them very reliable indicators of correct 'blind' tracheal placement. However, caution is advised, especially when single-use bougies are used. The hold-up sign can cause serious airway trauma or bronchospasm. In animal models, forces as small as 0.8 N (0.08 kg) can cause airway perforation and current evidence points against the use of this sign. Capnography after intubation remains the most reliable method for confirming tracheal tube placement.

Airway Trauma and Pitfalls

A complication rate of ≈5% has been reported with several bougies, including the Frova introducer. Bleeding is by far the commonest complication but epiglottic and glottic damage, tracheal and bronchial perforation, intensive care admissions and fatalities have been reported. A large majority of reports were associated with the single-use bougies most likely due to their increased stiffness.

As many available bougies have not been tested for their airway trauma potential great caution is needed: avoid untested devices, avoid insertion > 25 cm depth, avoid using the 'hold-up' sign and avoid using a hollow lumen bougie for oxygen delivery. Keeping the laryngoscope in place throughout airway instrumentation is also advised. Single-use bougies should not be used with double lumen tubes, as fragments have been found in the airway after their use.

The reusable Eschmann bougie is designed for a maximum of five uses. As it can only undergo low-level decontamination and tracking uses is difficult there are some concerns about cross-contamination risk, though no data are available to support or discourage their (re-)use.

Aid to Videolaryngoscope-Guided Intubation

The advantages of videolaryngoscopy in the management of the difficult airway are well documented, but airway adjuncts may be needed to aid the VL-guided intubation. Bougies or stylets may help guide the tube into the trachea when tube advancement is problematic despite a full view of the glottis, especially when a hyperangulated VL is used. A bougie may improve speed and success in up to one third of VL-guided intubations and some advocate routine use especially in emergency settings and in the pre-hospital setting. When used with a hyperangulated blade VL the bougie needs to be curved to match the blade profile (Figure 15.3), and the degree to which this curve is maintained during intubation will depend on the bougie and environmental factors such as temperature. The narrow external diameter of the bougie may improve manoeuvrability (compared with a styletted tracheal tube) but there are also reasons why the

rigidity of a stylet may be preferred for VL-guided intubation and this is discussed below. Stylets with a flexible tip may provide benefit but at present are under-evaluated (see Chapter 17).

Airway Trauma Associated with Combined Bougie and Videolaryngoscope Use

The incidence of bougie-related airway trauma during VL-guided intubation appears to be smaller than during direct laryngoscopy, with a reported incidence of 0.8% in a recent observational study of 543 intubations using a videolaryngoscope with the Frova bougie. The issue of the 'blind spot' and trauma during intubation is discussed in Chapter 17.

Bougies for Intubation through an SGA or for SGA Placement

Bougies have been used to aid intubation through an SGA. Techniques include blind bougie placement or combined with a flexible optical bronchoscope (FOB). Blind attempts at tracheal intubation via an SGA have very low success rates, risk airway trauma and are not

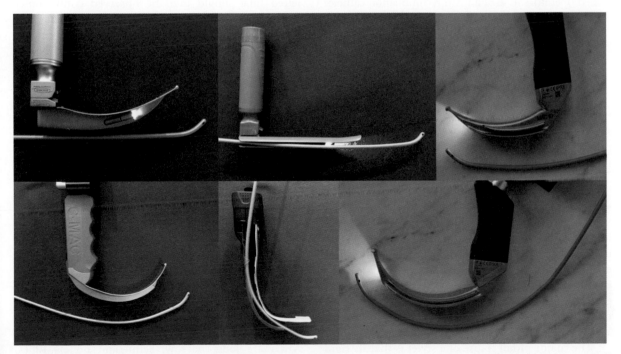

Figure 15.3 Assembling and shaping of tracheal introducers with different direct laryngoscopes (MacIntosh, Miller blade) and channelled/unchannelled videolaryngoscopes. In each of the lower figures the bougie must be curved to match the curve of the videolaryngoscope to achieve its goal.

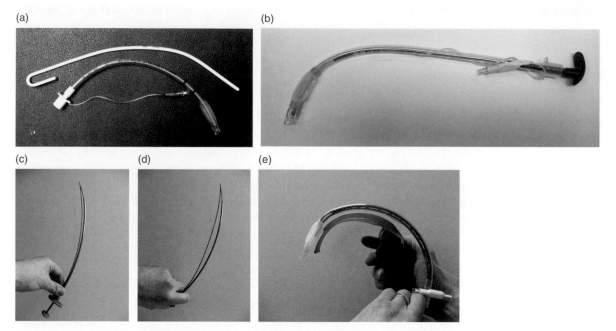

Figure 15.4 Stylets. (a) Standard malleable stylet, (b) preformed stylet for use with an angulated videolaryngoscope – inserted in tracheal tube, (c–e) a deformable stylet: it is supplied in its 'unactivated position' (c), and is activated by pushing the proximal end, which causes it to bow (d); when this is done with the stylet in the tracheal tube it curves the tube (e).

recommended. Bougie placement through an SGA with FOB guidance has a high success rate but requires two skilled operators. Use of an Aintree intubation catheter is likely a preferable technique – see Chapter 13.

A bougie may also be used to aid placement of the ProSeal LMA – this is described in Chapter 13.

Bougie Use during Emergency Front of Neck Airway (eFONA)

A number of national airway management guidelines promote the scalpel-bougie as a technique of choice for eFONA (this is described in Chapter 20).

Stylets

Stylets are rigid tracheal tube guides that are inserted into the tracheal tube before intubation. They may be used to curve straight or non-rigid tubes and also to accentuate the curve of curved tubes, especially during intubation with a hyperangulated VL. Traditionally bougies have been favoured in the UK and the stylet in many other parts of the world but especially in North America. With increased use of VLs this variation is reducing.

The major pitfall to use of a stylet is that its rigid tip may cause significant airway injury. To avoid this the distal tip of the stylet should never be inserted

further than the Murphy eye or ≈1.5 cm proximal to the tip of the tracheal tube. The passage of the styletted tube should then be observed continuously during its passage through the airway. When the tube tip reaches the glottis, the stylet should be progressively withdrawn as the tracheal tube is advanced, so that the stylet tip never reaches the glottic opening.

Standard stylets are plastic-covered pieces of malleable wire (Figure 15.4). Preformed, mostly rigid, stylets are increasingly produced by individual VL manufacturers and used during VL intubation (Figure 15.4). The stylets are designed so that the curve of the stylet matches the curve of the hyperangulated VL blade. This enables the styletted tube to run along the distal end of the VL blade during intubation, in a technique that greatly simplifies intubation (see Chapter 17).

Deformable stylets are available that can be deployed to create a 'dynamic' curve such that the curve of the tracheal tube matches that needed to achieve intubation (Figure 15.4).

Airway Exchange Catheters (AECs)

AECs are long, narrow, semi-rigid hollow tubes, inserted through an *in-situ* airway device in order to exchange one airway device (tracheal tube or SGA) for another or for management of 'at-risk' extubation. While bougies may be used for the same purpose they are generally too rigid and too short and AECs are better suited to the role. The hollow lumen of the AECs enables oxygen administration during or after the procedure but this is a high-risk strategy.

Tracheal Tube Exchange

AECs are made from a range of materials (including a combination of stiffer catheter body with a softer distal tip intended to reduce the risk of direct trauma) and vary in length and diameter (Table 15.2). AECs designed for double-lumen tube exchange are longer than those for single-lumen tubes ($\approx$100 cm vs. $\approx$80 cm).

Use during 'At-Risk' Extubation

An AEC may be placed in the airway prior to extubation of a patient with a difficult airway and may be tolerated by awake patients for up to 72 hours. Local anaesthetic may be placed on the AEC or administered through its lumen. If reintubation is required the tracheal tube is railroaded over the AEC using this as a guide. AEC-guided reintubation success rates are $\approx$85% with a risk of pneumothorax during the procedure of $\approx$1.5%. This is discussed further in Chapter 21.

Optimal Use of AECs

AEC use for tube exchange or safe extubation seems to be a safe and effective procedure if basic rules are followed.

- Lubricate the AEC before use.
- Insert the AEC no more than 20–24 cm orally and 27–30 cm nasally in an adult patient. This ensures the AEC sits within the tracheal tube with minimal or no protrusion beyond the tip of the tube and it does not reach the carina. Maintaining the AEC tip above the carina will reduce patient discomfort and trauma risk.
- During AEC use administer oxygen by face mask or nasal specs. Oxygen administration through the lumen of an AEC is associated with a significant risk of barotrauma and should be avoided unless there is clear benefit over standard administration routes.
- If oxygen is administered via an AEC it should be via a low-pressure source at low flow ($\leq$ 1 L min^{-1}).

- In the case of rapid decompensation of a patient with an AEC *in situ*, reintubation should be prioritised over oxygenation via the AEC.
- Use a tracheal tube with a tip designed to avoid impingement on the airway (e.g. ILMA tracheal tube, Parker tip tube) during railroading.
- Direct or videolaryngoscopy during intubation over an AEC (both during tube exchange and reintubation) is likely to facilitate the procedure and is recommended.
- Successful reintubation over an AEC should always be confirmed with capnography and a backup plan should be in place for failure.
- When used for 'at-risk' extubation, the patient should be nursed in high dependency or intensive care unit and the AEC only removed when the airway danger has resolved.

Airway Trauma Potential and Pitfalls

If used inappropriately, AECs have potential to cause serious airway injury. Due to their length, these devices are often inserted too far into the airway and this risks direct airway trauma. Oxygen administration via an AEC has an even higher potential to cause life-threatening or fatal airway injury. When the tip of the AEC is above the carina, oxygen administration through the AEC is unlikely to cause barotrauma whatever the oxygen flow rates. However, when inserted deeper into the airway to the first point of resistance oxygen administration from a high-pressure source (e.g. wall or cylinder) can cause barotrauma within few seconds even at oxygen flow rates as low as 2 L min^{-1}.

Bougies, stylets and AECs are simple and highly effective devices which when used appropriately have an important role in managing a range of airway challenges, from difficult intubation to tube exchange manoeuvres and safe extubation strategies. Complication rates are low when used correctly, but there is a risk of major harm if poor quality devices are used or technique is poor. Insertion of either device too far into the airway is the single greatest pitfall to avoid.

Further Reading

Axe R, Middleditch A, Kelly FE, Batchelor TJ, Cook TM. (2015). Macroscopic barotrauma caused by stiff and soft-tipped airway exchange catheters: an in vitro case series. *Anesthesia & Analgesia*, **120**, 355–361.

Table 15.2 Airway exchange catheters

Device	Material	Colour	Length (cm)	Outer diameter Fr (mm)	Hollow	DLTs	Notes
Endoguide (Teleflex Medical)	Tefloned PVC	White	525/700/830	15 Fr (5)	Yes	Yes (size limit)	Tin wire inside for modelling
VBM	PET	Light blue	80	11/14/19 Fr	Yes	Yes (size limit)	
Aintree intubation catheter (Cook Medical)	PET	Light blue	56	19 Fr	Yes (4.7 mm)	No	Special for FOB intubation
AEC (Cook Medical)	PET	Yellow	83	8/11/14/19 Fr	Yes (1.6/2.3/3/ 3.4 mm)	Yes (size limit)	
Arndt AEC (Cook Medical)	PET	Yellow	(50/65/78) 70	(8 Fr) 14 Fr	Yes (0.38 inch tip)	Yes (size limit)	Wire-guided, bronchoscope port
AEC soft-tip (Cook Medical)	PET/soft tip	Green-violet	100	11/14 Fr	Yes (2.3/3 mm)	Yes	Stiff body/soft tip
Tube Exchanger (DEAS)	PET	Blue	53.5/70	2/3.3/5	No	Yes (size limit)	
Cannula AEC (Cook Medical)	PET	Yellow	45	8 Fr	Yes	No	
Tracheostomy Cannula Exchange Guide (DEAS)	PVC	Transparent	40	6.0/7.0 mm	Yes	No	Rounded tip with lateral holes, depth markers
Staged Extubation (Cook Medical)	PET	Green-violet	83	14 Fr	Yes	Yes	0.0135 inch/145 cm guidewire and soft-tipped airway catheter

DLT, double-lumen tube; FOB, flexible optical bronchoscope; Fr, French; PET, polyethylene; PVC, polyvinyl chloride.

Driver BE, Prekker ME, Klein LR, et al. (2018). Effect of use of a bougie vs endotracheal tube and stylet on first-attempt intubation success among patients with difficult airways undergoing emergency intubation: a randomized clinical trial. *JAMA*, **319**, 2179–2189.

Duggan LV, Law JA, Murphy MF. (2011). Brief review: supplementing oxygen through an airway exchange catheter: efficacy, complications, and recommendations. *Canadian Journal of Anaesthesia*, **58**, 560–568.

Hodzovic I, Latto IP, Wilkes AR, Hall JE, Mapleson WW. (2004). Evaluation of Frova, single-use intubation introducer, in a manikin. Comparison with Eschmann multiple-use introducer and Portex single-use introducer. *Anaesthesia*, **59**, 811–816.

Nolan JP, Wilson ME. (1992). An evaluation of the gum elastic bougie. Intubation times and incidence of sore throat. *Anaesthesia*, **47**, 878–881.

Chapter 16

Tracheal Intubation Using the Flexible Optical Bronchoscope

P. Allan Klock, Jr, Mridula Rai and Mansukh Popat

Introduction

Flexible bronchoscopes and intubation scopes offer unparalleled utility for the safe management of patients with a difficult airway. Many centres have seen decreased use of flexible optical scopes after the introduction of videolaryngoscopes but it is imperative that anaesthesia providers gain and maintain skills in using this invaluable airway management tool. Modern flexible bronchoscopes use a video camera at the tip of the scope rather than glass fibres to transmit the image. The term flexible optical bronchoscopes (FOBs) is used here to describe devices including flexible fibre-optic and flexible videoscopes used for tracheal intubation.

FOBs figure prominently in most airway management algorithms (see Chapter 4).

The FOB has many characteristics which make it an ideal tool for tracheal intubation and some disadvantages that must be understood for optimal use. Both are described in Table 16.1.

Successful FOB intubation requires several elements:

- understanding the equipment
- learning basic manipulations and hand–eye coordination
- mastering upper airway endoscopy
- correct tube selection
- mastering tube delivery into the trachea

The Anatomy and Function of the FOB

The modern-day FOB consists of the following parts (Figure 16.1).

Body

This is held in the palm of either hand; the thumb of the same hand is used to manipulate the control lever and the index finger activates the suction

Table 16.1 Advantages and disadvantages of flexible optical bronchoscopic (FOB) intubation

Advantages

Flexibility conforms easily to normal and difficult airway anatomy

Continuous visualisation of airway during endoscopy

Less traumatic than rigid laryngoscopes:

- Does not require cervical spine movement
- Can steer around friable tissue or tumours
- Does not require significant pressure on airway structures, facilitating intubation using topical local anaesthetics and minimal or no sedation

Latest equipment is lightweight and portable

Can be used with other intubating techniques (e.g. direct or videolaryngoscopy)

Can be used with ventilatory devices (e.g. supraglottic airway (SGA))

Can be used for oral or nasal intubation

Can be used on patients of all age groups

Can be used with awake, sedated or anaesthetised patients

Can be used to determine or confirm tube position in trachea

Videoscopes facilitate teaching and assistance by other members of the care team

Disadvantages

Equipment is expensive to purchase and maintain

Many departments find a high cost of repairs

Special skills are needed to become proficient in FOB use

Regular use is needed to maintain high skill levels

The FOB does not create space in the airway, it can only navigate an already present pathway

The lens is easily soiled if blood, secretions or other fluids are in the airway

The tracheal tube is not directly seen as it passes through the vocal cords (though its position can be confirmed as the FOB is removed)

valve. The control lever is pressed down to move the tip of the scope anteriorly and up to move the tip posteriorly.

With traditional fibreoptic scopes, the body has an eyepiece, which can be focussed by a diopter ring to produce a sharp image. The eyepiece has a pointer which helps to orient the operator to the anterior direction of the tip. With videoscopes the image is projected on a video monitor. The body also has a port which accesses the working channel.

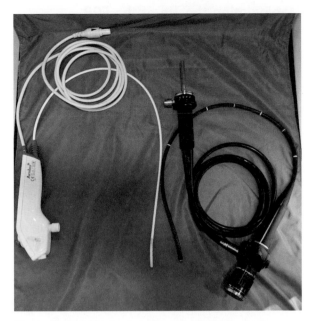

Figure 16.1 Flexible intubation scopes. The black scope is a fibreoptic bronchoscope that uses glass fibres to transmit the image from the objective lens at the end of the insertion cord to the eyepiece. The white scope is a single-use scope that uses a video camera chip at the end of the insertion cord and light emitting diodes to provide light.

Insertion cord

This part of the scope is steered into the airway and acts as a flexible guide over which the tracheal tube is advanced, facilitating intubation. The outer diameter of the insertion cord determines the size of the smallest tracheal tube that can be easily passed over it. Neonatal scopes have an outer diameter of 2.2 mm, paediatric scopes and scopes used for double-lumen tube placement range from 3.5 to 4.0 mm and adult scopes range from 5.0 to 6.3 mm. It is desirable to use a tracheal tube with an internal diameter at least 1 mm greater than the outer diameter of the insertion cord, e.g. most adult scopes with insertion cord diameter of 4 mm will allow a tracheal tube of 5 mm or larger to easily pass over it. Most insertion cords are 55–60 cm long to allow passage of the tracheal tube once its tip is positioned in the trachea.

The insertion cord contains

- In fibreoptic scopes: up to 10,000 image and light transmitting fibreoptic bundles
- In videoscopes: wires that energise the light emitting diodes (LEDs) at the tip and transmit the image from the camera tip to the image processor

- Mechanical wires connecting the control lever to the bending element, enabling anterior and posterior deflection of the tip

The Working Channel

This is a narrow channel that extends from a port in the body of the FOB to the distal end of the insertion cord. It can be used to insufflate oxygen or to instill drugs (especially local anaesthetics), to pass guidewires or (in larger FOBs) brushes or biopsy forceps. The effectiveness of the suction depends on the diameter of the channel. A typical adult scope has a 1.5 to 3.2 mm channel. Channels less than 2.0 mm are adequate but not very effective for removing viscous secretions.

Light Source

Traditional optical bronchoscopes have an external light source, usually a halogen lamp enclosed in a casing. This is connected to the body by a light guide cable. Videoscopes have LEDs at the tip of the scope to provide light.

Camera and Monitor

Traditional optical bronchoscopes may use a camera attached to the eyepiece which projects the image to a video monitor. Modern videoscopes have a camera chip at the tip of the scope which transmits the image directly to the video monitor. A video monitor facilitates training and optimises assistants' efforts as they can see if their jaw thrust or other manoeuvres are effective. In addition, it is easier to keep the insertion cord straight and under a small amount of tension with a videoscope because the eyepiece does not need to be near the operator's face.

Setting Up FOB Equipment

Here is an example of a simple checklist:

- Ensure the FOB has been cleaned and disinfected before use.
- Check that the tip moves in the appropriate direction when the control lever is moved and there is no slack between the control lever and tip motion.
- Attach the suction valve and catheter to the working channel port and ensure that the suction works when the suction valve is activated.

- Plug the light guide cable to the light source and switch it on.
- Defog the lens by wiping it with an alcohol swab.
- For fibreoptic scopes: hold the tip of the scope 1 cm from an object and adjust the diopter ring until the image is sharp. Attach the camera to the eyepiece and set up the video monitor.
- Lubricate the insertion cord (including the bending element but not the lens).
- Load the tracheal tube onto the insertion cord, pulling it up to the body of the FOB, and secure it with a small piece of tape.

The scope is now ready to use.

Learning Basic Manipulations and Hand–Eye Coordination Skills

Holding the FOB

The endoscopist holds the body of the scope in the palm of one hand using the thumb to manipulate the control lever and the index finger to activate the suction valve when required. The thumb and index finger of the other hand holds the insertion cord (Figure 16.2). It is important that the insertion cord is kept straight and slightly taut: if it becomes slack then rotation movements of the body are not effectively transmitted to the tip of the scope.

Manipulating the Tip of the FOB

There are three degrees of freedom the endoscopist can use to advance the tip of the FOB into the trachea (Figure 16.3). These are: scope advancement (or withdrawal); tip deflection; and whole scope rotation. Advancing the whole FOB moves it towards the target: withdrawal is required if the scope has been advanced too far. The control lever moves the tip of the FOB anteriorly or posteriorly only: downward movement of the control lever bends the tip anteriorly (or away from the endoscopist), and upward movement bends the tip posteriorly (or towards the endoscopist). Sideways movements of the tip are achieved by rotation of the entire FOB towards the target while maintaining tip deflection. Most operators find it helpful to move their body when trying to achieve full rotation of the scope. In practice, good endoscopy technique involves performing the three basic manipulations simultaneously in order to bring the tip of the FOB towards the target.

Position of the Endoscopist and the Patient

The operator will usually choose either to stand behind the patient's head with the patient supine (more common in anaesthetised patient) or to stand in front of and face to face with the patient who is sitting upright (common in the awake patient). The latter is helpful if the patient is dyspnoeic, has

(a)

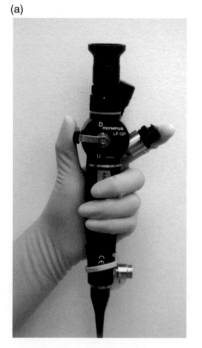

(b)

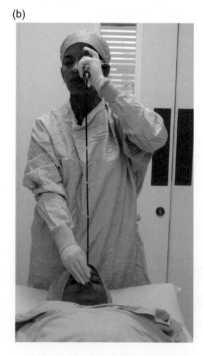

Figure 16.2 (a) The body of the intubation scope is held in the palm of one hand. The thumb manipulates the control lever and the index finger can be used to activate the suction valve. (b) The insertion cord is held straight and taut at all times, regardless of whether the scope uses video or fibreoptic technology.

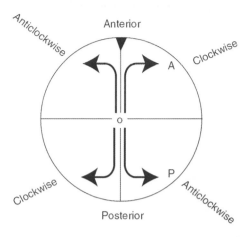

Figure 16.3 Two-dimensional illustration of tip manipulation. The visual field is represented by a circle with four quadrants. The orientation marker is at the 12 o'clock position. Anterior tip deflection and rotation of the body in the clockwise direction are required to move the tip of the FOB from O (neutral position) to target A and posterior tip deflection with anticlockwise rotation of the body will move the tip from O to target P.

a compromised airway from bleeding or oedema or has a full stomach. It is important to appreciate the differences in the observed anatomy when the operator is behind the patient rather than facing the patient.

The endoscopist should be comfortable when performing FOB endoscopy. Standing on a platform instead of standing on tip-toe may be useful to gain enough height to keep the insertion cord straight. If this is not done, the arms will fatigue rapidly and the insertion cord will slacken and bow.

Mastering Upper Airway Endoscopy

Use of the FOB is not intuitive. Practice is required to acquire and maintain a high skill level. Non anatomical trainers can be used during early learning phases. Anatomical manikins and virtual reality trainers can be used to acquire and maintain higher skill levels (Figure 16.4). However, while these tools are educationally valuable, they are not a substitute for practice on patients for acquiring and maintaining the necessary skills.

Flexible Optical Bronchoscopic Intubation

Intubation with an FOB involves guiding the tip of the FOB from the nose or the mouth into the trachea under continuous vision (Figure 16.5).

Nasal Route

The nasal approach prevents the possibility of the patient biting the scope and creates a straighter approach to the larynx than an oral approach. The vascular and sensitive lining of the nose requires application of topical vasoconstrictors (e.g. with xylometazoline, ephedrine or phenylephrine) before instrumentation in all patients and local anaesthesia in the awake patient (see Chapter 9).

Tips for Performing Nasopharyngeal Endoscopy (See Figure 16.5)

- Check the orientation of the image displayed is correct before entering the nostril.
- Insert the tip of the scope just inside each nostril (anterior rhinoscopy) and select the more patent nostril (Figure 16.5).
- Gently advance the tip of the scope and identify the triangular airspace bounded by the inferior turbinate, nasal septum and the floor of the nose.
- Follow the airspace, which generally gets bigger as the scope is advanced towards the nasopharynx until the posterior pharyngeal wall can be seen.
- In anaesthetised patients, a jaw thrust may be required at this point to open the airspace as the scope enters the oropharynx. The soft palate (and sometimes the uvula) and base of tongue come into view and the epiglottis can be seen at a distance.
- The tip is directed underneath the epiglottis and a full view of the laryngeal inlet is seen.
- The scope is advanced through the glottic opening into the trachea where the tracheal rings are identified and advanced to bring the carina into view.

Oral Route

When using an FOB for orotracheal intubation, the scope must be protected from the patient biting. The larger lateral dimension of the oral cavity may make it difficult to keep the FOB in the midline and negotiating the oral pharynx, posterior pharynx and larynx requires a large degree of scope curvature in a small distance. These problems are overcome by using an oral 'airway guide' such as the Berman, Ovassapian, VBM oropharyngeal airway or a supraglottic airway (SGA). The Berman airway is a commonly used device and is available in three adult sizes.

(a)

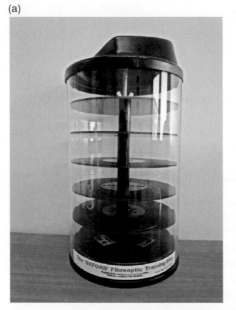

(b)

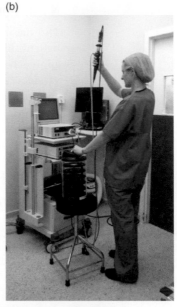

Figure 16.4 FOB training devices. (a) The 'Oxford' Fibreoptic Teaching Box. (b) A trainee practising FOB manipulation skills on the Oxford box. (c) Practice using the ORSIM (Auckland, New Zealand) virtual reality airway trainer.

(c)

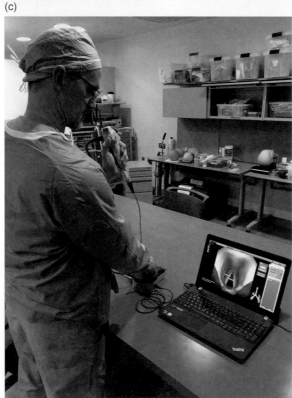

The FOB is passed through the airway guide and the epiglottis is visualised. The scope is advanced further through the glottis into the trachea and the tube is advanced into the trachea. The Berman airway can then be 'peeled' off the tracheal tube (Figure 16.6). In practice, because of its length the Berman airway often causes gagging in the awake patient: this can be avoided by cutting off the distal 1 to 1.5 cm.

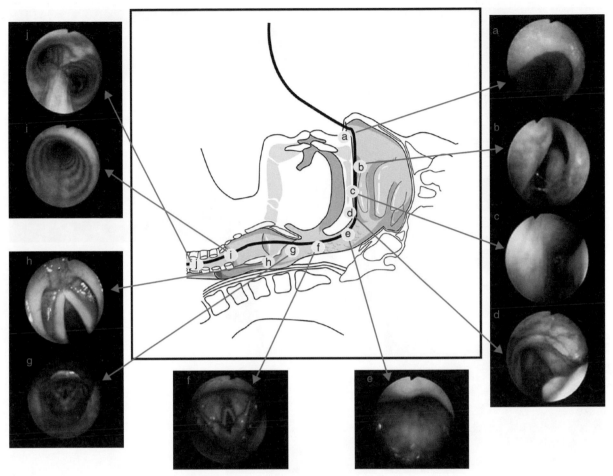

Figure 16.5 (centre) Upper airway anatomy during nasotracheal endoscopy. The endoscopist is standing behind a supine patient. (a) The right nostril is selected. (b) The tip of the FOB is advanced in the triangular space bounded by the nasal septum (left), inferior turbinate (bottom) and the lateral wall of the nose (right) of the visual field. (c) The FOB tip above the inferior turbinate, which is to the right of the visual field. (d) The posterior opening of the nasal cavity is indicated by the disappearance of the inferior turbinate (at the 5 o'clock) position. The posterior pharyngeal wall is seen at the centre of the visual field. (e) The soft palate is seen in the upper part and the base of the tongue in the lower part. (f) Epiglottis in view. (g) Laryngeal inlet with vocal folds, vocal cords, cuneiform and corniculate cartilages. (h) True and false vocal cords. (i) Trachea with tracheal rings. (j) Carina with openings of right and left main bronchi.

Tracheal Tube Selection, Tube Advancement and Hang-Up

The final stage of FOB intubation involves advancing the tracheal tube over the scope into the trachea and removing the FOB from the tube. Failure may occur due to impingement of the tube tip on anatomical structures (usually the right arytenoid cartilage) as it is advanced over the FOB. This is known as tube hang-up and has been reported in more than half of FOB intubations in one prospective study. Hang-up can be reduced by understanding its causes and overcome when encountered by using certain manoeuvres.

Big Scope – Small Tube

The larger the gap between the insertion cord and the tracheal tube the higher the risk of hang-up. This is particularly likely when a smaller scope (e.g. 4.0 mm) designed for management of double-lumen tubes or paediatric intubation is used with an adult-sized tracheal tube. The scope falls into the interarytenoid space (midline) and the tracheal tube tip impacts the right arytenoid cartilage. One should seek to use the smallest tracheal tube that is appropriate for the patient and the procedure and the largest FOB that will fit easily inside it.

145

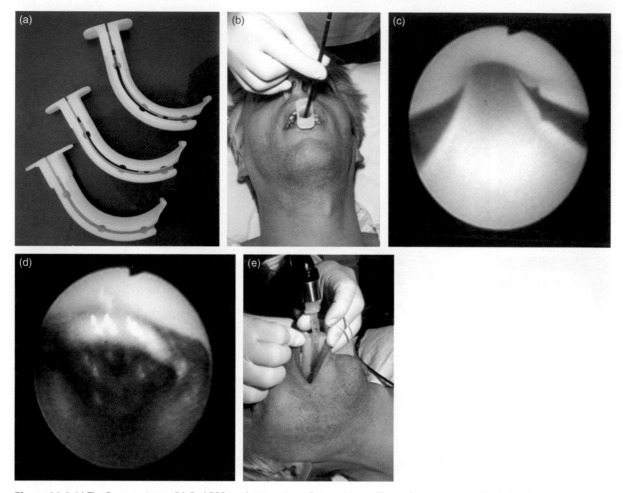

Figure 16.6 (a) The Berman airway. (b) Oral FOB intubation using a Berman airway. The endoscopist is standing behind a supine anaesthetised patient. The FOB is inserted through the lumen of the Berman airway. (c) (Internal view) FOB tip in the lumen of the Berman airway. (d) (Internal view) FOB exiting the lumen. The upper flange is seen lifting the epiglottis. (e) The Berman airway is peeled off once the tube has been railroaded over the FOB into the trachea.

Tracheal Tube Tip Design

Certain tracheal tubes such as the intubating laryngeal mask airway (ILMA) tube and the Gliderite with Parker-Flex Tip are easier to pass as the tip is tapered or curved (Figure 16.7). Softer flexible tubes such as flexometallics or warmed silicone tubes are preferable to rigid standard tubes. A size 6.0–6.5 mm ID may be suitable for nasal intubation and 6.0–7.0mm ID for oral intubation.

Technique of Tube Advancement

After the tip of the scope is well below the vocal cords and within 2–3 cm of the carina the tracheal tube is advanced into the trachea. The tracheal tube is customarily loaded with the tip of the tube facing the right side or 3 o'clock (neutral position). If there is any resistance to advancement of the tube (hang-up), withdraw the tube by 1–2 cm and rotate 90° anticlockwise and advance again (Figure 16.8). This will bring the tip of the tube to the 12 o'clock position and the bevel to the 6 o'clock position, preventing impact with the right arytenoid and enabling smooth advancement. In practice one can reduce hang-up by simply loading the tube onto the FOB with the tip at 12 o'clock when intubating from behind the patient. If the patient is awake, they can be instructed to breathe in deeply, which will abduct the vocal cords and reduce the risk of hang-up.

Before removing the FOB, place the tip at the carina, gently pinch the insertion cord with thumb and forefinger at the level of the 15 mm adaptor and withdraw the scope until the tip of the tube is visible on the FOB monitor. The distance between the operator's fingers and the 15 mm adaptor is the same as between the tip of the tube and the carina, which should ideally be 3–4 cm. If required, adjust the length of the tube in the trachea under direct visualisation.

Withdraw the scope, connect the tube to the anaesthetic circuit, and confirm position by capnography and auscultation of both lung fields.

Clinical Application of FOB Techniques in Difficult Airway Management

For the decision on when to choose an awake intubation and which techniques to use we refer to Chapters 4, 9 and 19.

There are numerous techniques that employ the FOB and may be suitable for difficult airway management. All may be performed awake or in an anaesthetised patient.

- Direct (oral or nasal)
- Via an SGA
- Combined techniques
- Retrograde FOB intubation

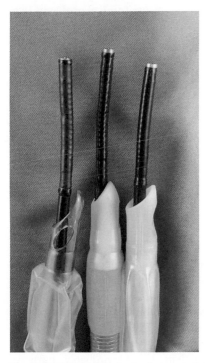

Figure 16.7 Tracheal tube tip designs. Left: Gliderite Gliderite (Parker-Flex Tip) tube, centre: tube for intubating LMA (ILMA), right: standard tracheal tube.

(a)

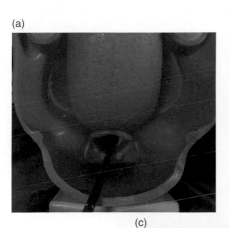

(b)

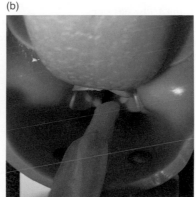

(c)

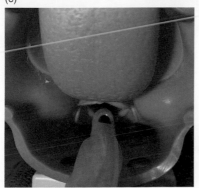

Figure 16.8 (a–c) Tube hang-up. (a) the FOB rests in the interarytenoid groove. (b) The tip of the tracheal tube hangs up on the right corniculate cartilage preventing passage into the glottis. (c) After withdrawing the tube and rotating 90° anticlockwise the presenting part of the tube is anterior and slips easily between the vocal cords.

Awake FOB intubation is perhaps the commonest and most important technique for management of the patient with a predicted difficult airway.

Awake FOB intubation

Although 'awake' FOB intubation is the common terminology used the patient is usually sedated. During this technique the airway is anaesthetised with local anaesthetic. This enables the patient to undergo FOB-assisted tracheal intubation with minimal discomfort, anxiety or pain.

The following considerations are important:

- Airway evaluation
- Airway strategy
- Explanation and consent
- Premedication
- Monitoring
- Oxygenation
- Level of sedation
- Topical anaesthesia of the airway

Airway Evaluation and Development of an Airway Strategy

Two questions need to be answered:

Does the patient need an awake intubation?

Is the awake FOB intubation going to be easy or difficult?

Patients with only bony anatomical problems (e.g. temporomandibular joint ankylosis and patients with ankylosing spondylitis) who are predicted to be difficult to intubate with conventional direct laryngoscopy (Figure 16.9) are often easy to intubate using FOB intubation.

Patients with some degree of soft tissue airway pathology, with or without bony abnormality, but with no clinical evidence of upper airway obstruction are generally easy to intubate, but may prove difficult due to the 'bulk' of tumour or as a result of previous surgery (Figure 16.10). Blood and secretions may be present and can make topical anaesthesia difficult. A novice operator may find these situations quite challenging.

Patients with soft tissue pathology and clinical signs of upper airway obstruction are the most difficult. The risk of complete airway obstruction due to a severely narrowed airway is relatively low. However, each patient has to be assessed individually, and in some cases an awake FOB intubation may be contra-indicated. If endoscopy reveals that the airway is so narrow that the endoscope will cause complete obstruction the patient should probably have an awake tracheostomy or cricothyroidotomy. Sedation should be avoided or given very cautiously in the patient with critical airway obstruction. If FOB intubation is chosen the person performing it must be an accomplished operator. A surgeon skilled at obtaining a front of neck airway (FONA) should be present and

(a)

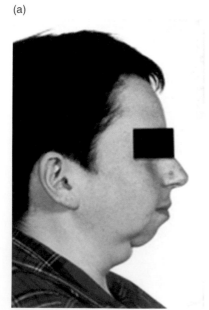

(b)

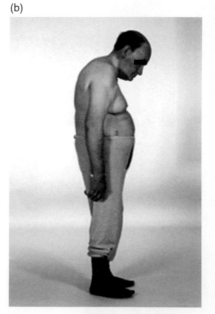

Figure 16.9 Anticipated difficult intubation: bony deformities. (a) Patient with Still's disease that required an awake oral FOB intubation to secure the airway prior to induction of general anaesthesia. (b) Patient with ankylosing spondylitis and severe spinal flexion deformity.

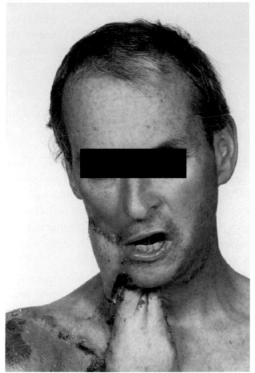

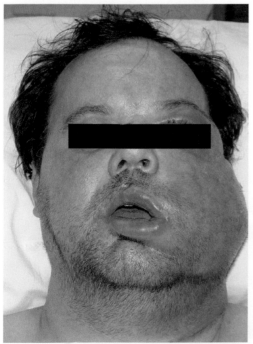

Figure 16.10 Anticipated difficult intubation: soft tissue deformities. (a) Patient with limited mouth opening due to oral cancer surgery and radiotherapy and multiple free flap procedures. (b) A dental abscess resulting in soft tissue oedema and restricted mouth opening.

ready in the room while the airway is being manipulated and the patient intubated.

Have an Airway Management Strategy

Never assume that awake FOB intubation will always be successful. It is vital to have a premeditated airway strategy: a logical progression of plans that will be used if particular problems are encountered (Chapter 4). A strategy might include involving a more senior colleague or a surgeon, employing airway adjuncts in combination with the FOB such as an SGA or videolaryngoscopy and the ultimate backup plan includes a FONA.

Explanation and Consent

It is useful to explain to the patient what intubation is, why is it needed and how it would usually be performed in a patient with a normal airway. Then explain the difficulties that would result if intubation were to be performed after induction of anaesthesia in their case and the safety of an awake FOB technique for them. If sedation is to be used, reassure the patient that they will be sedated and comfortable and that many patients have no recall of the event afterwards. Patients are often afraid they will be restrained and have a tube forced into their throat. Assure the patient that they can pause the procedure at any time to take a small break. Giving the patient this locus of control is comforting and often makes them much more agreeable to the procedure.

The local anaesthetic technique is explained carefully, including that this will reduce the discomfort of the procedure but not provide complete numbness. The patient is reassured that they will have a general anaesthetic once the tracheal tube is in place. The conversation not only explains the procedure, but establishes rapport.

The need for formal verbal or written consent for the procedure will depend on the local hospital policy.

Premedication

Anti-sialogogues such as hyoscine (0.2 mg IM) or glycopyrrolate (0.2 mg IM or IV) can be given 1 hour (if IM) or 20 minutes (if IV) before the procedure. A dry mouth assists topical anaesthesia in three ways: first, the drug is not diluted by saliva; second, a smaller fraction of drug is swallowed; and third, dry mucosa provides better contact between the tissue and the local anaesthetic. A dry mouth also reduces soiling of the lens as it traverses the most dependent parts of the airway.

Monitoring

Standard anaesthetic monitoring should be applied according to normal standards and does not differ from other anaesthetic settings. Continuous wave-form capnography should be used during moderate or deep sedation and to confirm successful tracheal intubation.

Sedation

The depth of sedation should be monitored. The goal of sedation is a relaxed and calm patient who is able to respond appropriately to verbal commands or mild physical stimuli. Over-sedation may lead to hypoventilation, airway obstruction, hypoxia and cardio-respiratory depression. This may result in a confused, restless or uncooperative patient. On the other hand, under-sedation and inadequate topical anaesthesia may also cause patient discomfort and restlessness. Sedation techniques for awake intubation are described in Chapter 9.

Oxygenation

Oxygenation techniques for awake intubation are described in Chapter 9.

Topical Anaesthesia of the Upper Airway

Topical anaesthesia of the upper airway above and below the vocal cords is essential to any awake intubation technique (Figure 16.11). Nerve blocks or direct topicalisation of the airway may be used – both are described in Chapter 9. To anaesthetise the airway below the vocal cords 2 mL 4% lidocaine can be delivered via a needle placed through the cricothyroid membrane. Alternatively, the spray as you go (SAYGO) technique may be used. When SAYGO is employed, the 0.5 mL aliquots of 4% lidocaine are delivered to the epiglottis and anterior commissure of the vocal cords, then 1 mL is delivered to the anterior wall of the larynx just below the cords.

FOB Intubation in the Anaesthetised Patient

Essential requirements are as follows:

- Maintain oxygenation, ventilation and adequate anaesthesia at all times. Anaesthesia may be best achieved by using a total intravenous technique.
- Abolish upper airway reflexes using general anaesthesia, supplemental local anaesthetics and/ or neuromuscular blockers.

FOB intubation may be performed after induction of general anaesthesia. This requires good pre-oxygenation, oxygenation throughout all phases of airway management (e.g. high flow nasal oxygen), careful monitoring and a skilled operator. The passage to the vocal cords may be improved with tongue retraction using gauze or Duval's forceps, jaw thrust or by use of an airway guide as described above.

FOB Intubation through an SGA

The FOB can also be used to guide a tracheal tube through an SGA, including some specifically designed for this purpose such as the ILMA. It may be used in an

(a)

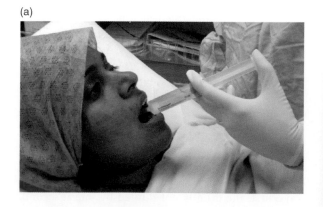

(b)

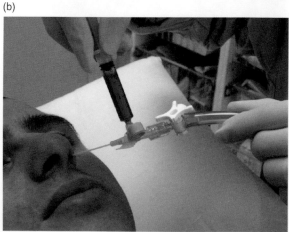

Figure 16.11 (a) Direct application of lidocaine gel to oral cavity via syringe. (b) Direct application of local anaesthetic using a 20G intravenous catheter connected to green oxygen tubing (McKenzie spray technique). Oxygen flowing at 2–4 L results in a fine jet spray and can be used to apply local anaesthetic to the mouth or nose.

anticipated difficult airway and is an excellent rescue technique after failure to intubate with conventional laryngoscopy: it is Plan B of the UK Difficult Airway Society guidelines for unanticipated difficult intubation. It can be performed awake but is more commonly undertaken in the anaesthetised patient.

There are three main advantages to this technique. The SGA can be used to oxygenate and ventilate the patient during the procedure; it moves tissues out of the way, creating a clear passage to the larynx; and it prevents soiling of the airway and FOB by blood or secretions from the nose or mouth.

Blind intubation via most SGAs, whether with a tracheal tube or bougie, has a low success rate and may cause trauma and bleeding rendering any subsequent FOB intubation difficult or impossible. For these reasons, blind intubation through SGAs other than those designed for this is not recommended. Even for the ILMA an FOB-guided technique is likely to improve success. FOB intubation through an SGA is a relatively simple technique, the success of which depends largely on choosing the right equipment.

Considerations for Intubation through an SGA

Tracheal Tube and SGA Stem Diameter

It is essential to choose a tracheal tube of sufficiently small *external* diameter so it will pass easily through the SGA stem. The latter varies widely according to the SGA type and size. For example, a 6.0 mm ID tracheal tube is likely the largest that will pass through a size 5 classic laryngeal mask airway (cLMA). The Air-Q has a larger diameter stem and a removable 15 mm adaptor, and the i-gel has a wide and relatively short stem: both are well suited for SGA-assisted FOB intubation. Conversely, the Supreme LMA and laryngeal tube devices have a narrow stem and small airway orifice, respectively, making them unsuitable for this technique.

Tube Length

The tracheal tube must also be sufficiently long to pass through the entire SGA, enter the trachea and for its cuff to lie below the cords. Many tracheal tubes, even uncut, are too short for this purpose: many are 27–28 cm long and will barely reach the vocal cords when passed through a cLMA. Some reinforced tubes are up to 33 cm in length but these tubes tend to have a thick wall and a relatively large external diameter, and are awkward to advance, lessening their value for this procedure. Other suitable tubes are the north

facing nasal RAE (approximately 32 cm in length) or microlaryngoscopy tube.

Tube Tip

As with other forms of FOB intubation, a tube with a curved tip is preferable to avoid hang-up on the SGA or the glottis.

Removal of the SGA

Unless the operator is using the ILMA, once the patient is intubated it is advisable to deflate the SGA cuff and leave it in place. Attempts to remove the SGA may result in extubation as the stem of the SGA is too short to permit this manoeuvre.

Overall, the technique requires a tracheal tube that is thin, long and with a non-bevelled tip and even then, removal of the SGA afterwards is often impractical. These techniques are often rather cumbersome. Most of the above disadvantages of FOB intubation through the SGA can be overcome by using a two-stage technique using an Aintree intubation catheter. This is described in Chapter 13.

Tips for Performing FOB Intubation through an SGA

- Prepare the FOB as before and load the tracheal tube onto the scope.
- Insert the SGA using optimal technique as it is essential the airway orifice sits over the larynx.
- Ensure that the SGA is seated well and the patient can be ventilated through it.
- Advance the FOB through the stem of the SGA.
  - If the glottis is seen, guide the FOB through the larynx and trachea until the carina is visible.
  - If the glottis is not seen, gently reposition the SGA from side to side or in and out to obtain a view of the glottis. If there is still no view remove all devices and start again.
- Railroad the tracheal tube over the FOB into the trachea.
- Confirm the position of the tube with the FOB and by capnography.
- Deflate the cuff and leave the SGA in place. Secure the tracheal tube so that it does not slide within the stem of the SGA.
- Note: it is important to ensure that there is sufficient lubricant between the FOB and the tracheal tube, and during railroading add gel to the tip of the tube to ensure that the tube slips smoothly over the scope and through the stem of the SGA.

FOB Intubation through the ILMA

The ILMA (Figure 16.12) is an SGA specifically designed to aid blind intubation. It has a reported first-pass success rate of around 75% and overall success rate of > 95%. However, in a small group of patients (10–14%) this can only be achieved after two to three attempts or occasionally not at all. Using the FOB with the ILMA can help to overcome this problem, and this technique has reported success rates of 100%. It is described in Chapter 13.

Combined Techniques

Occasionally copious secretions or massive haemorrhage (Chapter 32) in the airspace can interfere with FOB intubation due to soiling of the airway and FOB tip. In other cases, redundant soft tissue, macroglossia, extrinsic airway compression or abnormal anatomy may obliterate a natural passage to the vocal cords. In these cases, a direct or videolaryngoscope can augment the FOB. One study showed this is particularly helpful in patients with combined difficult airway anatomy and restricted cervical motion. These combined or hybrid techniques help overcome the main weaknesses of the FOB, namely soilage of the lens and inability to create an airway passage *de novo*. These techniques are discussed more in Chapter 19.

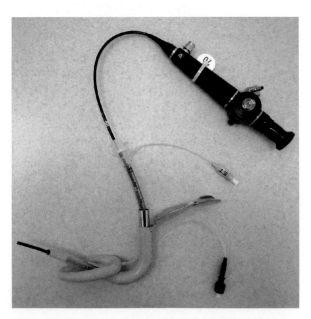

Figure 16.12 Intubating laryngeal mask airway (ILMA) with a dedicated ILMA tracheal tube. FOB-guided tracheal intubation through the ILMA has a high success rate and is the preferred technique.

Retrograde FOB Intubation

Rarely, when access to the upper airway is impossible a retrograde FOB intubation technique may be indicated. This consists of passing a guidewire through a 20G cannula inserted through the cricothyroid membrane. The guidewire is gently fed through the mouth and onto the distal end of the working channel of the FOB (with the tracheal tube already mounted on it) until it exits from the working channel port. The FOB is now passed under vision over the guidewire into the trachea, until the 20G cannula is visible. The cannula and the guidewire are slowly withdrawn, and the FOB is advanced to just above the carina. The tube is railroaded over the FOB as described above.

Conclusion

Understanding the equipment, knowledge of airway anatomy, good endoscopy skills, correct choice of tubes and techniques to advance the tube into the trachea are vital to the success of FOB intubation techniques. The technique may be difficult when there is serious tissue swelling or disruption, because endoscopy requires that there is an airspace and visibility can be reduced by blood or other fluids. Awake FOB intubation remains as the gold standard for intubation in a patient with an anticipated difficult airway.

Further Reading

Asai T, Shingu K. (2004). Difficulty in advancing a tracheal tube over a fibreoptic bronchoscope. Incidence, causes and solutions. *British Journal of Anaesthesia*, **92**, 870–881.

Du Rand IA, Blaikley J, Booton R, et al. (2013). British Thoracic Society guideline for diagnostic flexible bronchoscopy in adults: accredited by NICE. *Thorax*, **68** (Suppl 1), i1–i44.

Johnson DM, From AM, Smith RB, From RP, Maktabi MA. (2005). Endoscopic study of mechanisms of failure of endotracheal tube advancement into the trachea during awake fiberoptic orotracheal intubation. *Anesthesiology*, **102**, 910–914.

Law JA, Morris IR, Brousseau PA, de la Ronde S, Milne AD. (2015). The incidence, success rate, and complications of awake tracheal intubation in 1,554 patients over 12 years: an historical cohort study. *Canadian Journal of Anaesthesia*, **62**, 736–744.

Marfin AG, Iqbal R, Mihm F, et al. (2006). Determination of the site of tracheal tube impingement during nasotracheal fibreoptic intubation. *Anaesthesia*, **61**, 646–650.

Ovassapian A. (1996). *Fibreoptic Endoscopy and the Difficult Airway*. 2nd Ed. Philadelphia: Lippincott-Raven.

Videolaryngoscopy

Lorenz Theiler, Tim Cook and Michael Aziz

Introduction

Videolaryngoscopy has all but evolved to a gold standard for difficult laryngoscopy and intubation. A multitude of videolaryngoscope (VL) devices and designs are available. Videolaryngoscopes can be categorised into three main types according to their blade type:

- Macintosh-like blade
- hyperangulated blade
- blade with an integrated tracheal tube-guiding channel (i.e. a conduit)

Each of the three designs have their indications and each requires distinctive training and specialised handling. Related to VLs are video stylets, which are also briefly described in this chapter.

Videolaryngoscopy provides technical benefits and significant non-technical benefits to the intubation team. Consistently, VLs improve laryngeal view compared with direct laryngoscopy. The ability of other team members (or trainers) to observe what the primary intubator is seeing when using a VL fosters enhanced teamwork and learning.

Development

Traditionally, laryngeal structures can be visualised either indirectly, e.g. by using mirrors, or directly, by the use of standard laryngoscopes. For the last 20 years, with the recently expanding variety of VLs available, the anaesthesia community has gradually turned to indirect laryngoscopy as the favourite means to visualise the larynx. The impact of videolaryngoscopy on tracheal intubation is easily comparable to the introduction of Macintosh's laryngoscope blade in 1943. It may not be as revolutionary as the introduction of the supraglottic airway device, but it is arguably the most important advance in airway management in recent decades.

The concept of introducing not only light to the tracheal opening, but also a camera, was introduced to

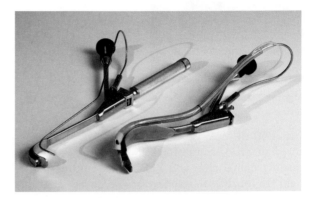

Figure 17.1 The Bullard scope. (Courtesy of Professor Paul Baker, Auckland Hospital, NZ.)

the anaesthesia community quite some time ago. A variety of flexible optical bronchoscopes (FOBs) (see Chapter 16) were in use since the 1970s and rigid optical scopes followed afterwards. One rigid optical scope, combined with a laryngoscope, is the Bullard laryngoscope (Figure 17.1). It features important characteristics of modern VLs with a hyperangulated blade: it provides an optical scope, albeit with the eye at the tip of the tracheal tube and not at the tip of the blade, and a very angulated blade to facilitate intubation around anatomical obstacles at the base of the tongue. As such, it did not require the alignment of the glottis on the same axis with the line of sight, which is a prerequisite for direct visualisation of the laryngeal structures.

At the beginning of the twenty-first century, the concept of placing a camera on the laryngoscope blade started to be marketed. First, on a standard Macintosh blade equipped with a fibreoptic scope (e.g. Laryflex by Acutronic, Hirzel, Switzerland, Figure 17.2, and Storz DCI Videolaryngoscope, Karl Storz, Tuttlingen, Germany). The cumbersome assembly and cleaning prohibited widespread use. Dr John Allen Pacey, a surgeon, introduced a sharply angulated blade with a digital camera in 2001, the GlideScope (Verathon,

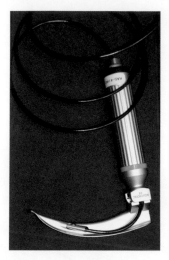

Figure 17.2 The Laryflex.

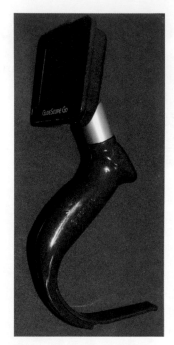

Figure 17.3 The GlideScope Go.

Inc., Bothell, WA, USA, Figure 17.3). This device featured a CMOS (complementary metal-oxide semiconductor) digital chip and LED (light emitting diode) light to enable portability and reduced assembly needs. Since then, a wide range of VLs have become available, with different features and designs.

Studies comparing the success rate of tracheal intubation between standard laryngoscopy and videolaryngoscopy are often insufficient because of inconsistent methodology. Hyperangulated blades are very different from Macintosh blades and also very different from blades with an integrated tube-guiding channel (conduit). Regardless of study limitations, there is ample evidence available to confirm VLs are superior to standard laryngoscopes in providing an improved laryngeal view.

Compared to standard laryngoscopy, tracheal tube advancement may be more difficult, especially with hyperangulated blades. This is most commonly due to the operator having inadequate knowledge or experience of videolaryngoscopy technique. Inadequate training or experience should not be confused with a limitation of the technique and it is important to understand that there is a learning curve for all VLs, but particularly for hyperangulated and conduited devices. When correctly performed, the use of videolaryngoscopy is associated with higher intubation first-attempt success rates, fewer oesophageal intubations and less sore throat and hoarseness.

An often-overlooked aspect of the use of VLs is one of the most important ones: using a screen to view the intubation procedure provides the opportunity to evolve the intubation procedure from a manoeuvre performed solely by one laryngoscopist to a task performed and guided by a team. The team approach may optimise intubation attempts (e.g. an assistant providing optimal external laryngeal pressure or adjusting cricoid force) and can help prevent errors such as oesophageal intubations, as helpful hands and eyes can support the intubation procedure. It is also possible to record the intubation process for teaching purposes and legal documentation. The record can now serve to document the ease or difficulty of the procedure and to confirm proper tube placement without signs of injury or aspiration.

Overview of Different Videolaryngoscopes

When choosing a VL, the type of blade is the most important decision (Figure 17.4). Several manufacturers offer both hyperangulated and Macintosh blades. Blades with conduits are routinely hyperangulated.

Furthermore, both single-use and reusable systems are available. While the performance is similar, differences regarding financial, logistic, environmental and hygienic issues guide purchase decisions.

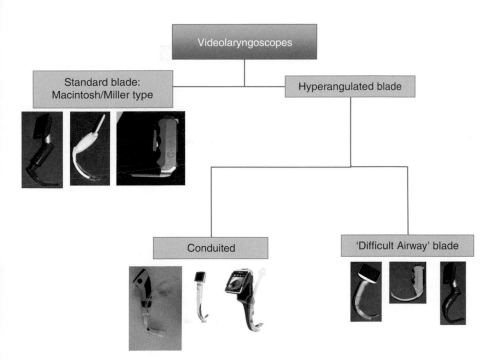

Figure 17.4 Overview of videolaryngoscope types.

Use of Videolaryngoscopes with a Macintosh-Type Blade

Videolaryngoscopy with a Macintosh-type blade closely resembles direct laryngoscopy. For practitioners experienced with standard laryngoscopy who are new to using VLs, it may be prudent to start with a Macintosh-type VL blade. The transition is much smoother and the early failure rate may be lower. Another advantage is the opportunity to readily switch back to direct laryngoscopy, e.g. in case of severe contamination of the lens or the presence of ambient light, especially in pre-hospital environments.

A 'patient–screen–patient' approach is recommended, just as in regional anaesthesia with ultrasound. Thus, the operator looks at the patient when advancing or moving the blade and then at the screen to observe the effect of that movement while holding the device still. Again, when inserting the tracheal tube, the operator does not look at the screen until the tube is advanced beyond the line of sight at the posterior pharynx. The advancing of the tube towards and beyond the glottic opening may be observed either directly as in standard laryngoscopy, or by observing the screen.

Intubation may be facilitated by using either a tracheal tube with a stylet inserted or an intubation aid (a 'bougie') (see Chapter 15).

Use of Videolaryngoscopes with a Hyperangulated Blade

The advantage of using a hyperangulated blade lies in the ability to look around obstacles at the oropharyngeal curve, such as a prominent base of the tongue, which would impede or defeat direct laryngoscopy. Hyperangulated blades may be inserted along the side of the tongue (like a Macintosh-type blade) or in the midline. In either case the tip of the blade should be placed in the vallecula. Minimal force should be needed to place the blade and this is one of its advantages.

In most circumstances a hyperangulated blade will improve the view of the larynx, compared with direct laryngoscopy. However, intubation may not necessarily become easier – though this is most commonly due to poor operator technique. When passing the tracheal tube, it must pass through the two curves of the upper airway: first anteriorly to meet the glottic inlet, then posteriorly to lie along the tracheal axis. This problem has been termed as 'you see that you fail': the tracheal tube is not passed despite a perfect view of the glottis. Successful intubation with a hyperangulated VL mandates a stylet (or another semi-rigid introducer) with an angulation resembling the angle of the blade. The manufacturers of the GlideScope and C-MAC devices each market their own rigid stylet with this preformed configuration. Once a tracheal tube has a stylet within it, it becomes more rigid and if care is not taken, the tube or stylet may injure the posterior wall of the pharynx (Figure 17.5). This complication is closely associated with hyperangulated blades and evidence supports an expected 1% event rate. The hyperangulated blade means it is inevitable that the tip of the tracheal tube will pass out of direct sight during insertion. It may not then appear on the VL screen until it is advanced a little further, meaning there is a 'blind spot' when the tube tip is visible neither directly nor indirectly. In practice this blind spot is very small. Also, if the tip of the tracheal tube is slid along the blade as it disappears from view this should minimise contact with the posterior pharyngeal wall and virtually eliminate the risk of injury.

During laryngoscopy itself, placing the VL tip beyond the epiglottis and lifting directly ('Miller style') is not advisable, as this may injure the fragile epiglottic structure. Also, this technique displaces the larynx further anterior, which makes tube passage more difficult.

There are several different views regarding optimising tube passage with a hyperangulated VL. Some take the view that when the anterior wall of the trachea becomes visible, the tip of the blade is too close to the glottis. In order to facilitate easier intubation, a less than ideal view of the glottic opening is adopted by partly withdrawing the blade, i.e. to achieve only a partial view of the glottic opening. An alternative approach is to consider the VL screen to be a 3 × 3 grid and ensure that the glottic opening is in the middle of this grid. If the styletted tracheal tube is then slid

along the blade in direct contact with the VL blade the tube will reliably enter the glottis. This technique relies on the fact that the VL camera is 'looking' straight down the blade and if the blade is optimally positioned over the glottis, simple optics mean passing the tube along the blade will direct it to the glottis. In some ways this technique is akin to treating the hyperangulated blade as if it were conduited (see below).

Once the tracheal tube reaches the glottis, however that is achieved, withdrawing the stylet may help facilitate further advancement of the tube down the tracheal axis as the tube 'unbends' and this is essential to minimise risk of injury. Other methods to assist tracheal tube passage include simultaneous rotation of the tracheal tube as it is advanced and 'reverse loading' of the tracheal tube on the stylet – i.e. inserting the curved stylet against the pre-shaped curve of the tracheal tube so that when the stylet is withdrawn the tube naturally projects posteriorly towards the tracheal axis. Choice of tracheal tube type may also impact on success and risk of injury: choosing a tracheal tube that is one size smaller than normal, one that is not rigidly curved or even is flexible, and one that has a bullet tip (e.g. Parker tip) may all assist. Finally, external laryngeal pressure may help align the trachea with the direction of the tracheal tube. It is, however, important to emphasise that with proper training and experience, difficulty passing the tracheal tube when using a hyperangulated VL blade should be both very uncommon and readily overcome.

Use of Videolaryngoscopes with a Conduit

Videolaryngoscopes with an integrated guiding channel are also hyperangulated blades. To ensure intubation, the glottic opening must be in the middle of the VL screen to enable advancing the tracheal tube. Thus, positioning of the VL is the technical part, while intubation itself will be comparably easy. These blades may be useful in awake videolaryngoscopic intubation (see below), and a bite block is integrated within the blade, protecting the tube. Beginners and incorrectly trained personnel tend to insert these blades too deep, which prevents optimal device positioning, making intubation impossible. The disadvantage of VLs with a conduit lies in the fact that the tracheal tube can only be advanced through the channel, alternative

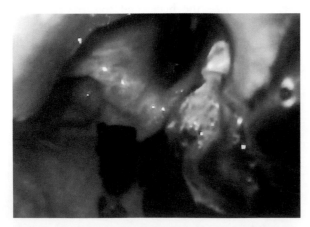

Figure 17.5 Pharyngeal injury using a hyperangulated blade with an inadequately pre-shaped tracheal tube (tube visible at the right side of the picture).

approaches to the glottis are not possible (e.g. nasal intubation). Furthermore, these blades tend to be a bit bulky, requiring a larger mouth opening.

Of note it is important to use the tracheal tube recommended by the manufacturer for a given conduited device. The devices are designed to facilitate intubation with the tracheal tube exiting the conduit aligned with the axis of the channel. If too small a tracheal tube is used it will 'cut across the curve' of the conduit, tending to exit the conduit facing posteriorly and intubation will fail. For the same reason, if intubation with a conduited VL is difficult, use of a bougie down the channel is unlikely to help.

Adjuncts to Videolaryngoscopes and Useful Combinations

Tracheal introducers (bougies) and stylets are discussed in Chapter 15. Bougies may be used with high success in a similar manner to that for direct laryngoscopy. The use of a bougie for videolaryngoscopy may be most beneficial with Macintosh-type blade designs. Bougies are unlikely to be of great value when using a hyperangulated VL if they are not malleable. They generally fail to maintain their curvature and therefore do not match the curvature of the VL blade. Stylets are well suited to use with hyperangulated VLs: either malleable ones that can be preformed to the required shape or manufacturers' own devices designed to use with a specific VL (e.g. GlideScope and C-Mac). Their use is described above. Recently a number of bougies which are semirigid or with deflectable ('steerable') tips have been described (Figure 17.6). These may be more suited to use with hyperangulated VLs than conventional bougies, but evidence to support this is awaited.

Videolaryngoscopes can easily be combined with other optical devices including flexible, rigid or semirigid video stylets. An example is the combination with FOB-guided intubation – video-assisted flexible intubation (VAFI) – and this is described in Chapter 19.

The Use of Videolaryngoscopes in Awake Patients

Awake videolaryngoscopic intubation is an increasingly accepted and taught technique. A variety of techniques are described. In most settings hyperangulated blades, including those with conduits, will be favoured as they generally require less force

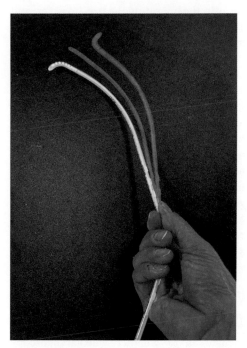

Figure 17.6 An example of a flexible-tipped stylet. The tip is flexed/extended by moving the thumb up/down.

and tissue distortion to achieve an excellent position over the larynx. Several studies have observed equivalent success rates with VLs compared to FOBs in awake patients, though in some of these studies deep sedation was used meaning they were not strictly 'awake' techniques. The topic is discussed further in Chapter 9.

The Use of Videolaryngoscopes in the Emergency Department and Out of Hospital

Emergency airway management out of the operating theatre and out of hospital is challenged by restricted time, physiologically compromised patients and often the limited experience of the airway practitioners involved. While true anatomical difficult airway per se is relatively rare, difficulties routinely arise from restricted range of motion of the head and neck by collars or manual in-line stabilisation and the presence of blood or gastric content in the oral cavity. The out-of-hospital environment may also pose difficulties due to intubation at night, in the rain, snow or cold and under bright sunlight. The fundamental principles of airway management are the same as in the operating theatre, however, and VLs are being used with great success in many prehospital services around the world. If available, the VL should be the first-line device, as many factors may make multiple attempts unsafe. There may be advantages to initially using a VL with a Macintosh-style blade, backed up by a hyperangulated blade. The former will be more familiar to less experienced operators and the user can revert to direct laryngoscopy if the monitor is rendered useless by blood or secretions on the camera or lighting conditions on the screen. Because of numerous challenges related to research in emergency environments, the literature is not fully supportive of videolaryngoscopy in the emergency environment despite robust observational data. Future research is needed to solidify the role of videolaryngoscopy in this environment.

Use of Videolaryngoscopes for Routine vs. for Difficult and Rescue Use?

There is debate as to whether videolaryngoscopy should be a routine and first-line technique or whether it should be reserved for those predicted or found to be difficult to intubate. The debate is unresolved, but only a small number of institutions have managed to adopt routine, or 'universal' videolaryngoscopy.

Elective and emergency airway algorithms increasingly emphasise the role of videolaryngoscopy in managing difficult intubation and failed direct laryngoscopy. They also emphasise the importance of operators being skilled and experienced in the use of the devices – which can only be achieved by regular use in easier settings.

The evidence indicates that most benefit of videolaryngoscopy is in those patients who are predicted or known to be difficult during direct laryngoscopy and intubation. However, it also indicates that multiple – even as few as two – attempts at intubation may increase the risk of harm to patients. Advocates of universal videolaryngoscopy suggest that routine use will ensure that the minimum number of attempts at intubation are used for each patient, will maximise operator skills and experience and will ensure the maximum human factor benefits are accrued by the team. Opponents of universal videolaryngoscopy may consider it unnecessary, costly and overcomplicating – by slowing down easy intubations and requiring adjuncts where these would otherwise not be needed.

If universal videolaryngoscopy is adopted there is an argument for choosing a Macintosh-type system, with a hyperangulated system held in reserve. The former will provide some operator and team benefits of videolaryngoscopy while also enabling training of novices in direct laryngoscopy and it will not slow down 'easy' intubations. The hyperangulated VL can be reserved for genuinely difficult cases.

When VL is adopted only for predicted difficulty and as a rescue device, some experts argue it makes little sense to use a Macintosh-type VL as direct laryngoscopy will already have failed. A hyperangulated VL is a more logical choice as it will provide additional proven benefits in the setting of difficult or failed direct laryngoscopy.

In addition to difficult airway management, routine use of VL has also been adopted in many departments for the placement of double-lumen tubes and tubes used for intraoperative neuromonitoring of the recurrent laryngeal nerve, which require exact placement between the vocal cords.

Rigid Optical Scopes (Video Stylets)

Video stylets are very distinctly separate from other videoscopes and several of them predate bladed VLs.

The Bonfils rigid optical scope (Figure 17.7a) is one of the more widely known devices and may be used via a midline or retromolar approach. This can be especially useful in patients with limited mouth opening in both asleep and awake patients. There are several closely related devices available. A less widely known variant is the SensaScope (Acutronic, Hirzel, Switzerland, Figure 17.7b). It consists of an S-shape rigid scope with a flexible tip. The advantage is the possibility to insert the device beyond the glottis, which makes subsequent insertion of the tracheal tube easier. Its main disadvantage is the unusual handling required, which includes a motion similar to a bartender filling a glass of beer. Very recently, Karl Storz introduced the C-MAC Video Stylet (Figure 17.7c), a rigid scope similar to the Bonfils, but with a flexible tip similar to the SensaScope, which facilitates tracheal intubation. The C-MAC Video Stylet thus combines the theoretical benefits of both older devices. So far, there are no randomised controlled trials available evaluating this technique. Rigid optical scopes may be used with or without a laryngoscope, and also in conjunction with a VL. In comparison to FOBs, they have a faster learning curve, including in oncological patients with rigid tissue caused by radiation therapy. Their main disadvantage that they can only be used via the oral route.

(a)

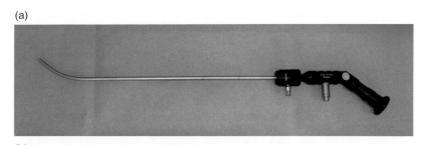

Figure 17.7 (a–c) Rigid and semi-rigid video stylets. (a) Bonfils. (b) SensaScope, upper inset: flexed tip; lower inset: extended tip. (c) Storz video stylet with deflectable tip.

(b)

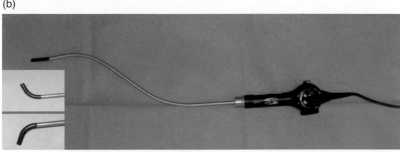

(c)

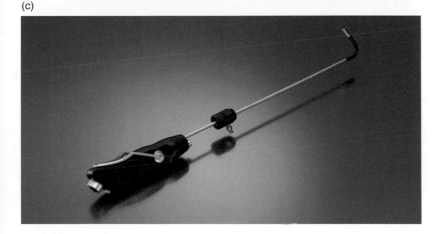

Documentation

Classic grading of intubating conditions used in direct laryngoscopy such as the Cormack and Lehane score may need to be adjusted when using indirect laryngoscopy, particularly if there is a good view of the larynx but difficulty intubating. Several scores have been proposed, such as the Intubation Difficulty Score, which also includes the force applied, external laryngeal manipulations and the position of the vocal cords. The Fremantle score includes laryngeal view, ease of tracheal tube passage, the device and any adjuncts. Regardless of the score used, it is vitally important to document whether a VL or a standard laryngoscope was used, which blade was used and whether or not advancing the tube into the trachea posed any difficulties. Ideally, both the view of the glottis on the monitor and via direct laryngoscopy are documented. Most VLs feature the possibility to directly record the intubation process. Photos and videos documenting successful, smooth intubation may benefit the intubating personnel if the tracheal tube dislocates at a later stage, raising the question of primary oesophageal intubation. Furthermore, videos may be used for teaching purposes.

Further Reading

Aziz MF, Brambrink AM, Healy DW, et al. (2016). Success of intubation rescue techniques after failed direct laryngoscopy in adults. A retrospective comparative analysis from the Multicenter Perioperative Outcomes Group. *Anesthesiology*, **125**, 656–666.

DeJong A, Molinari N, Conseil M, et al. (2014). Videolaryngoscopy versus direct laryngoscopy for orotracheal intubation in the intensive care unit: a systematic review and meta-analysis. *Intensive Care Medicine*, **40**, 629–639.

Kelly FE, Cook TM. (2016). Seeing is believing: getting the best out of videolaryngoscopy. *British Journal of Anaesthesia*, **117**(Suppl 1), i9–i13.

Lewis SR, Butler AR, Parker J, Cook TM, Smith AF. (2016). Videolaryngoscopy versus direct laryngoscopy for adult patients requiring tracheal intubation. *Cochrane Database of Systematic Reviews*, **11**, CD011136.

Pieters BMA, Maas EHA, Knape JTA, van Zundert AAJ. (2017). Videolaryngoscopy vs. direct laryngoscopy use by experienced anaesthetists in patients with known difficult airways: a systematic review and meta-analysis. *Anaesthesia*, **72**, 1532–1541.

Chapter 18

Expiratory Ventilation Assistance and Ventilation through Narrow Tubes

Michiel W.P. de Wolf and Michael Seltz Kristensen

Introduction

When ventilating through (artificial) small-diameter airways, decreasing the diameter increases the resistance to flow exponentially. Therefore, insufflation requires specialised equipment to generate high enough pressures. However, the elastic recoil of the lungs and thorax cannot always generate the required driving pressure to provide the same airflow back through the small-diameter airway.

Traditional insights therefore dictate that the patient's own airway must be non-obstructed or that expiration should be prolonged leading to a decrease in minute volume and carbon dioxide retention. Importantly, if expiration is incomplete, this will lead to air trapping with the potential for barotrauma, haemodynamic compromise and even death.

Expiratory Ventilation Assistance

Ventrain (Dr Enk, Ventinova Medical, Eindhoven, the Netherlands, Figure 18.1) is a manually operated, flow-controlled ventilator that, when combined with a high-pressure gas source, can generate the pressures needed to overcome the resistance to inspiratory flow of a small-diameter airway but also generate sufficient subatmospheric pressures to facilitate expiration through the same small-diameter airway. Thus, both inspiration and

expiration are active processes. This has been coined expiratory ventilation assistance (EVA).

Contrary to traditional means of ventilating through small-bore catheters or cannulae, an open airway to enable passive egress of air is therefore no longer a prerequisite when ventilating with Ventrain. In fact, airway obstruction improves ventilation with Ventrain as gas that is insufflated will not leak out through the upper airway, increasing the efficiency of intrapulmonary gas delivery and pressure build-up (for instance positive end-expiratory pressure (PEEP)).

Originally invented to be used through transtracheally placed cannulae in case of emergencies, Ventrain is now being used in other settings as well, both emergent and elective. In essence, any airway tube with a Luer lock could be used including intubating catheters, airway exchange catheters and bronchial blockers.

Mode of Mechanism

Ventilation with Ventrain works as follows: its gas tubing is connected to a high-pressure source, usually an oxygen flowmeter or an oxygen cylinder with a flow regulator. The tubing at the side port (located at the bottom of Ventrain) is attached to the patient's small-bore airway tube via a Luer lock connection. An additional connection is provided for sidestream capnometry.

Ventrain has two openings that can be occluded by the clinician's thumb and index finger. With both apertures open (Figure 18.2A), no relevant flow occurs to or from the patient (equilibration phase). With both apertures closed, flow is directed to the patient (inspiration, Figure 18.2B).

After releasing the upper opening (lifting the thumb) while keeping the index finger on the lower opening, air from the high-pressure source will preferentially flow forwards. Inside the Ventrain the tubing decreases in diameter. This results in an increased speed of airflow which according to Bernoulli's principle leads to a pressure drop. The resulting

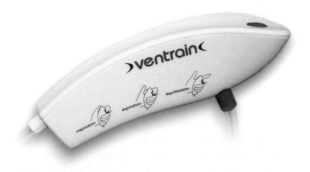

Figure 18.1 Ventrain.

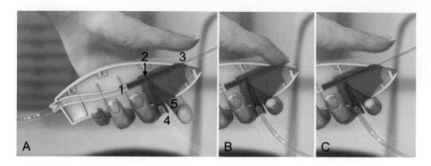

Figure 18.2 Mode of mechanism of Ventrain, see text for explanation.

subatmospheric pressure causes suction and therefore facilitates gas flow from the patient through the small-bore airway during expiration (EVA, Figure 18.2C).

Flow Control

Ventrain is a flow-controlled ventilation mode. Inspiratory volumes can be calculated from the set flow. For instance: at a flow of 15 L min⁻¹, during inspiration each second 250 mL is insufflated and with an inspiratory to expiratory (I:E) ratio of 1:1 this would theoretically lead to a minute volume of 7.5 L min⁻¹.

In clinical practice minute volume will also depend on other factors including pulmonary compliance, resistance to flow through the cannula, the degree of upper airway obstruction and the number of equilibration manoeuvres. Therefore, minute volumes are usually (slightly) lower than calculated.

The gas flow is set according to the patient's characteristics. Flows should be individualised, but the following settings can be used as guides: 12–15 L min⁻¹ for the adult, 4–6 L min⁻¹ if used to ventilate a collapsed lung through a bronchial blocker and 2–6 L min⁻¹ for paediatric patients through an airway exchange catheter or intubating catheter. Start with a low flow and increase as necessary.

Typically used I:E ratios in adults are 1:1, but in very small-diameter airways the resistance to flow might be increased to such an extent that the suction pressure will not be enough to accomplish complete expiration as quickly as inspiration is accomplished. It is therefore recommended to use longer expiration times compared to inspiration times when ventilating through paediatric intubating or airway exchange catheters, or through bronchial blockers.

Pitfalls and Safety Measures

The high-pressure source must be able to generate high enough pressures to vent gas through the high resistance of the tubing of Ventrain and of the small-diameter airway it is attached to. Typically, these are oxygen flowmeters ('wall oxygen') or oxygen cylinders with flow regulators, both of which can generate pressures of 4–6 atmospheres. When used correctly the patient's airway is exposed only to a fraction of this pressure, but the high-pressure source can be a source of barotrauma during misuse. Most oxygen outlets on anaesthesia machines cannot generate the required pressure.

When using a flowmeter, this should preferably be pressure compensated. If this is not the case, then the backpressure caused by Ventrain will compress gas in the flowmeter and displayed flow will be lower than actual delivered flow. If this is not recognised, the clinician might be inclined to increase the flow, which will lead to erroneous and potentially dangerous high settings. If a non-pressure compensated flowmeter is used, then Ventrain must be uncoupled from the flowmeter before flow is set. After connection, the flow reading can be expected to drop, but actual delivered flow will be the same as the flow that is set before attaching Ventrain to the flowmeter. If in doubt this problem can be overcome by using an oxygen cylinder with flow regulator.

Insufflated air is not humidified and therefore the time that a patient is ventilated with Ventrain should be minimised.

It is necessary to continuously observe the patient's chest. Besides observing for a chest rise during inspiration, it is equally important to let the chest fall to its original position during expiration to prevent hyperinflation. On the other hand, overly vigorous deflation might lead to subatmospheric intratracheal pressures and atelactasis. The I:E ratio should be adjusted as necessary. Releasing both the thumb and index finger from their respective openings (Figure 18.2A) will slowly let the patient's intrathoracic pressure equilibrate with the atmospheric pressure. It is recommended to perform this equilibration manoeuvre regularly during ventilation in completely obstructed airways to minimise the risk of unintended high or subatmospheric airway pressures.

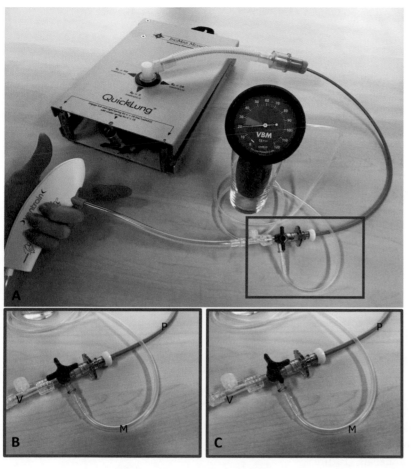

Figure 18.3 (A) Simulated set-up to enable intermittent intratracheal pressure measurements during Ventrain use in combination with a single-lumen catheter using a manometer. (B) Position of three-way stopcock during ventilation: manometer is functionally disconnected. (C) Position of three-way stopcock during intermittent intratracheal pressure measurement: Ventrain is functionally disconnected. V = tube to Ventrain; M = tube to Manometer; P = catheter to Patient.

Using a single small-bore lumen together with Ventrain, intratracheal pressures can be measured intermittently by attaching a manometer between the tube/catheter and Ventrain (Figure 18.3A). Measurements are done after functional disconnection of Ventrain (for instance by using a three-way stopcock, Figure 18.3A and 18.3C) during a ventilation pause, preferably at the end of an inspiration (peak pressure) or after an expiration (end-expiratory pressure). This can be done to guide flow settings and I:E ratios. During ventilation, pressures (which do not reflect intrapulmonary pressures) are high at this point and might damage the manometer. The manometer should therefore be functionally disconnected during Ventrain ventilation, using the three-way stopcock (Figure 18.3B).

Tritube

Tritube (Ventinova Medical) was developed for ventilation with Ventrain. It has three lumens: a 2.4 mm internal diameter ventilation lumen,

a lumen through which tracheal pressures can be continuously monitored (as opposed to intermittent pressure measurements described above) and a cuff lumen (Figure 18.4). Sealing the airway by cuff inflation will optimise oxygenation and ventilation, and continuous airway pressure measurement increases the safety of ventilation.

End-tidal carbon dioxide can be measured intermittently during an equilibration phase as described above (Figure 18.2A).

Importantly, when the cuff is inflated, care should be taken that the patient does not start to breathe spontaneously. If this were to occur, the subatmospheric intrathoracic pressure combined with an obstructed airway might lead to negative pressure oedema. Therefore, at the end of anaesthesia, the Tritube cuff should be deflated. Air can then still be insufflated with Ventrain and a leak should be expected. Also, ventilation with face mask can be done during recovery with Tritube in place and the cuff deflated.

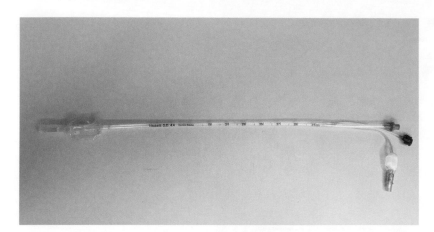

Figure 18.4 Tritube.

The small-diameter airway is tolerated very well in the awake patient, and it can be left intratracheally during recovery (cuff deflated!), as a safety measure should airway compromise occur postoperatively.

Evone an Expiratory Ventilation Assistance Automated Ventilator

The Evone ventilator (Ventinova Medical) is based on the same principle as Ventrain and should be used with Tritube. Automation of small lumen ventilation can be expected to increase ease and safety by displaying tidal volumes, continuous carbon dioxide monitoring, setting airway pressures and alarms (Figure 18.5). Ventilation with Evone is flow-controlled, and inspiratory and expiratory flows are constant, leading to a linear pressure increase and decrease respectively. Another difference from traditional ventilation modes that might confuse the clinician when getting accustomed to working with Evone is how to set ventilator variables: inspiratory and end-expiratory pressures will define tidal volumes according to the compliance of the respiratory system. Flow and I:E ratios will define minute volume. Respiratory frequency cannot be set but is a resultant of the set variables mentioned.

Evone also has a jet ventilation mode. This can be used during emergence from anaesthesia when the cuff will have to be deflated, as flow-controlled ventilation will be less efficient if the airway is no longer occluded.

Conclusion

Small-diameter tubes can enable ventilation of very narrow airways and may both optimise the surgeon's

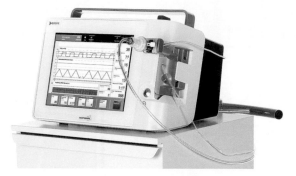

Figure 18.5 Evone ventilator.

view during airway surgery and decrease the incidence of airway trauma. However, their resistance to flow is increased. Expiratory ventilation assistance with the handheld Ventrain can aid management in this potentially difficult situation. It is easy to use but not a foolproof tool and proper training is imperative before use in a clinical situation. With the Tritube, ventilation with Ventrain can be optimised by electively sealing the airway and safety can be increased by continuous airway pressure monitoring. Recently, an automated small lumen ventilator (Evone) has been introduced which might increase safety further and expand the use of small-diameter airways in anaesthetic care.

Further Reading

Berry M, Tzeng Y, Marsland C. (2014). Percutaneous transtracheal ventilation in an obstructed airway model in post-apnoeic sheep. *British Journal of Anaesthesia*, **113**, 1039–1045.

Cook TM, Nolan JP, Cranshaw J, Magee P. (2007). Needle cricothyroidotomy. *Anaesthesia*, **62**, 289–290.

Hamaekers AE, Borg PA, Enk D. (2012). Ventrain: an ejector ventilator for emergency use. *British Journal of Anaesthesia*, **108**, 1017–1021.

Kristensen MS, de Wolf MWP, Rasmussen LS. (2017). Ventilation via the 2.4 mm internal diameter Tritube® with cuff – new possibilities in airway management. *Acta Anaesthesiologica Scandinavica*, **61**, 580–589.

Paxian M, Preussler NP, Reinz T, Schlueter A, Gottschall R. (2015). Transtracheal ventilation with a novel ejector-based device (Ventrain) in open, partly obstructed, or totally closed upper airways in pigs. *British Journal of Anaesthesia*, **115**, 308–316.

Willemsen MG, Noppens R, Mulder AL, Enk D. (2014). Ventilation with the Ventrain through a small lumen catheter in the failed paediatric airway: two case reports. *British Journal of Anaesthesia*, **112**, 946–947.

Chapter 19

Multimodal Techniques for Airway Management

Pierre Diemunsch, Pierre-Olivier Ludes and Carin A. Hagberg

Combination Techniques: Development and Advantages

As described in other chapters, all techniques in airway management may fail and this risks harm to the patient. Despite advances in techniques such as the development and evolution of supraglottic airways (SGAs) and different modes of laryngoscopy each of these may fail. As these new techniques have been developed there has been an increasing realisation that procedural success is not our prime aim, and that airway management is not an end in itself, but only a means of delivering oxygen to the patient. Hand in hand with this has been adoption of techniques to enhance oxygenation during airway procedures.

There has also been a move away from focussing exclusively on prediction of difficult intubation and towards an emphasis on how to manage it when it occurs. Current thinking focusses primarily on what to do in the event of difficulty, rather than simply knowing that something will have to be done.

Advances in mechanics, optics and ultrasonography, combined with the development of intelligent and intelligible algorithms by airway societies, have created multiple opportunities for the modern airway manager.

Accepting that each individual step of the process of airway management may fail offers the opportunity to combine techniques into 'combination techniques' that *use the specific advantages of one medical device to mitigate the limitations of another*.

The most obvious example is the use of a videolaryngoscope (VL) to facilitate intubation with a flexible optical bronchoscope (FOB). We will present this technique in detail.

Other multimodal approaches are based on a combination of FOB intubation with (i) direct laryngoscopy, (ii) an SGA or (iii) a specially designed face mask such as a Fibroxy or VBM mask. The latter

two combinations differ from those aimed solely at facilitating tracheal intubation in that they optimise the safety of the procedure by maintaining the delivery of oxygen to the patient. The combination of high flow nasal oxygen (HFNO) and bronchoscopy can be included in the same group. Further examples are included in the list of Further Reading.

The multimodal approach is also suitable for FOB training where textbook knowledge is combined with computer-based virtual reality training, and simulations encompassing the development of non-technical and teamwork skills before the student ultimately engages in clinical practice under the guidance of a tutor.

Difficulties in Routine Acquisition of Flexible Optical Bronchoscopy Skills

Awake FOB-guided intubation is still the standard technique for management of predictable difficulties in mask ventilation and tracheal intubation. Although the possibility of abandoning it in favour of videolaryngoscopy has been discussed on occasion, this has rightly now been largely dismissed in the recent literature and with increasing availability of relevant technology there is even the possibility to expand opportunities.

Despite anaesthetists being required to master FOB-guided intubation, opportunities for practice are limited: the absolute number of patients with a predicted difficult airway is low, and the availability and fragility of equipment, hygiene issues and the risk of transmitting infectious diseases have all been limiting factors. As a result, many anaesthetists complete their initial training without acquiring FOB skills properly and with few opportunities to practise and are in real danger of losing their skills.

There are various solutions to these training issues: the advent of single-use endoscopes has largely resolved the problems relating to equipment availability and hygiene. Extending the indications for FOB intubation beyond the scope of difficult airway management and cervical spine instability may be advisable as many patients with normal airways could benefit from the avoidance of the physiological stress of laryngoscopy (e.g. neonates and patients with hypertension, diabetes or cardiac disease).

Use of a multimodal approach is likely to increase the use of FOB-based intubation techniques, both benefitting patients and providing increased training and skill maintenance opportunities.

Learning the Multimodal Airway Management Concept with Virtual Reality

Traditionally the acquisition of FOB skills is based primarily on an understanding of the basic of scope manoeuvring (see Chapter 16) and on initial learning using a virtual reality simulator or navigator as a part-task trainer. Simulation optimises the subsequent clinical practice of FOB-guided intubation. High-fidelity simulators have limitations including cost and cumbersome logistics around their use. Low-fidelity simulators, such as home-made wooden panels with a selection of holes to choose from, are inexpensive and their educational effectiveness is comparable to that of high-fidelity devices. However, they still require logistic infrastructure including premises, a real FOB with connectors and

a display screen and a team of motivated instructors. They do not allow students to familiarise themselves with the endoscopic anatomy of the human upper airways.

Virtual endoscopic software overcomes these limitations by enabling users to browse inside three-dimensional reconstructions of human CT/MRI scans. They are developed using the multimodal bronchoscopy model. For instance, the VFI program (Karl Storz, Tuttlingen, Germany, Figure 19.1) provides on two lateral screens: the three-dimensional reconstructed image of the whole airway and the corresponding X-ray image. The location of the tip of the virtual FOB is indicated on these two images with a red arrow. The main screen provides the image collected by the virtual FOB. Using the computer mouse, the trainee can perform a virtual progression through the airways from either the mouth or the nose into the trachea. The trainee benefits from a part-task schedule since they can first get used to the endoscopic airway anatomy. They can then easily acquire endoscopic psychomotor skills, as they constantly follow the position of the FOB tip along with the view obtained from this tip. Indeed, this is the ideal preparation for the clinical multimodal VL-FOB approach to intubation, where the anaesthetist can follow on a VL screen the position of the FOB, from outside this FOB, as the FOB provides the main endoscopic view on its own screen and is progressively introduced towards the carina (see below).

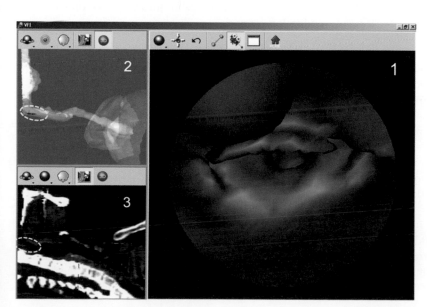

Figure 19.1 The VFI program enables practice of virtual bronchoscopies on CT scan or MRI-based reconstructions. The main screen (1) shows the image collected from the tip of the virtual flexible optical bronchoscope (FOB). The lateral screens show, from outside, the position of the tip of the virtual FOB as a red arrow (2) on a three-dimensional reconstruction of the airways and (3) on the X-ray image. The progression of the virtual FOB is followed in real time on the three screens. This creates a realistic simulation of the multimodal FOB bronchoscopy where the progression of the FOB is initially followed from outside on the videolaryngoscope screen along with the endoscopic view from the FOB (see text).

Limits of Videolaryngoscopes When Used Alone

The introduction of videolaryngoscopy was a decisive step forward in terms of both achieving intubation and facilitating the FOB approach. However, combining the two techniques is still underused. Videolaryngoscopy used alone has become an integral part of the recent recommendations of learned societies concerning difficult intubation but even VLs are associated with failures when used alone. They cannot reliably and completely replace FOB techniques.

For this reason, combining the advantages of videolaryngoscopy with the well-recognised benefits of FOB-guided intubation is an inherently appealing technique.

SGAs and Multimodal Airway Management

There are numerous SGAs that have been developed and marketed in the last decades to compete with the classic laryngeal mask airway. For many advantages are variable and debatable with some very quickly withdrawn from the market. Amongst several SGAs that are suitable for combined techniques for tracheal intubation the i-gel is a significant advance for multimodal techniques. It is a single-use, cuffless SGA device made of a gel-like thermoplastic elastomer. It has a short and wide stem and is easily inserted, where its airway orifice reliably sits over the glottis (see Chapter 13).

In difficult intubation algorithms, SGAs are generally placed in the second line after failure of intubation using direct and videolaryngoscopy. Blind tracheal intubation via an SGA is not recommended and intubation under visual control, with FOB-guided intubation using the SGA as a conduit, is recommended. This constitutes a multimodal technique and is recommended by both the American Society of Anesthesiologists (ASA) and the Difficult Airway Society (DAS). The technique used may be a one-step technique in which the FOB directly guides a tracheal tube into the trachea via the SGA, or the two-step technique in which first an Aintree intubation catheter is guided into the trachea before being replaced by a tracheal tube. The two techniques are described in Chapters 16 and 13, respectively.

Combined Videolaryngoscopy and Bronchoscopy as an Example of Multimodal Airway Management

Rigid VLs provide benefit during management of difficult intubations because they improve glottic exposure and improve the laryngoscopic grade compared with direct laryngoscopy.

However, despite improved laryngeal view, it is sometimes difficult to advance the tracheal tube towards the glottis and achieve intubation, particularly for those inexperienced with the technique. With increasing use of videolaryngoscopy this situation is increasing and it is likely that it is especially prevalent when videolaryngoscopy has been used in the belief that it alone could resolve all difficult intubation situations, when in fact a flexible device (such as an FOB with a steerable tip) was genuinely indicated.

Another risk associated with the use of videolaryngoscopy with devices that do not have a built-in conduit is tissue injury while the tracheal tube is advanced around the device's 'blind spot'. This is especially a risk when using a hyperangulated device (see Chapter 17). Advancing a tracheal tube, especially when combined with a rigid tube guide, can cause pharyngeal injuries, including to the soft palate, the tonsillar pillars and other structures.

For these reasons of efficacy and safety, it may be preferable to replace the rigid guide with a flexible, atraumatic guide or, better still, to combine the rigid videolaryngoscopy and FOB to benefit from the advantages of both techniques and overcome the limitations of each.

Practical Conduct of Combined Videolaryngoscopy and FOB Intubation

This combined technique can be undertaken awake or with general anaesthesia.

Oxygen should be provided throughout and HFNO may be suitable for the awake or apnoeic anaesthetised patient. After induction of general anaesthesia or after appropriate topical anaesthesia, the senior airway manager performing the intubation (the operator) starts by placing the VL in the patient's mouth until the best possible view of the glottis is obtained. The operator then takes the FOB, holding the distal end as if it were an intubation tube. The operator begins to insert the FOB under direct external vision, and then under indirect videolaryngoscopic vision, bringing it as close as possible to the glottic orifice. The assistant holds the handle of the FOB and actuates the control lever. On the operator's instructions, the assistant presses the control lever on the handle of the FOB in order to bend its tip upwards. This manoeuvre displays the glottis on the FOB screen, even if it was not visible on the VL screen. The operator then, under double visual (videolaryngoscopic and FOB) control, finishes inserting the FOB through the glottis and into the trachea until it approaches the carina, asking the assistant to angle the tip of the FOB as appropriate (upwards until the anterior commissure of the vocal cords is reached, then downwards towards the carina while remaining as centred as possible in the tracheal lumen) (Figure 19.2). The operator then completes tracheal intubation by railroading the tracheal tube, previously mounted over the FOB, down until its bevel is in the right position above the carina. Use of an appropriate tracheal tube with a curved bevel will facilitate intubation. The VL provides a view of the tube's passage into the laryngeal inlet. This may help resolve any difficulties at this point. Where appropriate, nasal intubation is possible using the same basic technique.

The described technique is that favoured by the authors, but it may also be achieved with the operator undertaking the FOB manipulation while the assistant opens the oral route using the VL (Figure 19.3). In this case, the operator can track the position of the FOB tip as it advances, on the VL screen. It is the operator who will successively direct the FOB down to the posterior wall of the oropharynx, then upwards to the anterior commissure of the vocal cords, and finally downwards towards the carina while remaining as perfectly centred in the tracheal lumen as possible. The rest of

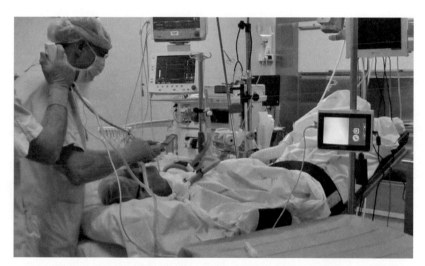

Figure 19.2 Multimodal bronchoscopic intubation using videolaryngoscopy and a flexible optical bronchoscope (FOB). The operator takes the distal end of the FOB as if it were a tracheal tube and inserts it into the mouth under direct and then videolaryngoscopic control. The assistant holds the FOB handle and bends the tip upon request as the progression of the device is followed on the screen of the FOB (see text).

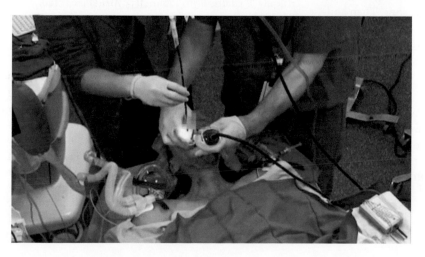

Figure 19.3 Multimodal bronchoscopic intubation using videolaryngoscopy and a flexible optical bronchoscope: alternative technique. The operator performs the endoscopy and the assistant facilitates the procedure with a videolaryngoscope (see text). (Image from AirwayOnDemand from Dr Will Rosenblatt : Use of videolaryngoscope and flexible intubation scope combo. July 26, 2018.)

the procedure is identical. This alternative technique is ideal for experienced endoscopists but seems a little less ergonomic than the first, as both the operator and the assistant are standing next to the patient's head.

Combining Direct Laryngoscopy and FOB-Guided Intubation

The combined use of direct laryngoscopy and flexible optical bronchoscopy has been reported in intensive care patients and as a means to support the learning of FOB-aided intubation skills.

In the authors' experience, videolaryngoscopy considerably facilitates bronchoscopy by keeping the oropharynx open and preventing lateral deviations of the FOB. The operator uses both the external view of the FOB tip on the VL screen, and the internal view of the airways on the FOB screen. Every step of the FOB insertion procedure is carried out under vision control, and using a combination of both techniques can also reduce the pressure exerted by the VL blade on the base of the tongue, thereby reducing the associated physiological stress. The combined technique can be used regardless of the VL or FOB chosen and it enables practitioners to reproduce, in a clinical setting, the perfectly controlled procedures learned by observing the various windows on the virtual bronchoscopy simulator screen (see above). It is suitable as a 'best first attempt' method in the event of predictable difficulty. It has regularly been used with success following failed intubation attempts with either videolaryngoscopy or FOB alone.

The combined videolaryngoscopy and FOB technique may also be used for tracheal tube exchange, particularly when this is expected to be difficult for either anatomical or physiological reasons. Then ability to observe the glottis (with the VL) and the internal airways (with the FOB) adds a level of control not possible with other techniques.

Conclusion

A constructive approach to the problem of difficult intubation consists in combining available techniques to take advantage of their respective strengths, rather than using them individually in a manner that does not eliminate their specific shortcomings.

Based on reflection, rather than the iterative substitution of devices, the multimodal management of difficult intubation is an increasingly popular solution among anaesthetists and intensivists. It can be applied to a large number of devices intended for airway visualisation, tracheal intubation and patient oxygenation.

The multimodal approach is particularly useful for the vast majority of practitioners who only occasionally carry out bronchoscopy. It facilitates high quality care of patients, education and training, and overcomes technical procedural problems thereby preventing complications and avoiding failures.

Further Reading

Boet S, Bould MD, Schaeffer R, et al. (2010). Learning fibreoptic intubation with a virtual computer program transfers to 'hands on' improvement. *European Journal of Anaesthesiology*, **27**, 31–35.

Giglioli S, Boet S, De Gaudio AR, et al. (2012). Self-directed deliberate practice with virtual fiberoptic intubation improves initial skills for anesthesia residents. *Minerva Anestesiologica*, **78**, 456–461.

Gil K, Diemunsch P. (2018). Flexible scope intubation techniques. In: Hagberg CA, Artime CA, Aziz MF (Eds.), *Hagberg and Benumof's Airway Management*. 4th ed. Philadelphia: Elsevier. pp. 428–470.

Greib N, Stojeba N, Dow WA, Henderson J, Diemunsch PA. (2007). A combined rigid videolaryngoscopy-flexible fibrescopy intubation technique under general anesthesia. *Canadian Journal of Anaesthesia*, **54**, 492–493.

Higgs A, McGrath BA, Goddard C, et al.; Difficult Airway Society; Intensive Care Society; Faculty of Intensive Care Medicine; Royal College of Anaesthetists. (2018). Guidelines for the management of tracheal intubation in critically ill adults. *British Journal of Anaesthesia*, **120**, 323–352.

Lenhardt R, Burkhart MT, Brock GN, et al. (2014). Is video laryngoscope-assisted flexible tracheoscope intubation feasible for patients with predicted difficult airway? A prospective, randomized clinical trial. *Anesthesia & Analgesia*, **118**, 1259–1265.

Quintard H, l'Her E, Pottecher J, et al. (2017). Intubation and extubation of the ICU patient. *Anaesthesia Critical Care & Pain Medicine*, **36**, 327–341.

Vlassakov K. (2016). Multimodal airway management: combining advanced airway techniques can be better. *Anesthesiology News Airway Management*, **13**, 53–59.

Front of Neck Airway (FONA)

Paul A. Baker, Laura V. Duggan and Dietmar Enk

Introduction

The clinical situation where a patient's trachea cannot be intubated and other methods to ventilate the lungs fail is traditionally termed the 'cannot intubate, cannot ventilate' (CICV) situation. However, to emphasise the importance of oxygenation in this setting, the term 'cannot intubate, cannot oxygenate' (CICO) is now preferred. It poses a rare, life-threatening event. CICO requires an emergency front of neck airway (eFONA) to avoid hypoxic brain damage or death. Immediate action with a clear plan, appropriate equipment and skills is essential. The ability to efficiently perform eFONA is a fundamental requirement for any practitioner engaged in advanced airway management. This chapter will consider the risk factors and management of CICO and the eFONA procedure.

Incidence

Some anaesthetists may never be required to perform an eFONA procedure. In a Danish airway audit, eFONA occurred in 1:17,000 anaesthetics. In the United Kingdom NAP4 audit, eFONA was performed in 1:50,000 anaesthetics. Of the six patients who died during NAP4, three died after failed emergency airway access. The incidence of eFONA is much higher in the emergency department and community retrieval medicine and may be as high as 1:200 attempted intubations.

Predictors

Percutaneous palpation of the cricothyroid membrane (CTM) can be difficult when performed under stressful conditions, particularly in obese patients and women (pregnant and non-pregnant), where success rates are consistently less than 50%. This is a concern when using any technique that relies on palpation of neck landmarks as a first step. Palpation difficulty is also more likely in patients with a fixed cervical flexion, thick immobile neck, deviated airway, previous radiotherapy and inflammation or induration of the neck.

Indications and Contraindications for eFONA

The most common indication for eFONA is CICO. This may occur acutely where the need for an eFONA is immediately apparent. Conversely, it might evolve insidiously after multiple upper airway manoeuvres; a presentation often difficult to recognise, leading to delayed management. Team training in situation awareness and communication aims to address this delay.

Contraindications for eFONA include total distal airway obstruction or transection and the use of cricothyroidotomy in infants (≤ 12 months old) due to CTM size and fragility.

Pre-eFONA Management

Due to the invasive nature, technical difficulty and potential for failure, avoidance of eFONA is perhaps the most important safety message, and steps should be taken to safely avoid the *need* for it (acknowledging that when it is indicated it must be undertaken without delay). For example, careful assessment and planning might lead to the decision to perform an awake intubation. Other alternatives could include deferring the case, inserting an elective cricothyroid cannula or calling for help to establish an awake eFONA.

Attempts at supraglottic airway (SGA) management should be optimised and limited. Muscle relaxants can improve airway management for many patients with functional airway obstruction including laryngospasm and opioid-induced muscle rigidity. Conversely, patients with distal airway obstruction, including tracheomalacia and mediastinal masses, should **not** be paralysed. In these cases, paralysis can lead to extrinsic large airway compression, elimination of diaphragmatic movement and decreased expiratory flow.

Avoiding hypoxia, although intuitively obvious, may not be prioritised and hypoxia may even go unnoticed as the team struggles with tracheal intubation. Hypoxia risk can be mitigated by attention to pre-oxygenation and oxygenation during intubation attempts. Options include pre-oxygenation by face mask and low flow nasal oxygen (< 15 L min^{-1}) or heated humidified high flow nasal oxygen (up to 70 L min^{-1} in adults) (see Chapter 8). During an eFONA procedure, efforts to oxygenate via the upper airway should continue.

eFONA Management

Practice guidelines clearly describe recommended steps required to manage a CICO situation and eFONA. Recognition is the most important step. Delays in managing CICO events lead to a poor outcome in over 60% of cases. Delays have been attributed to human factors including fixation error with multiple intubation attempts, poor situation awareness (losing track of time and/or failure to recognise urgency or seriousness), lack of available functioning equipment and lack of eFONA skills. Cognitive aids, checklists, cohesive practised teamwork and time checks can help to mitigate these problems.

Time can be saved by preoperatively extending the patient's neck and identifying the trachea and CTM with the aid of ultrasound. Marking the CTM is a visual indicator that eFONA is an anticipated potential outcome and part of the predetermined team-reviewed plan. When the possible need for eFONA is anticipated a 'double set-up' may also be useful: one team managing the airway conventionally with a second team prepared and ready to perform eFONA if required.

The most expert airway practitioner available should perform eFONA. Ideally, that clinician will be a skilled airway surgeon. In their absence, other appropriately skilled surgeons may be called to establish eFONA, but anaesthetists must also be prepared to act. Precious time should not be wasted waiting for a surgeon.

eFONA Techniques

The ideal eFONA technique should have the following features:

- a high success rate
- a low complication rate
- easy to learn

- involves only a few steps
- provides protection against aspiration
- enables adequate ventilation regardless of upper airway obstruction

Three main techniques have evolved for eFONA using various ventilation devices, both 'home-made' and commercial. These are:

Needle cricothyroidotomy (i.e. small-bore cannula (2–3 mm inner diameter (ID)). This requires a high-pressure gas source (wall or cylinder pressure, e.g. up to 4 bar = 58 psi = 400 kPa) to overcome cannula flow resistance. A sufficiently patent upper airway is important to allow passive expiration and avoid barotrauma.

Large-bore cannula (> 4 mm ID). This technique is used in various commercial kits. Some use a Seldinger (wire-guided) technique. A cuffed cannula facilitates positive pressure ventilation. The cannula may allow for adequate passive expiration in the presence of upper airway obstruction.

Surgical airway. This enables placement of a large-bore tracheal tube. A cuffed tube enables conventional positive pressure ventilation in the presence of upper airway obstruction and establishes protection against aspiration.

Needle Cricothyroidotomy and Corresponding Equipment

Needle cricothyroidotomy requires identification of the CTM. If right-handed the operator stands on the patient's left side and if left-handed on the right side). Using the laryngeal handshake technique with an optimally extended neck, the fingers and thumb of the non-dominant hand then move down the lateral borders of the thyroid cartilage to the cricoid cartilage, the index finger then moves to the midline in an attempt to palpate the CTM (Figure 20.1).

Needle cricothyroidotomy is ideally performed with a purpose-made transtracheal cannula attached to a saline-filled syringe (e.g. Emergency Transtracheal Airway Catheter, Cook Medical, Bloomington, IN, USA; Cricath, Ventinova Medical, Eindhoven, the Netherlands; Ravussin cannula, VBM Medizintechnik, Sulz a. N., Germany, Figure 20.2). These cannulae are less likely to kink compared to intravenous cannulae.

A preliminary skin incision may improve the accuracy of cannula insertion. The needle is inserted through the skin by the dominant hand and caudally directed at a 45° angle while aspirating until a loss of

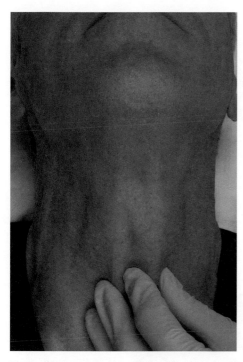

Figure 20.1 Laryngeal handshake.

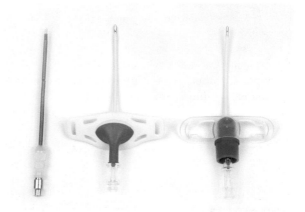

Figure 20.2 Emergency transtracheal cannulae (left to right, Patil, Cricath and Ravussin).

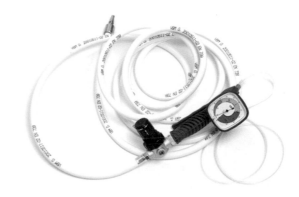

Figure 20.3 Manujet III pressure-regulated jet-ventilator.

resistance is felt and air bubbles appear in the saline-filled syringe. With the needle stabilised by the dominant hand, the cannula is advanced off the needle by the non-dominant hand and the needle is subsequently removed. A second aspiration test is performed to confirm correct placement of the cannula before commencing oxygenation. Presence of air can also occur in the hypopharynx and oesophagus creating a false positive air aspiration test.

Ventilation through a small-bore cannula requires a high-pressure gas source to overcome the resistance of the cannula. Various options have been proposed to manage cannula ventilation (Figures 20.3–20.6). Devices either provide pressure- or flow-regulated ventilation.

High-pressure source ventilation in the presence of small lung volumes and outflow obstruction can quickly deliver potentially dangerous airway pressures leading to barotrauma.

A manual jet-ventilator such as the Manujet III (VBM) is an example of a *pressure-regulated device* (Figure 20.3). It includes pressure ranges on the regulator for different age groups:

baby 0–1 bar (0–14.5 psi = 0–100 kPa);

infant 1–2.5 bar (14.5–36.3 psi = 100–250 kPa);

adult 2.5–4 bar (36.3–58 psi = 250–400 kPa) (Figure 20.4).

It is essential to start with a low pressure (maximum 0.5 bar (0–7.3 psi = 0–50 kPa)) when first operating the manual jet-ventilator while firmly holding the cannula and observing chest movement and palpating for surgical emphysema. Inspiratory time is kept to a minimum (usually 1 second using a manual jet-ventilator). Respiratory rate is determined by the witnessed time taken for chest recoil. Manual jet-ventilators are associated with a high incidence of complications and are relatively contraindicated for use in neonates, infants or any patient with upper airway obstruction.

Advice: start with minimum pressure and increase pressure until chest movement can be seen. Focus should be on the chest, with a goal to restore oxygenation rather than ventilation. Given the risk of haemodynamic deterioration caused by high intrathoracic

173

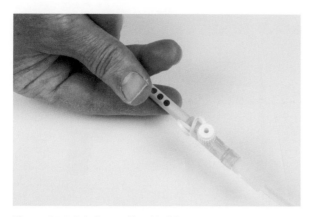

Figure 20.4 Enk Oxygen Flow Modulator.

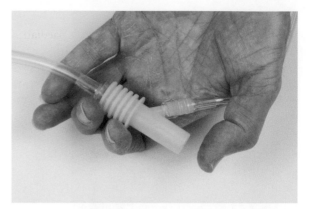

Figure 20.5 Rapid O₂.

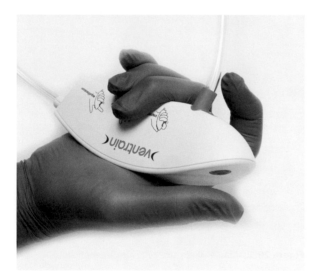

Figure 20.6 Ventrain flow-regulated ventilator.

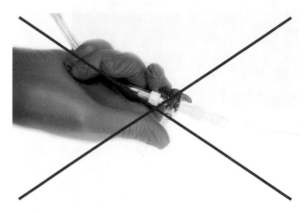

Figure 20.7 Thee-way tap - generally not recommended.

pressure, opening the upper airway using jaw thrust or airway adjuncts such as oro- or nasopharyngeal airways or SGAs is recommended.

Flow-regulated devices that rely on passive expiration include the Enk Oxygen Flow Modulator (Cook Medical, Figure 20.4) and the Rapid O₂ insufflator (Meditech Systems, Figure 20.5). These are both Y-connector variants with equivalent outflow diameters. There are very few reports of these devices being used for eFONA.

For children the Advanced Paediatric Life Support (APLS) guidelines recommend that oxygen flow should be initiated at 1 L min^{-1} year of age^{-1} and an inspiratory to expiratory (I:E) ratio of 1:4 at a rate of 12 breaths min^{-1}. These recommendations should be modified to suit the patient.

The Ventrain (Ventinova Medical, Figure 20.6) is a flow-regulated ventilation device providing assisted expiration by actively withdrawing gas during the expiratory phase by Bernoulli's principle (see Chapter 18). It is capable of limiting high intrathoracic pressure and is supported by clinical and experimental evidence.

Advice: a thorough understanding of these flow-regulated devices is required prior to use.

Self-made devices for emergency cannula ventilation are inherently dangerous. Three-way taps in the oxygen line for ventilation are unsafe due to uncontrolled continuous inflation, even with the side port open to the atmosphere (Figure 20.7). This can rapidly lead to barotrauma because of inadequate flow release, even when several serial three-way taps are used.

Bag-valve-mask (BVM) ventilation through a cannula is inadequate to support oxygenation in adults.

Needle Cricothyroidotomy in Children

There are only seven cases of emergency paediatric transtracheal needle ventilation reported since 1950. Despite the reported difficulty and complications associated with infant cannula cricothyroidotomy, many medical organisations continue to recommend this technique for emergency airway access in children.

Advice: it is not advisable to intubate through the CTM in a neonate or infant due to the difficulty of identifying this very small landmark and fragility of the cartilages, which can lead to injury to these structures. Similarly, cannula tracheotomy is also difficult to perform and is associated with low success and high complication rates. An open tracheotomy is the preferred entry point for neonates and infants (see below).

Large-Bore Cannula Cricothyroidotomy Kits

Large-bore cannula cricothyroidotomy kits are available in both cuffed and uncuffed varieties (Figure 20.8). These kits may involve a Seldinger (wire-guided) or direct insertion technique. The Seldinger technique starts with a small 1.5 cm skin incision at the level of the CTM. A finder needle is then placed through the CTM into the trachea, followed by a wire advanced through the finder needle. The wire then guides a dilator/cannula assembly. The dilator is removed leaving only the cannula in the trachea.

Advice: although intuitive to those practised in Seldinger techniques there is no evidence that cricothyroidotomy kits are superior to a scalpel cricothyroidotomy technique. There are also several

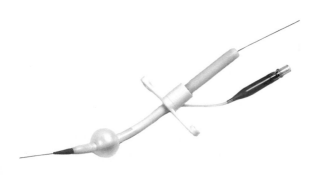

Figure 20.8 Melker cuffed cricothyroidotomy kit.

reports in the literature regarding wire kinking in eFONA situations leading to failure. Therefore, this technique is not recommended by the authors.

Scalpel-Bougie Technique in Adults

One option for a surgical cricothyroidotomy is the scalpel-bougie technique. There are several variants, but the following procedure is recommended as the standardised approach for an eFONA in the UK Difficult Airway Society 2015 guidelines for management of the unanticipated difficult intubation and is supported by these authors.

The operator stands, and uses the laryngeal handshake to identify the CTM, both as described above. A curved (size 10 or 20) scalpel blade, held transversely with the dominant hand, is placed through the CTM. The blade is then rotated 90° into a longitudinal plane with the cutting edge of the blade directed caudally. The operator changes hands, picks up a bougie with the dominant hand and holds the scalpel in the non-dominant hand. While keeping the scalpel in a vertical plane, the operator gently pulls the scalpel toward themselves to create a triangular opening through which the coudé tip of the bougie can be inserted. The bougie is run down the face of the scalpel and directed into the trachea. The scalpel is kept vertical to avoid directing the bougie laterally. The scalpel is removed and a size 6.0 mm ID cuffed tracheal tube is railroaded over the bougie and into the trachea. The bougie is removed and the patient is oxygenated and ventilated with BVM or an anaesthesia circuit.

Advice: if the CTM cannot be located by palpation, an up to 8–10 cm vertical incision is made. Blunt digital dissection can be used to identify anatomical structures and the non-dominant hand stabilises the larynx. Having located the CTM by palpation, a scalpel-bougie procedure is completed as described above. In patients where the trachea may not be in the midline (tumours, bleeding, infection, post-surgery etc.) it is of utmost importance to identify the trachea and the CTM *before* the need for an eFONA arises because otherwise even a longitudinal incision may only cause trauma and no access to the airway.

Advice for paediatrics: for a scalpel-bougie technique, the size of the bougie selected will dictate the size of the tracheal tube. For an adult or child ≥ 12 years, a 6.0 mm ID tube is the smallest tube that will pass over many adult bougies (external diameter 4.5–5 mm). A paediatric bougie (approximately 2.5 mm external diameter) can easily accommodate a size 4.0 mm ID tracheal tube. The width of a size 10 scalpel blade is 7 mm, which is appropriate for an adult but too wide for an infant or neonate. The size 15 blade is 4 mm wide and 12 mm long. This blade length is just adequate for the tracheal 10 mm depth of an 18-month-old child as measured by ultrasound.

The scalpel-bougie technique, with an option to proceed to an open cricothyroidotomy/tracheotomy, largely satisfies the ideal eFONA technique.

Emergency Surgical Tracheotomy in Children

The surgical tracheotomy technique, based on a study using 10 kg piglet cadaver models, may be used as the standard operating procedure for all paediatric age groups by trained operators. It requires surgical equipment and therefore can only be performed with preparation.

Initially, a midline scalpel incision through skin and subcutaneous tissue is made. The incision extends from below the thyroid cartilage to the sternal notch to allow blunt digital dissection down to the trachea. Next, an assistant grasps the wound edges with two towel forceps and exposes the base of the wound. The trachea is identified by blunt digital dissection. A third towel forceps now holds the upper trachea from side to side to stabilise it. A pair of scissors is then used to open the anterior wall of the trachea, 1–2 cm caudal to the larynx. The sharp tip of the scissors cuts caudally and longitudinally through two tracheal rings. Finally, tracheal intubation is performed under direct vision.

Obesity and eFONA

Obesity increases the risk of airway difficulty, the need for rescue techniques and the likelihood of failure. This includes eFONA (see Chapter 24).

Identifying front of neck landmarks is crucial for successful eFONA and is reliably more difficult in the obese. Numerous studies show success rates for identification of the CTM by palpation to be < 50% and as low as 39% for obese women in labour. Recognition of this problem preoperatively allows sufficient time to identify and mark the CTM with the aid of ultrasound.

The CTM is often impalpable and a longitudinal incision technique, as described above, is likely to be necessary.

The disproportionally higher number of obese patients presenting with difficult airways justifies use of specific training techniques to simulate difficulty in obese patients.

Summary

eFONA is a skill required by all practitioners involved in advanced airway management. Successful outcome requires a standardised approach, quick action with immediate access to equipment. Training as a team should be part of a comprehensive airway management education and simulation programme (see Chapter 36). Quality assurance requires ongoing reporting with analysis.

Further Reading

Duggan LV, Ballantyne Scott B, Law JA, et al. (2016). Transtracheal jet ventilation in the 'can't intubate can't oxygenate' emergency: a systematic review. *British Journal of Anaesthesia*, **117**(Suppl 1), i28–i38.

Duggan LV, Lockhart SL, Cook TM, et al. (2018). The Airway App: exploring the role of smartphone technology to capture emergency front-of-neck airway experiences internationally. *Anaesthesia*, **73**, 703–710.

Frerk C, Mitchell VS, McNarry AF, et al. (2015). Difficult Airway Society 2015 guidelines for management of unanticipated difficult intubation in adults. *British Journal of Anaesthesia*, **115**, 827–848.

Johansen K, Holm-Knudsen RJ, Charabi B, Kristensen MS, Rasmussen LS. (2010). Cannot ventilate-cannot intubate an infant: surgical tracheotomy or transtracheal cannula? *Paediatric Anaesthesia*, **20**, 987–993.

Kristensen MS, Teoh WH, Baker PA. (2015). Percutaneous emergency airway access; prevention, preparation, technique and training. *British Journal of Anaesthesia*, **114**, 357–361.

Law JA. (2016). Deficiencies in locating the cricothyroid membrane by palpation: we can't and the surgeons can't, so what now for the emergency surgical airway? *Canadian Journal of Anaesthesia*, **63**, 791–796.

Peterson GN, Domino KB, Caplan RA, et al. (2005). Management of the difficult airway: a closed claims analysis. *Anesthesiology*, **103**, 33–39.

Chapter 21

Extubation

Viki Mitchell and Richard Cooper

Introduction

Extubation is a critical moment which few anaesthetists approach with total confidence, fearing patient harm and the potential for professional embarrassment. Until recently, discussions about airway management have concentrated on laryngoscopy and intubation. Complications associated with extubation were either ignored or thought to be unavoidable. Minor issues such as coughing and breath-holding are common; more serious complications are rare and often preventable with proper planning. Maintaining oxygenation of the patient's lungs is the priority during and after extubation.

Prevalence of Problems

The UK 4th National Audit Project (NAP4) reported that 28% of very serious airway complications occurred at emergence or following extubation. Of the 38 reported cases, 5 patients suffered a hypoxic cardiac arrest, 10 required an emergency surgical airway and 13 had post-obstructive pulmonary oedema.

Adverse respiratory events are the leading cause of malpractice claims in the USA, disproportionately leading to death and brain injury. The American Society of Anesthesiologists' Closed Claims database identified 18 claims associated with extubation either in the operating or recovery area. Most of the claims subsequent to extubation were associated with a difficult airway, obesity or obstructive sleep apnoea (OSA) and sadly the data fail to demonstrate any reduction in claims relating to extubation between 1985–92 and 1993–9.

Failed extubation (i.e. the necessity to reintubate shortly after) occurs in approximately 0.1–0.2% of general anaesthetics administered for a wide range of surgical procedures involving adults. The prevalence increases roughly 10-fold for patients having procedures involving their airway and 10-fold again for patients extubated in critical care areas. Patients with OSA may be at 10 times the risk of requiring reintubation.

The Nature of Problems at Extubation

Although removal of the tracheal tube is usually uneventful, a smooth extubation is of special importance for some patients and in particular situations. Airway obstruction after extubation is the commonest cause of major complications at this time. There is increased risk in patients with obesity or sleep apnoea, residual anaesthesia or muscle weakness, surgery which involves the airway or compromises respiratory mechanics, prior airway difficulties and prolonged head-down positioning. Airway stimulation may result in the activation of reflexes such as coughing, laryngospasm or breath-holding. In some patients, even transient hypertension, tachycardia, increased pressures (venous, intra-gastric, intraocular or intracranial) may be problematic. Thus, the risks involved and the strategies chosen to achieve an uneventful extubation depend on the clinical context.

Problems Related to Reduced Airway Tone and Impaired Airway Reflexes

A number of factors may contribute to reduced pharyngeal tone, causing collapse and airway obstruction. This is a particular problem in obese patients, especially when accompanied by OSA with increased sensitivity to opioids and residual anaesthesia. Protective laryngotracheal reflexes are impaired after extubation for several hours and vomiting or regurgitation may result in aspiration. Blood in the airway, especially when concealed in the nasopharynx ('coroner's clot') increases the risk as inhalation of blood clots can cause complete airway obstruction.

Inadequate Reversal of Neuromuscular Blockade

Inadequate reversal of neuromuscular blockade increases the incidence of post-operative respiratory complications. Train of four (TOF) ratios of less than

0.9 are associated with adverse respiratory events. Clinical tests and qualitative assessment of TOF recovery after neostigmine reversal are unreliable and may result in incomplete neuromuscular recovery. As clinicians cannot detect fade with a TOF ratio > 0.7 and cannot distinguish clinically between ratios of 0.4 to 0.7 there is a strong argument for routine use of quantitative neuromuscular monitoring to ensure adequate reversal whenever a neuromuscular blocking agent is used. Sugammadex provides rapid and effective reversal of neuromuscular blockade.

Aspiration

Patients with increased gastric volume, reduced gastrointestinal motility, reduced lower oesophageal sphincter tone or impaired reflexes are at greater risk of aspiration. It is a leading cause of adverse respiratory complications.

Problems Related to Airway Stimulation

Any noxious stimulus applied during emergence from general anaesthesia can trigger laryngospasm, a sustained adduction of the true vocal cords, vestibular folds and/or aryepiglottic folds. Children are particularly predisposed to this maladaptive response (see Chapter 23).

Laryngospasm is an exaggeration of the normal glottic closure reflex, usually in response to airway stimulation. Although animal studies have suggested that hypoxia and hypercapnia may have an inhibitory effect on laryngospasm, it is untrue that the vocal cords will open before brain injury or death occurs.

Partial laryngospasm presents with a characteristic inspiratory 'crowing' sound but complete obstruction is silent. Laryngospasm may lead to post-obstructive pulmonary oedema and can progress to hypoxic cardiac arrest and death.

The risk of laryngospasm is greatest if extubation is attempted in a lighter plane of anaesthesia (i.e. between deep anaesthesia and being fully awake). Before extubation, airway suction should be performed under direct vision with the patient deeply anaesthetised, to clear the airway of debris. Further stimulation should be avoided until the patient is awake. Topical lidocaine sprayed onto the vocal cords at induction can reduce the risk after short procedures. Airway reactivity varies with anaesthetic agent, with sevoflurane and propofol being the least irritating. Treatment is shown in Box 21.1.

Post-obstructive Pulmonary Oedema

Post-obstructive pulmonary oedema occurs after 0.1% of all general anaesthetics, more commonly in young muscular adult males. Forceful inspiratory efforts against an obstructed airway create high negative intrathoracic pressure which can lead to pulmonary oedema. The commonest cause is laryngospasm, but it can also occur if a patient forcibly bites on a tracheal tube or supraglottic airway (SGA) occluding its lumen. It presents with dyspnoea, agitation, cough, pink frothy

---

Box 21.1 Treatment of laryngospasm

Initial actions

Call for help

Apply continuous positive airway pressure with 100% oxygen using a reservoir bag and face mask, ensuring the upper airway is patent. Avoid airway stimulation

Larson's manoeuvre: place the middle finger of each hand in the 'laryngospasm notch' between the posterior border of the mandible and the mastoid process whilst also displacing the mandible forward in a jaw thrust. Deep pressure at this point may help relieve laryngospasm

Low-dose propofol e.g. 0.25 mg kg^{-1} intravenously

Low-dose suxamethonium 0.1 mg kg^{-1} intravenously

If laryngospasm persists and/or oxygen saturation is falling:

A larger dose of propofol may be needed (1–2 mg kg^{-1} intravenously)

Suxamethonium 1 mg kg^{-1} intravenously

In the absence of intravenous access suxamethonium can be given intramuscularly (2–4 mg kg^{-1}), intralingually (2–4 mg kg^{-1}) or intraosseously (1 mg kg^{-1})

Atropine may be required to treat bradycardia

In extremis, a front of neck airway is indicated

> **Box 21.2** Management of post-obstructive pulmonary oedema
>
> Relieve the airway obstruction
>
> Administer 100% oxygen with full facial continuous positive airway pressure (CPAP) mask
>
> Sit the patient upright
>
> Tracheal intubation and ventilatory support may be required
>
> Opioids and diuretics may provide comfort and accelerate recovery
>
> A chest X-ray should be obtained to exclude other airway complications
>
> Critical care admission may be required

sputum and low oxygen saturations. The radiograph may show diffuse, bilateral alveolar opacities consistent with pulmonary oedema. Prompt recognition and management usually result in rapid resolution. Death is rare and usually attributable to hypoxic brain injury.

A bite block should always be used during emergence to prevent post-obstructive pulmonary oedema. If the patient does bite down on the tube, deflating the cuff may enable some inward gas flow and reduce the extent of subatmospheric intrathoracic pressure. Management of post-obstructive pulmonary oedema is shown in Box 21.2.

Conduct of Extubation

Intubation is a skill; extubation is an art. Extubation is elective and should always be planned and carefully executed. Production pressure often competes with the need for a carefully controlled emergence but the process should minimise noxious stimuli and distractions from patient care. Backup plans to ensure adequate oxygenation and reintubation if required should always be in place and communicated to the airway team.

A four-step approach to extubation supports robust decision making and safe management (Figures 21.1–21.3).

Step 1. Plan Extubation

A plan for extubation should be considered before induction of anaesthesia, reviewed and refined as the case dictates.

Airway Risk Factors

Pre-existing airway difficulties
- Causes include abnormal airway anatomy, obesity, OSA and patients at risk of aspiration of gastric contents

Airway deterioration

- Due to distorted anatomy, bleeding or swelling whether due to anaesthesia or surgery

Restricted access to the airway
- For example, halo-fixation, maxillo-mandibular wiring, cervical spine fixation or instability

General Risk Factors

Physiological factors
- These include limited cardiorespiratory reserve, neurological or neuromuscular impairment, hypo or hyperthermia, acid–base or electrolyte disturbances

Contextual considerations
- Coughing or straining may compromise the airway resulting in a neck haematoma formation or raised intracranial or intraocular pressure. Limited resources including inexperienced personnel or backup equipment

Step 2. Preparing for Extubation

This step involves the final optimisation of airway, general and logistical factors to provide the best possible conditions for success.

Reversal of neuromuscular blockade should be quantitatively confirmed with a nerve stimulator. The patient's general status should be reviewed including body temperature, acid–base balance, cardiovascular stability and analgesic adequacy. It is essential to bear in mind that an airway successfully managed under the optimal conditions of a controlled anaesthetic induction could be entirely different in an emergency. A deteriorating patient may create operator stress that impairs individual and team performance. Safe extubation requires the same level of monitoring and vigilance as induction and intubation. Good communication with the theatre team is important to avoid distractions and ensure that help is available if needed.

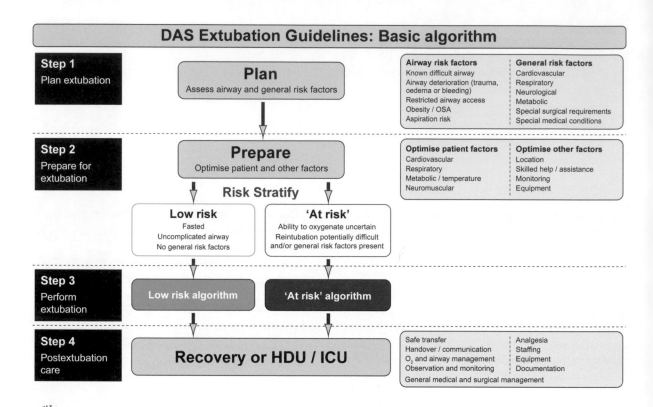

Difficult Airway Society Extubation Algorithm 2011

Figure 21.1 DAS extubation algorithm: basic. (Reproduced from Popat M, Mitchell V, Dravid R, Patel A, Swampillai C, Higgs A. Difficult Airway Society Guidelines for the management of tracheal extubation. *Anaesthesia* 2012; 67: 318–340, with permission from the Association of Anaesthetists of Great Britain & Ireland/Blackwell Publishing Ltd.)

Risk Stratification of Extubation

Together with planning, preparation enables the risk stratification of extubation along a 'low-risk' to 'at-risk' continuum. Extra care is needed for the latter and special techniques may be appropriate.

Step 3. Performing Extubation

Timing of Extubation: Deep vs. Awake vs. Deferred

The overriding consideration regarding the timing of extubation should be safety, not speed.

Deep extubation is an inappropriate technique in patients with anatomically difficult airways. It should only be considered if avoiding the stimulation of tracheal tube removal exceeds the risks of airway obstruction, breath-holding and aspiration. Most adult patients are extubated after they are awake, obeying instructions and demonstrating adequate spontaneous ventilation and oxygenation. Extubation should be performed when the patient

is either deep or awake – not between these two states.

When awake extubation is planned it is wise to inform the patient preoperatively and explain the process. This may improve cooperation and avoid rare occurrences where a patient later recalls awake extubation and reports 'awareness'.

In some situations, it may be safest to postpone extubation and manage the patient on a critical care unit for some hours or even days. Considerations include the potential for airway swelling, the risk of other physiological compromise, an anticipated need for return to theatre within a short period or the immediate availability of skilled assistance (Figures 21.2 and 21.3).

Pharmacological Agents

Opioids such as alfentanil, fentanyl, morphine and a low-dose remifentanil infusion have been used to suppress the cough reflex. Topical, intravenous or

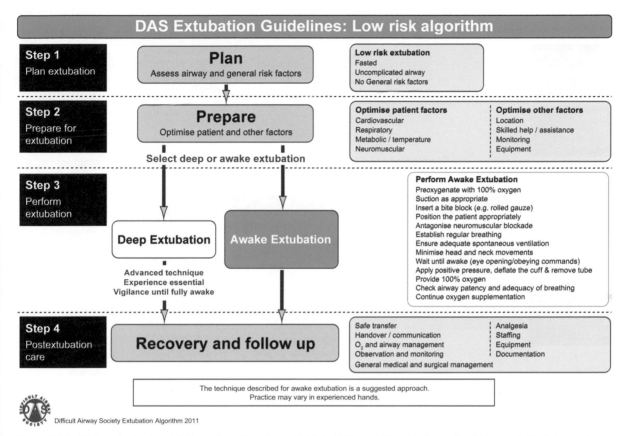

Figure 21.2 DAS extubation: low risk. (Reproduced from Popat M, Mitchell V, Dravid R, Patel A, Swampillai C, Higgs A. Difficult Airway Society Guidelines for the management of tracheal extubation. *Anaesthesia* 2012; 67: 318–340, with permission from the Association of Anaesthetists of Great Britain & Ireland/Blackwell Publishing Ltd.)

intracuff lidocaine may help to reduce coughing. Other pharmacological agents can attenuate the cardiovascular and respiratory changes associated with extubation, including opioids, calcium channel antagonists, magnesium, clonidine, ketamine and beta blockers.

Emergence and extubation are generally smoother following intravenous anaesthesia with propofol compared with anaesthesia with volatile agents.

Exchanging the Tracheal Tube for an SGA

An SGA is better tolerated than a tracheal tube and less likely to result in coughing or haemodynamic instability. It also sequesters secretions, permits assessment of spontaneous ventilation, permits control of the depth of anaesthesia, enables supplementation of ventilation and controlled bronchoscopic airway evaluation. Because of the risk of airway loss, the substitution of a tracheal tube with an SGA is regarded as an advanced technique. Such a substitution should only be performed under deep anaesthesia.

Many SGAs are designed such that they can be placed behind a tracheal tube without removing the tracheal tube. Once its position is satisfactory the tracheal tube can be removed and the SGA immediately maintains the airway. This is known as the Bailey manoeuvre.

Special Techniques for Extubation of the Difficult Airway
Remifentanil and Opioids

An intravenous infusion of remifentanil can be used to reduce undesirable cardiovascular and respiratory responses. The patient may remain more tolerant of the tracheal tube without significant respiratory depression after consciousness has returned and can be extubated smoothly once able to obey verbal commands.

Airway Exchange Catheters

Airway exchange catheters (AECs) can be used for patients with difficult airways, providing a conduit

181

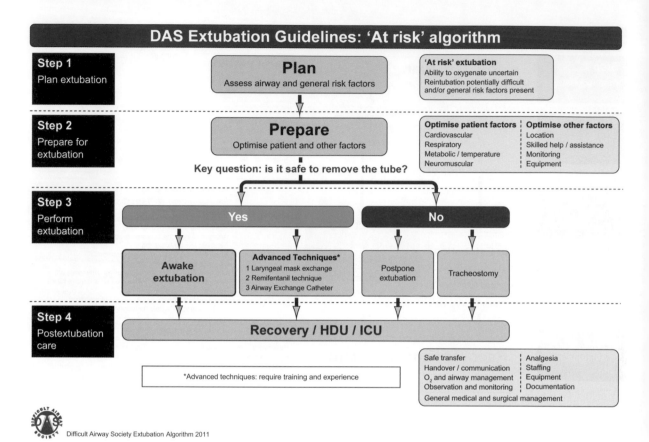

Difficult Airway Society Extubation Algorithm 2011

Figure 21.3 DAS extubation: at risk. (Reproduced from Popat M, Mitchell V, Dravid R, Patel A, Swampillai C, Higgs A. Difficult Airway Society Guidelines for the management of tracheal extubation. *Anaesthesia* 2012; 67: 318–340, with permission from the Association of Anaesthetists of Great Britain & Ireland/Blackwell Publishing Ltd.)

over which a tracheal tube can be passed should re-intubation be required.

The AEC is a long hollow tube designed to be placed through the tracheal tube prior to tracheal tube removal. After removal another tracheal tube can be railroaded over the AEC (tube exchange) or the AEC may be left in place as the patient wakes (AEC-assisted extubation). AECs are available with different outer diameters and different lengths depending upon the intended use. The AEC must be at least twice the length of the tube being removed or replaced (Figure 21.4).

The main risk with an AEC is of airway stimulation. Trauma may occur if the AEC is inserted to or beyond the carina. An AEC with a softened distal tip has been developed for double-lumen tube exchange but there is no evidence that this reduces the risk of trauma. The administration of supplemental oxygen from a high-pressure source should be avoided unless it is required for life-threatening hypoxaemia. Even oxygen insufflation at relatively low flow rates (2–4 L

min^{-1}) has been associated with barotrauma. This is more likely to occur with distal placement of the AEC or upper airway obstruction limiting the egress of gas. To avoid this the AEC tip should never lie distal to the carina (i.e. approximately 23–25 cm from the lips).

Sequence for Use of an AEC

- When the patient is ready for extubation, insert the AEC into the tracheal tube such that the distance markings on the two devices are aligned. The distance at the teeth (or naris) is noted.
- Suction the pharynx prior to deflation of the tracheal tube cuff.
- Remove the tracheal tube over the AEC, attempting to avoid advancement of the AEC. If advancement has occurred, this should be corrected.
- An orally positioned AEC should be secured with four-point fixation. Midline placement reduces the tendency for the AEC to be dislodged by the

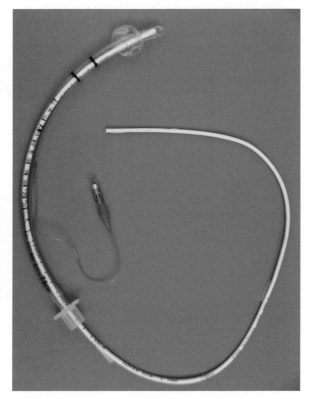

Figure 21.4 Cook airway exchange catheter (AEC) placed in an tracheal tube.

patient's tongue. If supplemental oxygen is provided by a face mask, a slit can be made in the mask through which the AEC can be passed. For a nasally positioned AEC, care should be taken to avoid pressure on the nasal ala.

- Record the depth at the teeth or naris in the notes.
- The patient should be able to breathe, talk or cough with the AEC *in situ*. It is generally well tolerated without requiring local anaesthesia or sedation.
- Clearly label the AEC and ensure that staff understand that this is not a nasogastric tube.
- Nurse the patient in a high dependency or critical care unit familiar with such devices.
- Oxygen can be given via a face mask, nasal cannula or CPAP mask. Oxygen insufflation, manual and jet ventilation should only be used in life-threatening situations due to the risk of barotrauma even in expert hands. If ventilation is required, consider using an active inflation/deflation device (Ventrain, see Chapter 18).

- Intolerance should prompt a reassessment of the depth of insertion. Most AECs are radio-opaque.
- The patient should remain nil by mouth until the AEC is removed.
- Remove the AEC when the airway is no longer at risk. Premature removal is a common error. Reintubation of a difficult airway in the absence of an AEC significantly increases the risk of morbidity.
- Alternatively, a staged extubation kit (Cook Medical) can be used. This entails extubation over an amplatz guidewire (see below).

Sequence for Use of an AEC for Reintubation

- Position the patient appropriately.
- Apply 100% oxygen with CPAP via a face mask.
- Attempt to minimise the discrepancy between the inner and outer diameters of the tracheal tube and AEC. A soft, blunt bevelled tipped tracheal tube should be considered (e.g. LMA Fastrach TT or Parker FlexTip).
- Administer anaesthetic, neuromuscular blockers or topical agents as indicated.
- Laryngoscopy will provide tongue retraction while videolaryngoscopy may allow visualisation of tracheal tube advancement, avoidance of arytenoid impaction and immediate confirmation of success. If a staged extubation kit was used, a tapered AEC is advanced over the guidewire and the tracheal tube is 'railroaded' over that.
- After reintubation, confirm the tube position with capnography and auscultation.

Step 4. Post-extubation Care and Follow-Up

Following difficulties with tracheal intubation or reintubation, there is a risk of mediastinitis resulting from soft tissue penetration. Early diagnosis requires a high clinical suspicion and is vital as there is a significant risk of mortality. The symptoms and signs include the triad of

- pain: retrosternal, cervical or sore throat
- pyrexia
- crepitus

Treatment includes broad spectrum antibiotics, urgent surgical referral, nil by mouth and imaging.

Airway Alert Form

Any difficulties with airway management should be explained to the patient in person and in writing, documented on the anaesthetic chart and in the main hospital clinical record. An airway alert, such as the DAS Difficult Airway Alert Form, with a standard template with prompts for documentation and communication should be used (see Chapter 34).

Summary

Extubation is a high-risk phase of anaesthesia. An extubation strategy should be in place for every anaesthetic. Extubation in a deep plane of anaesthesia is an advanced technique. If there is doubt about airway control, think about special strategies to minimise risk. Low-dose remifentanil may improve conditions during awake extubation. An airway exchange catheter is a useful aid. Follow-up and documentation are essential if airway difficulties have been encountered.

Further Reading

Asai T, Koga K, Vaughan RS. (1998). Respiratory complications associated with tracheal intubation and extubation. *British Journal of Anaesthesia*, **80**, 767–775.

Cavallone LF, Vannucci A. (2013). Review article: extubation of the difficult airway and extubation failure. *Anesthesia & Analgesia*, **116**, 368–383.

Cook TM, Woodall N, Frerk C; Fourth National Audit Project. (2011). Major complications of airway management in the UK: results of the Fourth National Audit Project of the Royal College of Anaesthetists and the Difficult Airway Society. Part 1: anaesthesia. *British Journal of Anaesthesia*, **106**, 617–631.

Cooper RM. (2018). Extubation and reintubation of the difficult airway. In: Hagberg CA, Artime CA, Aziz MF (Eds.), *Hagberg and Benumof's Airway Management*. 4th ed. Philadelphia: Elsevier. pp. 844–867.

Duggan LV, Law JA, Murphy MF. (2011). Brief review: Supplementing oxygen through an airway exchange catheter: efficacy, complications, and recommendations. *Canadian Journal of Anaesthesia*, **58**, 560–568.

Karmarkar S, Varshney S. (2008). Tracheal extubation. *Continuing Education in Anaesthesia Critical Care & Pain*, **8**, 214–220.

Peterson GN, Domino KB, Caplan RA, et al. (2005). Management of the difficult airway: a closed claims analysis. *Anesthesiology*, **103**, 33–39.

Popat M, Mitchell V, Dravid R, et al. (2012). Difficult Airway Society Guidelines for the management of tracheal extubation. *Anaesthesia*, **67**, 318–340.

Chapter

22

The Airway in Obstetrics

Wendy H. Teoh and Mary C. Mushambi

Introduction

'Physiological changes in pregnancy, active labour and isolated location increase the complexity of management of airway complications when they occur.' This was one of the key learning points from the 4th National Audit Project (NAP4) of the Royal College of Anaesthetists (RCoA) and Difficult Airway Society (DAS). The presence of the fetus means that severe hypoxia during difficult airway management can potentially compromise two lives. Many anaesthetists worry about the airway in obstetrics and this worry goes back over many years to the high number of cases of difficult and failed intubation and/or failed ventilation that regularly used to feature in the Reports on Confidential Enquiries into Maternal Deaths. Since the early 1980s, such incidences have reduced considerably and this is partly as a result of better training, staffing, equipment and facilities, and partly through greater use of regional anaesthesia in obstetrics. However, the risk of failed intubation remains and there is concern that changes in anaesthetic training as well as reduced number of general anaesthesia for caesarean sections have led to reduced exposure of trainees to general anaesthesia for caesarean section. A recent UK report on maternal mortality stated that effective management of failed tracheal intubation is a core anaesthetic skill which should be taught and rehearsed regularly and strongly recommended the use of simulation for teaching and rehearsing failed intubation. Recent publication of the obstetric difficult airway guidelines by the Obstetric Anaesthetists Association (OAA) and DAS includes an algorithm for 'Safe obstetric general anaesthetic'. This algorithm is designed to be used as a teaching tool to update and standardise the conduct of general anaesthesia for the pregnant woman.

Incidence of Morbidity and Mortality

Failed intubation in obstetrics is still higher than failed intubation in the general population and has remained unchanged over three decades at 1:390 for obstetric general anaesthetics (GAs) and 1:443 GAs for caesarean sections. Morbidity and mortality following failed intubation are similarly higher in the obstetric patient than the general population. Maternal mortality from failed intubation is approximately 2.3 per 100,000 GAs for caesarean section (1 death per 90–102 failed intubations) compared with 0.6 per 100,000 GAs for the general population in the NAP4 report. The incidence of front of neck airway (FONA) procedures was similarly higher at 3.4 per 100,000 compared with 2 per 100,000. When there is failed intubation during anaesthesia for caesarean section, it is very difficult to separate the effects on the fetus of the failed intubation from the underlying compromise that might be the reason for the caesarean section. However, in a large UK study, neonatal intensive care unit (ICU) admission was higher in the failed intubation group (34%) than in those who underwent uncomplicated general anaesthesia (20%), though this was not statistically significant. Multivariate analysis identified failed intubation and the lowest maternal oxygen saturation as independent predictors of neonatal ICU admission. The key message is that maternal hypoxia during airway difficulty may influence neonatal outcome.

Airway Assessment in Obstetrics

Prediction of difficult airway is notoriously inaccurate and is covered in detail in Chapter 5. While factors that predict difficulty in pregnancy are the same as for non-pregnant patients, the airway should be reassessed during labour because repeated straining during contractions, oxytocin and intravenous fluids may all cause airway oedema.

Table 22.1 Factors contributing to difficulty with the airway in pregnancy

Anatomical and physiological changes of pregnancy
- Weight gain
- Breast enlargement, hindering laryngoscope blade insertion
- Increased risk of airway oedema and engorgement during labour
- Worsened airway oedema from pre-eclampsia, use of large amounts of intravenous fluids, straining and pushing in labour
- Rapid onset of hypoxia during apnoea due to reduced functional residual capacity and increased oxygen consumption
- Reduced lower oesophageal barrier pressure and increased risk of regurgitation and aspiration
- Reduced gastric emptying in labour

Training issues
- Reduced clinical experience of anaesthetic trainees
- Reduced clinical experience of anaesthetic assistants
- Reduced use of general anaesthesia for caesarean sections
- Incorrect application of cricoid force particularly on a tilted table

Situation and human factors
- Urgency of situation and time pressure to deliver the baby
- Remote location means that it takes longer to get help when needed
- Lack of/poor communication between labour ward and theatre team members
- Anxiety or panic of the patient, partner or other staff members
- Poor decision-making and fixation error by clinicians during critical situations

Pregnant women with a potentially difficult airway should be identified as early as possible in pregnancy so that the anaesthetist can formulate an airway management and anaesthetic plan. Many obstetric units have antenatal anaesthetic clinics and each unit should have a checklist to assist midwives and obstetricians to identify women who should be referred to the anaesthetic clinic. Good communication and documentation are extremely important to ensure details of any airway management plan are available to the team involved in the final care of the patient.

Causes of Difficult Airway in the Obstetric Patient

These can be classified into anatomical and physiological changes of pregnancy, training issues and situation/human factors and are listed in Table 22.1.

General Anaesthesia

It has long been recognised that the obstetric rapid sequence induction (RSI) is outdated and that it needed to reflect current practice in the non-pregnant population. The OAA/DAS obstetric difficult airway guidelines provide an algorithm to support a modern safe approach to general anaesthesia in the obstetric patient (Figure 22.1).

There is emphasis on the planning and preparation, which include airway assessment, fasting and antacid prophylaxis and, where appropriate, intrauterine fetal resuscitation. When planning with the team, in addition to the routine WHO checklist which is now advocated prior to all surgical procedures, the obstetric team briefing should include team discussion and decision as to whether to wake the mother or proceed with anaesthesia in the event of failed intubation. This decision is influenced by several factors which relate to the woman, fetus, anaesthetist's experience and clinical situation. The majority of these factors are present prior to induction of general anaesthesia and are outlined in the OAA/DAS obstetric difficult airway guidelines (Figure 22.2).

Unfortunately, although the information in Figure 22.2 is useful in this very difficult decision-making process, it has some limitations. First, the lack of weighting of each factor means the team has no objective guidance on which of these factors are more important, and should therefore be prioritised. However, it is important to recognise that the mother's well-being has primacy in this decision-making process. The second limitation is that the final decision to wake or proceed will invariably be made during a very stressful time. As a result, human factors and situation awareness will play a significant role in the anaesthetist's final decision.

The use of thiopental for induction during RSI is declining whilst that of propofol is increasing. The 5th National Audit Project of the RCoA (NAP5) found a higher incidence of awareness in obstetric GA, during RSI and with the use of thiopental. In addition to reducing awareness the use of propofol for obstetric RSI has several advantages such as familiarity, availability, reduced drug errors and better suppression of

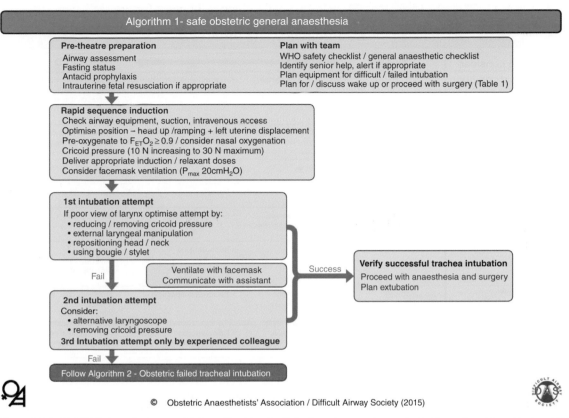

Figure 22.1 OAA/DAS obstetric airway guidelines. Algorithm 1 – Safe obstetric general anaesthesia. (Reproduced from Mushambi MC, Kinsella SM, Popat M, Swales H, Ramaswamy KK, Winton AL, Quinn AC. Obstetric Anaesthetists' Association and Difficult Airway Society guidelines for the management of difficult and failed tracheal intubation in obstetrics. *Anaesthesia* 2015; 70: 1286–1306, with permission from Obstetric Anaesthetists' Association/Difficult Airway Society.)

airway reflexes when compared with thiopental. In contrast, suxamethonium is still commonly used despite the advantages of using rocuronium with 'sugammadex backup'. This may be due to the cost of routine use of sugammadex. Recent recommendations include the use of mask ventilation prior to intubation (with maximum peak inspiratory airway pressure of 20 cmH$_2$0), the use of apnoeic oxygenation via nasal cannulae either as low flow (5–15 L min^{-1}) or as high flow humidified oxygen (up to 60 L min^{-1}), to prolong safe apnoea time. The routine use of head-up position and the early reduction or release of cricoid force should airway difficulty be encountered during the first laryngoscopy attempt are also recommended. NAP5 also found a higher incidence of awareness during difficult airway management at induction. It is therefore recommended that additional induction agent should always be available and be administered should a difficult airway be encountered. There is no consensus whether short-acting opiates should be used routinely in obstetrics or reserved for specific situations such as pre-eclampsia or patients with cardiac disease.

The choice of laryngoscope can influence success rate of tracheal intubation. There is now compelling evidence that, provided the anaesthetist is trained, videolaryngoscopes should be used as first line devices, as they provide better views of the larynx, have higher success rates of tracheal intubation and provide better teaching tool than direct laryngoscopes.

Table 1 - proceed with surgery?

Factors to consider		WAKE ⟷			PROCEED
Prior to induction	**Maternal condition**	• No compromise	• Mild acute compromise	• Haemorrhage responsive to resuscitation	• Hypovolaemia requiring corrrective surgery • Critical cardiac or respiratory compromise, cardiac arest
	Fetalcondition	• No compromise	• Compromise corrected with intrauterine resuscitation, pH < 7.2 but > 7.15	• Continuing fetal heart rate abnormally despite intrauterine resuscitation, pH < 7.15	• Sustained bradycaedia • Fetal haemorrhage • Suspected uterine rupture
	Anaesthetist	• Novice	• Junior trainee	• Senior trainee	• Consultant / specialsit
	Obesity	• Supermorbid	• Morbid	• Obese	• Normal
	Surgical factors	• Complex surgery or major haemorrhage anticipated	• Multiple uterine scars • Some surgical difficulties expected	• Single uterine scar	• No risk factors
	Aspiration risk	• Recent food	• No recent food • In labour • Opioids given • Antacids not given	• No recent food • In labour • Opioids not given • Antacids given	• Fasted • Not in labour • Antacids given
	Alternative anaesthesia regional securing airway awake	• No anticipated difficultly	• Predicted difficlutly	• Relatively contrainicated	• Absolutely contraindicated or has failed • Surgery started
After failed intubation	**Airway device / ventilation**	• Difficult facemask ventilation • Front-of-neck	• Adequate facemask ventilation	• First generation supraglottic airway device	• Seconf generation supraglottic airway device
	Airway hazards	• Laryngeal oedema • Stridor	• Bleeding • Trauma	• Secretions	• None evident

Obstetric Anaesthetists'Association / Difficult Airway Society (2015)
Criteria to be used in decision to wake or proceed following failed tracheal intubation. In any individual patient, some factors may suggest waking and others proceeding. The final decision will depend on the anaesthetist's clinical judgement.

Figure 22.2 OAA/DAS obstetric airway guidelines – Table 1 – proceed with surgery? Criteria to be used in the decision to wake or proceed following failed tracheal intubation. (Reproduced from Mushambi MC, Kinsella SM, Popat M, Swales H, Ramaswamy KK, Winton AL, Quinn AC. Obstetric Anaesthetists' Association and Difficult Airway Society guidelines for the management of difficult and failed tracheal intubation in obstetrics. *Anaesthesia* 2015; 70: 1286–1306, with permission from Obstetric Anaesthetists' Association/Difficult Airway Society.)

Unexpected Difficult and Failed Intubation

When tracheal intubation is unsuccessful after the first attempt, mask ventilation should be carried out whilst communicating with the team. The second intubation attempt should be by the most senior anaesthetist present, using a different laryngoscope and with the cricoid force removed. A maximum of two intubation attempts are recommended with a third attempt rarely indicated and reserved for a more senior anaesthetist. The physiological changes of pregnancy mean that airway swelling can develop very rapidly and can so convert a 'can oxygenate, cannot intubate' situation to a 'cannot intubate, cannot oxygenate' situation (CICO).

The OAA/DAS obstetric airway guidelines failed intubation algorithm is shown in Figure 22.3.

Once failed intubation has occurred, the priority is to ensure that the woman is well oxygenated using either a face mask or a second generation supraglottic airway device (SGA). If face mask ventilation was difficult before intubation attempts and if proceeding with surgery was the choice at pre-induction team decision, then immediate insertion of the SGA is the preferred rescue strategy. Once oxygenation is established, the final decision needs to be made whether to proceed with the anaesthetic or wake the patient. This will depend on the pre-induction decision (although some factors such as fetal and maternal condition and anaesthetist grade might have changed from the pre-induction state) and the airway

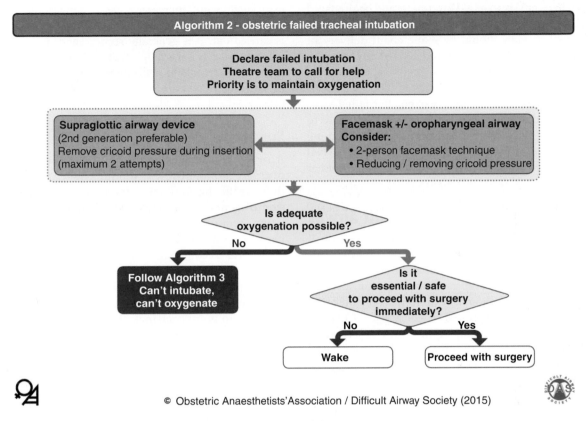

Figure 22.3 OAA/DAS obstetric airway guidelines – Algorithm 2 – obstetric failed tracheal intubation. (Reproduced from Mushambi MC, Kinsella SM, Popat M, Swales H, Ramaswamy KK, Winton AL, Quinn AC. Obstetric Anaesthetists' Association and Difficult Airway Society guidelines for the management of difficult and failed tracheal intubation in obstetrics. *Anaesthesia* 2015; 70: 1286–1306, with permission from Obstetric Anaesthetists' Association/Difficult Airway Society.)

device *in situ* and airway status. If the attempt to oxygenate the woman fails, then the CICO scenario is managed in a similar way to the non-pregnant patient as described in detail in Chapters 4 and 20. However, in a pregnant woman, if cardiac arrest occurs, as part of maternal resuscitation, a perimortem caesarean section should be carried out if the fundus is at the umbilicus or higher and this should be completed within 4 minutes of cardiac arrest.

Management after Failed Intubation

Previous guidelines on the management of failed intubation in obstetrics have focussed mainly on the management of the failed intubation, and

seldom discussed management of the woman after failed intubation once oxygenation has been established, particularly if the baby is still undelivered. Waking the mother up may not be an option. Therefore, continuing the anaesthetic needs to be conducted safely. Ventilation can be maintained either spontaneously or by controlled ventilation with or without additional muscle relaxant. Aspiration risk should be reduced by aspirating the gastric tube of the second generation SGA and minimising fundal pressure at delivery. If cricoid force is not impeding ventilation, it may be continued until the baby is delivered, accepting that applying consistent cricoid force for more than 4 minutes is not possible. The team should anticipate and plan in case a CICO scenario develops. If the decision is to wake the woman, the anaesthetist must reverse any muscle paralysis to avoid awareness and be prepared in case laryngeal spasm and a CICO scenario develop. A plan should be made about delivery of the baby if the baby is still undelivered after waking the woman up. This may entail regional anaesthesia or awake intubation (Chapter 9). However, a woman who has just been woken after failed intubation under general anaesthesia may be unable to cooperate fully for an awake procedure, making these more challenging. It is prudent to have two experienced anaesthetists for airway management at this stage.

Extubation following a Difficult Airway

Care must also be taken with extubation, especially if there is a risk of laryngeal oedema, perhaps exacerbated by either multiple intubation attempts or in patients with pre-eclampsia. In this situation, an extubation algorithm should be followed (Chapter 21). Delay in extubation should be considered if there is any concern with swelling of the airway. Observation and monitoring of the patient by appropriately trained recovery staff should continue postoperatively.

Management of the Known Difficult Airway Case

Women with a known difficult airway need careful multidisciplinary planning. In cases of severe airway difficulty, this may include the choice of an elective caesarean section, in order to avoid the woman presenting out of hours when appropriate staff and equipment may not be available. An elective caesarean section enables provision of optimum staff skill mix and necessary airway equipment. There has been debate whether a patient presenting for surgery with known airway difficulty should be managed with regional anaesthesia, thereby avoiding the need for intubation, or with awake intubation, thereby avoiding the possibility that control of the airway might be needed in an emergency and once surgery has started. Advocates of the former point out the apparent absurdity of meeting a difficult problem head-on when it can be simply avoided, whereas those of the latter highlight the small but serious risk of high regional block. Awake intubation itself is along standard lines, bearing in mind that the mother may be terrified and require careful sedation. Pregnancy is associated with increased nasal congestion and a significant risk of nasal bleeding if nasal intubation is carried out. It is generally recommended to avoid using cocaine as a nasal decongestant as it may interfere with placental blood flow and the systemic effects of vasoconstrictors are potentially hazardous in preeclampsia.

Summary

Airway management and failed intubation in the pregnant woman present unique challenges which differ from the non-pregnant patient. The provision of general anaesthesia in the obstetric population requires additional considerations which necessitate a rapid decision-making process that takes into account the safe outcome of mother and baby. It is important to use simulation to practise safe obstetric general anaesthesia, difficult and failed intubation: regularly and in a multidisciplinary setting. Before induction of general anaesthesia, the team briefing in obstetrics should consider whether to wake the patient or proceed with surgery in the event of failed intubation. Management after failed intubation should include strategies for either waking the woman or proceeding with surgery. All extubations in obstetrics should be considered as 'at-risk' extubation and the DAS extubation guidelines should be followed.

Further Reading

Cantwell R, Clutton-Brock T, Cooper G, et al. (2011). Saving mothers' lives: Reviewing maternal deaths to make motherhood safer: 2006–2008. The Eighth Report of the Confidential Enquiries into Maternal Deaths in the United Kingdom. *British Journal of Obstetrics and Gynaecology*, **118** (Suppl 1), 1–203.

Kinsella SM, Winton ALS, Mushambi MC, et al. (2015). Failed tracheal intubation during obstetric general anaesthesia: a literature review. *International Journal of Obstetric Anesthesia*, **24**, 356–374.

Mushambi MC, Kinsella SM, Popat M, et al. (2015). Obstetric Anaesthetists' Association and Difficult Airway Society guidelines for the management of difficult and failed tracheal intubation in obstetrics. *Anaesthesia*, **70**, 1286–1306.

Mushambi MC, Athanassoglou V, Kinsella SM. (2020). Anticipated difficult airway during obstetric general anaesthesia: narrative literature review and management recommendations. *Anaesthesia*, 75, 852–5.

Platt F, Lucas N, Bogod DG. (2014). Awareness in obstetrics. In: *Fifth National Audit Project of the Royal College of Anaesthetists and Association of Anaesthetists of Great Britian and Ireland: Accidental awareness during general anaesthesia in the UK and Ireland.* Editors Pandit JJ,

Cook TM. London: Royal College of Anaesthetists. pp. 133–143. ISBN 978-1-900936-11-8. Available at: https://www.nationalauditprojects.org.uk/NAP5report#pt.

Quinn AC, Milne D, Columb M, Gorton H, Knight M. (2013). Failed tracheal intubation in obstetric anaesthesia: 2 yr national case-control study in the UK. *British Journal of Anaesthesia*, 110, 74–80.

Chapter 23

The Paediatric Airway

Morten Bøttger and Narasimhan Jagannathan

Introduction

This chapter aims to provide the anaesthetist with practical skills to be more comfortable during paediatric airway management. Incorporating some of the techniques described in this chapter may help with airway management but it should be remembered that anaesthetising infants and children with severe co-morbidity is associated with numerous potential complications and requires management by experts.

Anatomical and Physiological Differences

The child displays a number of unique anatomical and physiological properties that diminish over time and develop towards adult anatomy and physiology. Neonates are aged less than 1 month and infants less than 1 year. A child may variously be defined as less than 16 years or less than 18 years but in terms of airway management at age 8 years the child can generally be managed using adult techniques.

The protruding occiput of the neonate causes the neck to flex in the supine position. Use of padding under the shoulders during airway management helps prevent upper airway obstruction, which is caused partly by the relatively large tongue, narrow nasal cavity and cephalad larynx.

Reduced functional residual capacity, higher closing capacity and a relatively high baseline oxygen consumption result in rapid desaturation. High quality pre-oxygenation of the infant prevents desaturation for about 30 seconds in the healthy child, hence gentle positive pressure ventilation may be needed during rapid sequence induction. Hypoxaemia is the most common complication occurring during paediatric airway management and pre-oxygenation is warranted for all infants and small children. When hypoxia occurs severe bradycardia and cardiovascular collapse may occur early.

During laryngoscopy, the relatively large tongue and the long, floppy, omega-shaped epiglottis can hamper gaining a direct view of the glottis. The cephalad, and flexible larynx may be mobilised, to improve the view and facilitate intubation. The angled nature of the glottic opening can make tracheal tube insertion more difficult especially in passing the anterior commissure.

During intubation, resistance may be noticed distal to the vocal cords, as the elliptical aperture of the cricoid cartilage is reached. This non-distensible structure is functionally the narrowest site of the paediatric airway and choice of tube size is designed around avoiding trauma and oedema here. Neonates have a short and collapsible trachea of about 5 cm in length and accidental endobronchial intubation is a significant risk.

Oedema of the larynx and trachea, due to traumatic intubation, can have dramatic consequences. A small amount of airway swelling may have a critical impact on the calibre of the infant airway: a 1 mm circumferential oedema can reduce cross-sectional area by 75% and increase airway resistance 16-fold.

Basics of Paediatric Airway Management

Airway Assessment

History

Information on prior anaesthetics and adverse reactions is relevant. Are there any obvious signs of airway compromise at home – any snoring, wheezing or sleep apnoea? History of recent upper airway infection and/or passive smoking should be obtained as it increases risk of laryngospasm during anaesthesia.

Airway Examination

As small children are uncooperative, formal airway tests are impractical (and not validated) and it is necessary to rely on history and clinical impression. What is the global appearance of the child? Does the child look normal or do they have syndromic features? Older children (> 3–4 years old) can cooperate with a more formal airway assessment.

Incidence of Difficult Airway

Craniofacial syndromes are the most common *reason* for difficult airways in the paediatric population. Micrognathia is the most common *physical finding* associated with difficult laryngoscopy in an infant.

In children, the difficult airway is less common than in adults and is particularly uncommon in healthy children. Some studies show an incidence of difficult mask ventilation in children of 0.2% compared with 1.4% in adults. Difficult laryngoscopy in children may be 2- to 20-fold less common than in adults but infants are more likely to have a difficult laryngoscopy with around 5% having a Cormack and Lehane Grade 3 or 4.

Preparing for Anaesthesia

The Challenge of Different Sizes: Drugs and Equipment

Selecting the correct equipment and drug doses, especially in the emergency setting, is one of the core challenges of paediatric anaesthesia. Relevant paediatric anaesthesia practice guidelines should be available at all times and these include those based on height or weight. Using smartphones or tablets, entering the weight (or estimated weight) in various apps prompts age/weight-specific vital signs, equipment and drug dose recommendations (e.g. Copenhagen Paediatric Emergency App).

Preparing for Emergencies: Laryngospasm

Reflex spasm of the intrinsic muscles of the larynx is a common complication in paediatric anaesthesia. The overall incidence is less than 1%, but is more frequent in young children and during ENT anaesthesia. Knowledge of risk factors is paramount. Hypersensitivity of the airway (e.g. caused by passive smoking, current or recent upper airway infection or asthma) increases risk up to 10-fold. An inexperienced airway manager is also an independent risk factor, probably due to likelihood of ill-timed airway management.

Pre-drawn syringes with suxamethonium (gold standard) and/or propofol should be prepared and placed at a predefined location known to all anaesthesia team members.

Initial management strategies include 100% oxygen, jaw thrust and mask continuous positive airway pressure (CPAP; 5–15 cmH$_2$O) followed by administration of propofol (1 mg kg^{-1}) and/or suxamethonium IV (0.1–0.5 mg kg^{-1}) or IM (4 mg kg^{-1}).

Keeping the Airway Open

Positioning

Correct positioning of the patient, aligning the axes of the mouth, hypopharynx and trachea, is key to improving the chances of successful mask ventilation and intubation. Positioning of the patient differs based on the age:

- Infant and child less than 2 years old: padding under shoulder to compensate for a large occiput
- Young child (2–8 years old): lying flat on their back
- Older child (> 8 years old): some level of head support to achieve 'sniffing' position

Practical Face Mask Ventilation

Select a mask of the correct size – the mask should enclose the nose and mouth but not cover the eyes (Figure 23.1). Using a uniform *three-step technique* enhances chances of successful face mask ventilation.

1. *Open the patient's mouth.* This usually clears the tongue from resting on the palate – a classic cause of airway obstruction in small children.
2. *Place the mask.* Maintaining mouth opening, the mask is placed, base first, on the jaw then the mask apex is rested on the bridge of the nose.
3. *Apply jaw thrust.* Jaw thrust effectively moves the base of the tongue away from the posterior wall of the oropharynx.

Consider omitting chin lift as this may lead to pressure applied at the submental region causing partial or complete airway obstruction.

Other practical tips:

- Supporting the weight of the anaesthesia circuit prevents traction on the face mask.
- Occasionally a two-person technique is needed when maintaining a tight mask seal and jaw thrust. The assistant (or the ventilator) does the 'bagging'.
- Placing the child in the lateral position during mask ventilation can be helpful, especially in children with micrognathia.
- Upper airway obstruction (e.g. hypertrophic tonsils) can usually be relieved by applying CPAP

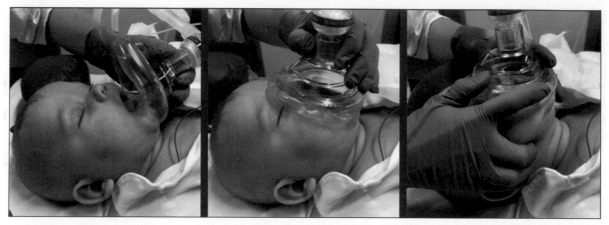

Figure 23.1 Appropriate technique for securing an open airway with a face mask.

of 5–15 cmH$_2$O. Splinting the airway in this way pushes soft tissue aside, and is a valuable and atraumatic strategy that should be used before insertion of airway adjuncts.

The Oropharyngeal Airway

The oropharyngeal airway is helpful in obtaining 'tongue control' in patients with no gag reflexes.

Sizing: the base of the oropharyngeal airway is positioned at the angle of the mouth; the tip should almost reach the angle of the jaw. If the oropharyngeal airway is too small, it will fail to 'cup' the base of the tongue and relieve the upper airway obstruction. If too large, it may cause hypopharyngeal trauma and/or laryngospasm.

Insertion: the standard technique is to use a tongue depressor, followed by 'tip down' atraumatic introduction. Alternatively, it can be inserted 'tip up' and rotated 180° on reaching the soft palate, before advancing into its final position.

The Nasopharyngeal Airway

The nasopharyngeal airway is a powerful tool in paediatric airway management during induction as well as recovery and readily overcomes supraglottic obstruction when correctly placed.

Commercial nasopharyngeal airways exist but soft uncuffed tracheal tubes (e.g. Portex Ivory) can be also be used for this purpose (see Figure 23.2).

Sizing: nasopharyngeal airway size should match the child's tracheal tube size estimate. Insertion depth is estimated by the distance from the nares to the ipsilateral tragus of the ear.

Insertion: the lubricated nasopharyngeal airway can be inserted for immediate relief of upper airway

obstruction, as it is much better tolerated by a child than the oropharyngeal airway. As target depth is approached, listening for breath sounds is advised. Gentle manipulation helps determine optimum positioning. Care must be taken to ensure a nasopharyngeal airway without a flange does not migrate inwards and get lost!

Laryngoscopy and Intubation

Basic Laryngoscopy

A selection of laryngoscope blades and handles exist, and for the healthy child most are effective. Introduction of the blade should be gentle and under direct vision at all times. Passing the base of the tongue, the rate of blade advancement should be reduced and finalised in small increments until optimum position is reached. Never use the laryngoscope as a fulcrum as gum and/or teeth damage can result.

One-person technique: hold the laryngoscope close to the hinge; this provides great control and makes your fifth finger available for external laryngeal manipulation in neonates, leaving the right hand available for tube insertion.

Two-person technique: sitting down, resting elbows on the operating table, the left hand supports the laryngoscope and the right hand can be used to manipulate the larynx. As direct vision of the glottis is established, the anaesthetist shifts the torso to one side, elbows still in place. An assistant confirms view of the cords and intubates the trachea.

Curved (Macintosh) blade laryngoscopy: this curved blade can be used in all age groups. The tip is placed in the vallecula and gentle ventral force is

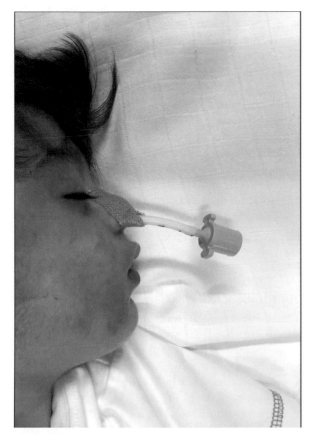

Figure 23.2 A shortened uncuffed tracheal tube (Portex Ivory) used as a nasopharyngeal airway in a child after removal of adenoid vegetations.

applied, to mobilise the epiglottis, facilitating direct vision of the cords and intubation. This technique can be challenging in neonatal airway management due to the high position of the larynx, and the long and floppy nature of the epiglottis. Failure to mobilise the epiglottis may necessitate gentle direct lifting of the epiglottis, if a straight Miller blade is not available.

Straight (Miller) blade laryngoscopy: the straight Miller blade is designed for airway management of the neonate and small child. The blade is advanced carefully over the body of the tongue, or in the right gutter of the mouth, aiming for the midline and the epiglottis. As the epiglottis is reached and lifted the glottis is exposed. The tracheal tube is either introduced 'free hand' or slid down the concave groove of the Miller blade and 'railroaded' into position.

The Tracheal Tube

These are classified according to internal diameter (ID) measured in millimetres. The smallest uncuffed tracheal tube measures 2.0 mm ID and the smallest cuffed equivalent is 3.0 mm ID, with both types increasing in size by 0.5 mm increments.

Importantly the outer diameter (OD) reflects the amount of space taken up by the tracheal tube once placed in the airway. The relation of ID and OD varies greatly depending on tracheal tube type. The OD of the uncuffed tracheal tube is only modestly greater than the ID whereas the cuffed tracheal tube has a thicker wall (housing the cuff inflation canal) and larger OD. A flexible tracheal tube has a wire-reinforced wall and correspondingly large OD.

In patients with airway pathology, it is advisable to specifically consider OD as part of the tube selection process.

The uncuffed tracheal tube: the uncuffed tracheal tube has traditionally been chosen in children younger than 8 years. High reintubation rates (as high as 30%) and risk of endothelial damage due to the snug fitting of the circular tracheal tube in the elliptical cricoid aperture are real drawbacks.

The cuffed tracheal tube: the cuffed tracheal tube has gained popularity in recent years for many reasons. Modern paediatric cuffed tubes have very soft high-volume low-pressure cuffs. It can be used in neonatal airway management, with minimal risk of post-extubation stridor, providing cuff pressure is kept low (preferably < 15 cmH$_2$O, never above 30 cmH$_2$O). The cuff provides a good seal protecting against aspiration, and enabling controlled ventilation in the presence of poor lung compliance or high airway resistance. A smaller tracheal tube (usually by 0.5–1.0 mm) than usual can be selected (see below).

Sizing

Diameter: a conservative approach to tube selection size should be taken to minimise the risk of airway trauma. Following these recommendations only 1% of patients need reintubation/change of initial tube.

Uncuffed tracheal tube size (ID in mm)

Preterm 1000 g:	2.5
Preterm 1000–2500 g:	3.0
Neonate to 6 months:	3.0–3.5
6 months to 1 year:	3.5–4.0
Children 1 to 2 years:	4.0–5.0
Children 2 to 8 years:	Age (year)/4 + 4

Cuffed tracheal tube size (ID in mm)

Term infants < 1 year:	3.0
Children 1 to 2 years:	3.5
Children 2 to 8 years:	Age (year)/4 + **3**

For preparation, it is advised to pick three tracheal tubes: one of the estimated size and one each of one size smaller and larger.

Insertion depth: the aim should be to stop advancing the tracheal tube as the cricoid is passed. Some tracheal tubes have insertion depth markers to aid insertion. In any case an insertion depth estimate is practical. Consider using the following equations:

Intubation insertion depth estimate (all ages)

Oral Or (> 2 years):	uncuffed tracheal tube ID (mm) × 3
Oral:	age (year)/2 + 12
Nasal:	age (year)/2 + 15

Some preformed oral tracheal tubes such as the Ring–Adair–Elwyn tube have a bend-to-tip distance that may be critical. These may be used during tonsillectomy and there is a danger, particularly if a larger tube is used, that compression by the Boyle–Davis mouth gag (see Chapter 26) could advance the tube causing endobronchial intubation.

Fixation

Although many techniques exist, none is emphasised here. The key point is that securing the tracheal tube (to prevent displacement *and* advancement into the main bronchus) is vital, especially in difficult airway management. In any episode of perioperative desaturation, accidental tracheal tube displacement and endobronchial intubation should be considered.

The 'DOPES' Mnemonic

Due to the unique anatomy and physiology, the child is at particular risk of perioperative complications. *DOPES* is a mnemonic, aiding systematic assessment of perioperative desaturation and/or high airway pressure in the intubated child.

Displacement: tracheal tube displacement is critical and must be identified without delay. Extubation results in loss of capnography trace. Endobronchial intubation causes reduced tidal volume in pressure-controlled ventilation or elevated airway pressure during volume-controlled ventilation.

Obstruction: secretions must be cleared. The Boyle–Davis mouth gag may cause compression or obstruction by kinking. Kinking also may occur under a hot air warming device as the soft plastic of the tracheal tube warms and softens.

Pneumothorax: may complicate neonatal resuscitation and is infrequently seen in paediatric trauma. Early diagnosis (ultrasound assessment looking for lung sliding may be beneficial) and decompression is required as soon as possible.

Equipment: if anaesthesia apparatus failure is suspected, ventilation with auxiliary equipment must follow for immediate relief and safe problem solving.

Stomach: difficult bagging can cause massive accumulation of air in the stomach. Routine gastric decompression is advised. If forgotten difficult ventilation may ensue. Decompress immediately.

Supraglottic Airway Devices (SGAs)

The classic laryngeal mask airway, cLMA, was introduced for paediatric use in the late 1980s, as a downscaled version of the adult cLMAs. Second generation SGAs (i-gel, ProSeal LMA, LMA Supreme, Ambu AuraGain) are available with a wide array of specifications (Table 23.1). Use of an SGA as a conduit for intubation is more common in children than in adults. When using an SGA with an air-filled cuff a manometer should always be used to measure cuff pressure (never exceed 60 cmH$_2$O). The appropriate size for a given age or weight is not standardised across different SGAs so it is important to consult manufacturer's instructions for use when selecting a paediatric SGA. In the presence of airway leak during controlled ventilation with an SGA it is useful to consider 'up-sizing' the device.

Insertion and Removal

SGAs can be placed in lighter planes of anaesthesia than a tracheal tube, including during spontaneous breathing, but insertion during too light anaesthesia risks complications. Insertion should always be atraumatic to avoid laryngospasm and/or airway trauma.

The cLMA is inserted with a fully deflated cuff and the aperture pointing caudad. Reaching the posterior wall of the oropharynx resistance is often felt. Applying gentle caudad pressure to the tip of the LMA, easy advancement is usually possible. Other techniques include inserting the cLMA semi-rotated or inverted until the soft palate is reached, at which

Table 23.1 Supraglottic airways for use in the paediatric population

Supraglottic airway device	Advantages	Disadvantages
Classic LMA/LMA Unique	• Long history of safety and efficacy • Large evidence base	• In infants (< 10 kg): delayed airway obstruction may occur • Have to modify when using for FOB intubation • No drain tube
air-Q	• Designed for tracheal intubation • Large evidence base for difficult airway management • Can accommodate cuffed tracheal tube • Stable in small children	• No drain tube
ProSeal LMA	• Long history of safety and efficacy • Large evidence base • Higher leak pressure than cLMA • Stable in small children • Drain tube	• No single-use version • Less suitable for FOB intubation (narrow airway tube)
Supreme LMA	• Single use • Higher leak pressure than cLMA • Drain tube	• Not suitable for FOB intubation (narrow airway tube)
i-gel	• Higher leak pressures than cLMA • Favourable FOB views • Drain tube	• Unstable in small children • Laryngeal bulging observed in small children • Small sizes (#1, #1.5) cannot accommodate cuffed tracheal tube
Ambu AuraGain	• Short shaft, anatomical shape • Favourable FOB views • Accommodates cuffed tracheal tube • Stable in small children • Gastric drain tube	• Bulky bite block

FOB, flexible optical bronchoscope.

point the device is rotated 'around the corner' and into its final position with its tip lying at the top of the oesophagus (see Chapter 13).

Controversy exists whether SGAs should be removed in a deep plane of anaesthesia or once the child is awake. The former decreases the risk of airway reactivity (i.e. coughing and laryngospasm) but may risk airway obstruction if the child is not appropriately managed during recovery. Certainly, removing the SGA in a light plane of anaesthesia (e.g. swallowing or just moving) but before the child is awake should be avoided as this has the disadvantages for both techniques and the advantages of neither.

Role of the SGA

Primary airway: SGAs are ideal for short-term anaesthesia, particularly in combination with peripheral nerve blocks or for non-surgical anaesthesia, during which spontaneous breathing can be maintained. The atraumatic properties of SGAs are particularly attractive when anaesthetising children with subglottic inflammation, e.g. croup.

Some SGAs are prone to rotate and this risks displacement: care must be taken to secure the SGA after placement. Positive pressure ventilation may be feasible but gastric insufflation can occur, particularly with first generation SGAs, potentially causing impaired breathing and hypoxia.

Rescue/emergency airway: the SGA has an important role in management of the difficult paediatric airway. They have the potential to push away soft tissue causing upper airway obstruction, thereby aiding ventilation. The SGA can be placed at light planes of anaesthesia and may be removed awake, adding to the usefulness of the device.

Conduit of intubation: aiming for a secure airway, the properly inserted SGA can be used as a conduit for flexible optical bronchoscope (FOB)-guided intubation. Some SGAs (e.g. air-Q, Ambu AuraGain) have wider diameters and shorter shafts and are designed to be conduits for tracheal intubation with FOBs.

Extubation

Lateral Positioning

Extubation with the patient lying on their side has certain benefits: secretions from the hypopharynx are cleared passively and base of tongue airway obstruction is prevented.

If mask CPAP is necessary this is easily done applying the three-step approach described above. One hand keeps the mask in place: as shown in Figure 23.3, the palm of the hand rests on the child's temple while the thumb applies jaw thrust and fingers two and three are positioned in a V-grip to apply uniform pressure to the centre of the mask to ensure a good seal.

Deep Extubation

Extubation during a deep plane of anaesthesia is preferred in children by many anaesthetists. Benefits include reduced patient agitation and ease of overall management. A nasopharyngeal airway may be a useful adjunct to deep extubation and lateral positioning, but the risk of airway obstruction clearly exists until recovery from anaesthesia. It is therefore an absolute prerequisite that the recovery room is nearby with appropriate resources and trained staffing for full paediatric airway monitoring and intervention.

With experience, combining lateral positioning and use of the nasopharyngeal airway may be beneficial to the anaesthetist managing extubation of patients with difficult airways, including upper airway secretions.

CPAP during Extubation

Administration of CPAP (20–30 cmH$_2$O) immediately before extubation causes a jet of air to escape the tracheal tree during removal of the tracheal tube. This will clear secretions from the glottis and may prevent laryngospasm.

Advanced Airway Management

Airway Assessment

A known difficult airway history is key in planning airway management. Review of the patient's medical record is mandatory and airway examining by colleagues in otorhinolaryngology may be a valuable addition.

The genesis of airway difficulty is heterogenic: congenital, infectious, inflammatory, metabolic, traumatic and iatrogenic. Detailed knowledge of the challenge at hand is crucial. Some syndromes and diseases worsen over time in contrast to the assumption that children outgrow their airway problems. Importantly the suspected location of any airway pathology, be it supraglottic, glottic and/or subglottic, has an impact on the airway management plan. Table 23.2 lists some of the challenging conditions linked to functional classification and location of pathology.

Independent risk factors associated with complications *during* management of the paediatric difficult airway include:

- Short thyromental distance (micrognathia)
- Weight less than 10 kg
- More than two tracheal intubation attempts
- Three direct laryngoscopy attempts before an indirect technique

Keeping the Airway Open

In many cases the ability to mask ventilate is uncertain and the airway must be secured during spontaneous ventilation. In younger children, or children with cognitive impairment the following approach is widely applied.

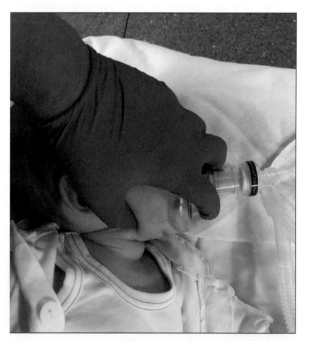

Figure 23.3 Lateral recumbent position mask CPAP in a 1.5-year-old child immediately after extubation.

Table 23.2 Suspected location of airway pathology in various conditions

Classification	Condition
Supraglottic pathology	**Maxillary hypoplasia**
	Apert syndrome
	Crouzon syndrome
	Pfeiffer syndrome
	Choanal atresia
	CHARGE association
	Mandibular hypoplasia (micrognathia)
	Pierre Robin sequence
	Treacher Collins syndrome
	Goldenhar syndrome
	Stickler syndrome
	Moebius syndrome
	Macroglossia
	Beckwith–Wiedemann syndrome
	Trisomi 21 (Down syndrome)
	Vascular malformation
	Metabolic disease
	Laryngomalacia
	Infection
	Peritonsillar/parapharyngeal/retropharyngeal
	Epiglottitis
	Masses of neck/parapharynx
Glottic pathology	**Glottic stenosis**
	Iatrogenic (intubation sequelae)
	Congenital
	Infection (e.g. papilloma)
	Neuromuscular (e.g. recurrent laryngeal nerve paresis)
Subglottic pathology	**Subglottic stenosis**
	Iatrogenic (intubation sequelae)
	Tracheal inflammation (e.g. tracheitis)
	Tracheal stenosis
	Tracheomalacia
Whole airway pathology	**Mucopolysaccharidoses**
	Hurler syndrome
	Hunter syndrome
	Sanfilippo syndrome
	Morquio syndrome
	Maroteaux–Lamy syndrome

Table 23.2 (cont.)

Classification	Condition
	Vascular lesions
	Lymphatic malformation
	Haemangioma
	Inflammation
	Trauma
	Foreign bodies
	Burns
Reduced mobility	Freeman–Sheldon syndrome
Mouth	Noonan syndrome
Jaw	Spinal fusion
Neck	Cervical stenosis
	Cervical instability
	Perioperative instrumentation – reduced post-op mobility

Induction: Spontaneous Ventilation

Mask (gaseous) induction with sevoflurane is a predictable and safe strategy. Bradypnoea may occur but has a predictably slow onset.

If venous access is established, a propofol induction and/or maintenance regimen may be used. Most children under 5 years maintain spontaneous ventilation after a propofol bolus of 2–3 mg kg^{-1} and a propofol infusion at 10 mg kg^{-1} h^{-1} maintains spontaneous ventilation. Low-dose remifentanil infusion or fentanyl boluses of 1 µg kg^{-1} may be needed especially in patients arriving from critical care areas sedated in the operating theatre.

Induction: Supraglottic Airway

Oxygen supply is provided via a nasopharyngeal airway (using a tracheal tube), SGA or bronchoscopy mask. The anaesthetic circuit is connected to the airway device as attention is directed at adjustable pressure limiting (APL) valve/pop-off valve setting. If a nasopharyngeal airway is used patency is dependent on correct depth of insertion and preventing it from kinking. Where there is considerable airway leak, the capnography may be flat due to the 'open' nature of the airway: look, listen and feel at all times!

Induction: Local Anaesthesia

Topicalisation of the larynx with 4% lidocaine reduces risk of laryngospasm and coughing during intubation. Gentle introduction of a videolaryngoscope enables an optimal view of the larynx with minimal tissue compression and autonomic response while also facilitating confirming the optimum position of the nasopharyngeal airway, early assessment of airway anatomy and spraying the glottis using an atomiser (e.g. MADgic, Teleflex) or bend-into-shape metal suction tip. Local anaesthesia can also be applied via the working channel of a flexible optical bronchoscope 'spray-as-you-go' style.

With the child anaesthetised and ventilating spontaneously and the airway topicalised there are several options for intubation, as follows.

Videolaryngoscopy and Other 'Indirect Laryngoscopes'

A large number of 'indirect laryngoscopes' exist based on video chip or light deflection technology (Table 23.3) (also see Chapter 17). Glottic view is generally improved though introducing the tracheal tube into the trachea can be a challenge, especially during training. Curved blade designs seem to be of particular benefit in management of severe micrognathia.

Straight and Macintosh bladed videolaryngoscopes can be used for direct laryngoscopy and videolaryngoscopy if there is a separate screen. A shared view of the airway is useful for difficult airway management and also during basic airway management training.

A *four-step approach* has been proposed using a non-channelled laryngoscope, minimising risk of airway trauma, as the technique emphasises the importance of visual guidance at all times.

The Four Steps of Indirect Laryngoscopy

Step 1: The laryngoscope is introduced in the midline of the mouth. Under direct vision, the tip of the scope is advanced to the base of the tongue.

Step 2: Under guidance of the monitor or eyepiece, the laryngoscope is advanced to its final position overlooking the glottis.

Step 3: The tracheal tube, with a malleable stylet inside, is advanced gently and under direct vision until the tip disappears behind the base of the tongue.

Step 4: Under guidance of the monitor/eyepiece, the tracheal tube is introduced into the trachea.

Table 23.3 Videolaryngoscopes and other 'indirect laryngoscopes' for use in the paediatric population

Indirect vision laryngoscopes	Features
C-MAC C-MAC Pocket Monitor	Videolaryngoscope Reusable blades • Miller 0 and 1, Mac 0, 2 and 3 • D blade paediatric – curved (child) Image and video capture (high definition) Price ++++
GlideScope AVL	Videolaryngoscope Single-use blades – curved • Size 0 (infant), 1, 2 and 2.5 (child) Image and video capture Price +++
McGrath MAC	Videolaryngoscope Single-use blades • Mac 1, 2, 3 • X2 (curved – limited availability) No image/video capture Price ++
King Vision	Videolaryngoscope Single-use blades – curved (channelled optional) • Size 1: infant • Size 2: child • Size 3: larger child Video out port (capture not included) Price: ++
Truview PCD	Optical laryngoscope Reusable blades – curved • Size O (neonate), 2, 3 and 4 (child) Continuous oxygen supply functionality Optional video capture capability (add-on) Price ++
Airtraq	Optical laryngoscope – channelled device Single-use design – curved Size 0: infant (tracheal tube 2.5–3.5) Size 1: child (tracheal tube 4.0–5.5) Optional video capture capability (add-on) Price +

If there is difficulty with step 4 a number of solutions exist:

'Hockey stick': the tracheal tube is shaped into an ice hockey stick shape. As the tip of the tracheal tube is

(a)   (b)

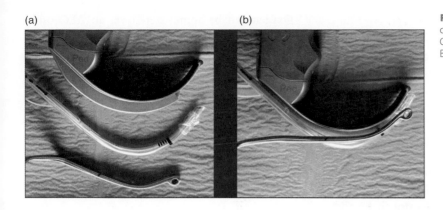

Figure 23.4 (a) Correct pre-use shaping of the tracheal tube when using a Storz C-MAC D-blade laryngoscope. (b) Boedeker forceps (Both Storz GmBh).

aligned with the glottis, it is slid over the stylet and into the trachea.

'Blade curve': the tracheal tube is shaped in a curve similar to the laryngoscope blade used (see Figure 23.4). The tip of the tracheal tube is placed directly into the glottic opening. As the stylet is retracted the tracheal tube is introduced into the trachea. If the tracheal tube is stuck at the glottic level, rotation 180–360° usually helps. If not, consider downsizing the tracheal tube.

Nasal intubation can also be managed during indirect laryngoscopy. Tube tip control in the hypopharynx is achieved using curved forceps, such as the Magills or Storz Boedeker curved forceps (Figure 23.4).

Flexible Optical Bronchoscope (FOB)-Guided Intubation

FOB-guided intubation remains the gold standard in management of the difficult airway.

Direct FOB-Guided Intubation

Modern video chip scopes offer superior image quality, mobility and slim design accommodating intubation with a 3.0 mm ID tracheal tube. FOBs can be even smaller and accommodate intubation with a 2.5 mm ID tracheal tube, but they lack the image quality of video chip devices.

The FOB, pre-fitted with the tracheal tube of choice, is introduced carefully and in small increments into the airway and advanced to the level of the carina. The tracheal tube is advanced over the scope. Resistance may be felt as the tracheal tube reaches the narrow parts of the airway: rotating the tracheal tube usually helps. The 'carina to tracheal tube tip distance' can be measured by advancing the FOB to the carina and then measuring how far it is withdrawn before the lumen of the tracheal tube is seen.

Indirect FOB-Guided Intubation

This technique enables FOB-guided intubation in small children using larger adult FOBs with a working channel, a guidewire and an 8 Fr airway exchange catheter (AEC). The scope is manoeuvred into position with its tip proximal to the glottis. A suitable soft tip guidewire is introduced carefully into the trachea via the working channel of the scope. As the scope is withdrawn, the guidewire is left in place. Next, the AEC is slid over the guidewire and then a tracheal tube is railroaded over the AEC. Finally, the AEC and guidewire are removed together and successful tracheal intubation is confirmed with capnography.

Route of FOB-Guided Intubation

Nasal intubation is the preferred route in cases of limited mouth opening. Other advantages include a straightforward path to the larynx and ease of tube fixation. *Oral intubation* is technically more difficult, but offers a shorter path to the larynx. Using an SGA as a conduit, passage is cleared to the larynx. This latter technique is very effective in overcoming upper airway obstruction and excessive soft tissues as are seen for example in patients with mucopolysaccharidoses.

Tube Delivery Aids

In selected cases probing the airway with a flexible stylet or bougie may be helpful. The 5 Fr Portex Tracheal Tube Guide fits through any tracheal tube of 2.0 mm ID or larger and is a valuable aid in stenotic and infant airway management.

Rigid Straight Laryngoscopy and Bronchoscopy

These tools may also be useful, ideally operated by an ENT surgeon, during difficult paediatric intubation.

Novel Techniques

Normal Tidal Volume Ventilation via a Small Lumen Tube

In extreme cases, airway access may be a small lumen AEC, or similar device, only. Conventional positive pressure ventilation will be futile due to delayed expiration. The Ventrain is a novel device that can enable oxygenation and ventilation via a very narrow airway device. Its mechanism of action is described in Chapter 18. As airway pressure can only be measured intermittently, using a three-way stopcock and a manometer, during Ventrain use, close observation of chest movement is strongly advised, to avoid barotrauma and circulatory instability.

Nasal High Flow Oxygen during Apnoea

This technique delivers weight-specific high flow humidified oxygen via nasal prongs and can be used before induction (during spontaneous ventilation) and after (during apnoea). The safe apnoea time is significantly extended, which may be beneficial during early airway management and during post-extubation stabilisation. In contrast to adults, high flow nasal oxygenation during apnoea offers relatively poor carbon dioxide elimination, which limits its safe duration of use.

Difficult Extubation

Airway management at extubation requires the same degree of attention as at induction. Initial and backup strategies should be clear to all team members, and certainly the route for reintubation should be highlighted.

Evaluation of potential supraglottic, glottic and subglottic challenges should be made. Airway oedema is a classic cause of problems in small airways and early steroid therapy should be considered.

Surgery can dramatically alter airway access (e.g. halo, maxillofacial surgery) having a great impact on the available reintubation plan. This should be identified beforehand.

Challenging cases can be managed by introducing an AEC into the tracheal tube before extubation. As the tracheal tube is removed the AEC is left in place as a conduit for reintubation. To avoid coughing the trachea can be primed with instillation of lidocaine (maximum 4 mg kg^{-1}).

Oxygen can be administered via an AEC using a catheter adaptor, but there is an important danger of barotrauma, especially if the AEC advances beyond the carina and particular caution should be taken (see Chapter 15).

A small size (8 Fr) AEC fits into a 3.0 mm ID tracheal tube. An alternative to the AEC, which itself may cause partial airway obstruction and stridor, is to exchange the AEC for a guidewire. While a 'staged extubation' kit comprising this equipment exists for adult practice, no such pre-prepared kit exists for paediatric airway management.

Emergencies

Paediatric Emergency Front of Neck Airway (eFONA)

eFONA is an extreme challenge in paediatric anaesthesia, though the need is fortunately rare. As the child grows, the challenge diminishes as adolescence is reached, approximating the challenge of the adult emergency airway. In adult anaesthesia, multiple techniques and equipment packs are available – this is not the case in paediatric anaesthesia. The rare and extreme nature of eFONA calls for training and simulation no matter the strategy chosen – whether needle or surgical approach.

The Small Child (< 8 Years)

Classic surgical cricothyroidotomy is virtually impossible due to the narrow cricothyroid membrane, measuring only a few millimetres in the neonate. Access is further hindered by the overlying hyoid bone.

Needle and cannula techniques

The difficulty of surgical cricothyroidotomy gives rise to the recommendation by some authors to perform eFONA with a needle at the cricothyroid or tracheal level. A few commercially available kits exist but efficacy is unproven. Introduction of the needle into the soft, collapsible and narrow infant airway is a major challenge. There is a significant risk of passing the needle 'through-and-through' (i.e. into and beyond the trachea) or into a paratracheal position.

Successful introduction of a small lumen catheter into the airway provides the opportunity to oxygenate by insufflation of high flow oxygen. Lack of a secure airway, risk of barotrauma and the inability to ventilate are major drawbacks to this approach, with risks even higher than in adult practice (see Chapter 20).

Surgical Techniques

Challenges of a surgical approach include lack of competency with a scalpel, risk of vascular damage etc. There is growing focus on eFONA techniques caudal to the cricoid as these bypass the narrowest part of the paediatric airway – the cricoid cartilage.

Minimising scalpel use and relying on palpation rather than direct vision, colleagues at Copenhagen University Hospital Rigshospitalet propose the *rapid five-step technique*. It may be better than needle techniques but supporting evidence is only from animal cadaver studies.

Rapid Five-Step Technique (Figure 23.5)

The equipment needed is readily available at most operation theatres: scalpel, towel forceps (three pairs), pair of scissors with a sharp tip and an adequately sized cuffed tracheal tube.

Step 1: Palpate the trachea and larynx and make a longitudinal skin incision upwards from the jugular notch up to the proximal larynx.

Step 2: Grasp the lateral edges of the wound with a towel forceps on either side and pull gently to the sides, then palpate the laryngeal structures to identifying the proximal trachea.

Step 3: Grasp the proximal trachea with the third towel forceps and pull gently anteriorly and cranially.

Step 4: Maintaining traction, penetrate the trachea with the pointy tip of the scissors and cut two to three tracheal rings.

Step 5: Still maintaining traction, pass a cuffed tracheal tube through the slit-type opening in the trachea. Stop advancing as the cuff enters the trachea. Inflate the cuff. Ventilate looking for chest movement and, if available, capnography.

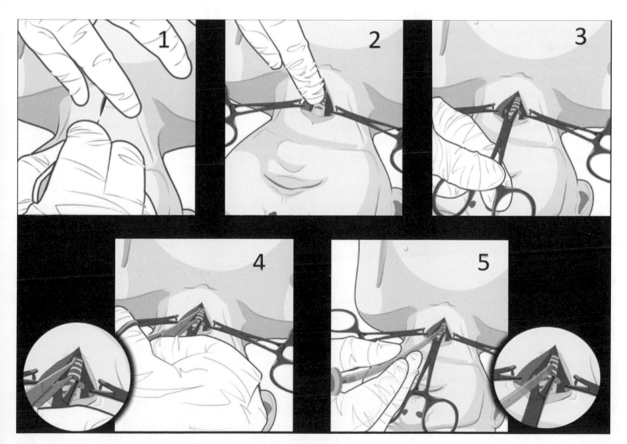

Figure 23.5 The rapid-5-step technique for paediatric emergency front of neck airway (eFONA).

Any eFONA technique requires training and must be practised on a regular basis on airway models. '*We train as we fight and fight as we train.*'

The Older Child (> 8 Years)

The older child exhibits anatomy and physiology similar to the adult patient and an adult approach is advised. The cricothyroid membrane is generally palpable and problems due to gross obesity are less frequent than in adults.

Airway Obstruction from a Foreign Body

Airway obstruction due to inhalation of a foreign body is the leading accidental cause of death in infants. Management of these cases is highly challenging and successful management is a team effort and may require collaboration between ENT and thoracic surgery as well as paediatric anaesthesia.

A strategy is ideally agreed before such emergencies present, but certainly should be rapidly communicated and agreed when the relevant staff assemble. The strategy may involve sedation and spontaneous ventilation or general anaesthesia and controlled ventilation and either may accommodate flexible or rigid bronchoscopy. There is no proven 'best technique' but a logical approach is presented here.

It is essential to determine the 'what, when and where' of foreign body obstruction. A fast and focussed pre-anaesthesia assessment is undertaken. Venous access must be secured immediately. A calm and structured approach is required as the child, parents and team members are likely to be stressed.

Particular difficulty may arise when a foreign body has been present for some time and organic matter has become friable, making removal very difficult, or when secondary pneumonia or secondary hyperexpansion distal to the foreign body has developed.

Partial Airway Obstruction

It is vital that spontaneous ventilation is maintained.

Adequate sedation/anaesthesia must be achieved before probing the airway as this could cause coughing or laryngospasm and prevent maintenance of spontaneous ventilation.

Initial 'priming of the airway' with nebulised adrenaline (200 µg kg^{-1}) and lidocaine (maximum 4–5 mg kg^{-1}) reduces the need for sedatives during initial flexible optical bronchoscopy. Consider administration of an anti-sialogue.

Initial sedation can be achieved with sevoflurane. Take into account the possibility of reduced tidal volumes and prolonged induction time. Alternatives include small repeated doses of propofol (0.5–1 mg kg^{-1}).

Passing the flexible bronchoscope through a bronchoscopy mask makes early assessment possible. A foreign body in the hypopharynx can be removed using direct or videolaryngoscopy and Boedeker forceps. A subglottic foreign body may be removed using a ureter-stone basket or similar equipment. A fexible bronchoscope enables foreign body removal as far as the level of the lobar bronchi. If a rigid bronchoscope is used an adaptor must be used to enable maintenance of oxygenation and volatile-based anaesthesia. Total intravenous anaesthesia (TIVA) may also be used.

Some prefer deep general anaesthesia as the risk of coughing and bucking is reduced. This is of particular benefit during rigid bronchoscopy, as tracheal lesions are associated with significant morbidity. Maintaining spontaneous ventilation may be challenging but reduces the risk of further advancing the foreign body with positive pressure ventilation.

Total Airway Obstruction

This should be treated according to Basic Life Support algorithms. In the conscious child this calls for immediate back blows and chest or abdominal thrusts. Failure to clear the airway will rapidly render the patient unconscious and may lead to cardiac arrest necessitating cardiopulmonary resuscitation.

Total airway obstruction calls for rapid action and maximum control of the airway. Immediate induction of anaesthesia is required including maintenance with TIVA and neuromuscular blockade.

A foreign body at the glottic level may be removed during laryngoscopy with the Boedeker or McGill forceps. Failure of immediate removal is potentially detrimental and eFONA should be considered.

If a subglottic foreign body causing total airway obstruction is suspected intubation should be avoided. An SGA is placed and attempts are made to positive pressure ventilate the patient. If successful, a flexible bronchoscope is introduced, via the SGA, and foreign body removal is attempted. Alternatives include rigid bronchoscopy.

In extremis – total obstruction, with a foreign body that is not extractable – pushing the obstruction into a main-stem bronchus may be the only option. Ideally, ventilation is now possible via the non-obstructed main-stem bronchus. eFONA will not resolve the situation and is not advised. Having secured immediate survival this way, planning for removal of the foreign body at main-stem bronchus level follows.

In extreme cases extracorporeal membrane oxygenation (ECMO) may be the last resort. This takes time and is not readily available at most centres.

Recovery/Post-Operative

Early discharge several hours after uncomplicated bronchoscopy is possible but admission until the next day is common in most centres. The level of post-operative dependency is directed by the case severity and potential for airway compromise. Especially in young children, the resulting airway trauma causes oedema that may necessitate tracheal intubation and steroid therapy.

Conclusions

Oxygenation is the cornerstone of paediatric airway management. Cuffed tracheal tubes can be used in all children. SGAs are important aids in emergency airway control. Skills in indirect laryngoscopy and flexible optical bronchoscopy must be maintained. Airway management of small children and children with co-morbidity requires expert skills. eFONA is extremely rare and different techniques than those used in adults are required.

Further Reading

Cote CJ, Hartnick CJ. (2009). Pediatric transtracheal and cricothyrotomy airway devices for emergency use: which are appropriate for infants and children? *Paediatric Anaesthesia*, **19**, 66–76.

Fidkowaki CW, Zheng H, Firth PG. (2010). The anesthetic considerations of tracheobronchial foreign bodies in children: a literature review of 12,979 cases. *Anesthesia & Analgesia*, **111**, 1016–1025.

Habre W, Disma N, Virag K, et al.; APRICOT Group of the European Society of Anaesthesiology Clinical Trial Network. (2017), Incidence of severe critical events in paediatric anaesthesia (APRICOT): a prospective multicentre observational study in 261 hospitals in Europe. *Lancet Respiratory Medicine*, **5**, 412–425.

Holm-Knudsen RJ, Rasmussen LS, Charabi B, Bøttger M, Kristensen MS. (2012). Emergency airway access in children – transtracheal cannulas and tracheotomy assessed in a porcine model. *Paediatric Anaesthesia*, **22**, 1159–1165.

Jagannathan N, Sequera-Ramos L, Sohn L, et al. (2014). Elective use of supraglottic airway devices for primary airway management in children with difficult airways. *British Journal of Anaesthesia*, **112**, 742–748.

Weiss M, Engelhart T. (2010). Proposal for the management of the unexpected difficult pediatric airway. *Paediatric Anaesthesia*, **20**, 454–464.

Airway Management in Obesity

Daniela Godoroja, Marie Louise Rovsing and Jay B. Brodsky

Chapter 24

Introduction

The World Health Organization (WHO) defines obesity as an abnormal/excessive accumulation of fat presenting a risk to health. Obesity is categorised according to body mass index (BMI), i.e. weight (kg) divided by the square of height (m) (kg m^{-2}), and has been divided into three classes.

Class 1	BMI 30 to < 35 kg m^{-2}
Class 2	BMI 35 to < 40 kg m^{-2}
Class 3	BMI ≥ 40 kg m^{-2}
Class 3 is also termed 'morbid', 'extreme' or 'severe' obesity.	

Anaesthetists are encountering increasing numbers of obese patients and airway management is a major concern in these patients. This chapter provides key points on safe airway management of this clinically demanding group.

Pulmonary Pathophysiology

Functional residual capacity (FRC) decreases as BMI increases, mostly due to a fall in expiratory reserve volume (ERV). Breathing at low lung volume promotes airway closure in dependent lung zones, causing decreased ventilation in the lung bases (atelectasis) with hypoventilation and ventilation–perfusion mismatch (shunt). The diminished lung volume also reduces airway calibre. Obesity is a pro-inflammatory condition causing airway hyper-reactivity. Obese patients have a high resting metabolic rate with increased oxygen demand. Oxygen consumption is increased because of the increased work of breathing. All these factors increase risk of hypoxaemia.

Preoperative Airway Assessment

Sleep-Disordered Breathing

Sleep-disordered breathing, typically obstructive sleep apnoea (OSA), occurs in 10–20% of Class 2 and Class 3 patients, and is undiagnosed in the majority of patients. OSA is associated with difficult mask ventilation, difficult direct laryngoscopy and upper airway obstruction following minimal sedation. Patients with OSA are prone to very rapid arterial oxygen desaturation during and immediately after induction of general anaesthesia and in the postoperative period. Untreated OSA may progress to obesity hypoventilation syndrome (OHS), a triad of severe obesity, daytime hypoventilation with hypercapnia, and sleep-disordered breathing. Chronic hypoxaemia and hypercapnia cause increased sensitivity to the effects of anaesthetic agents and opioids, which can progress to hypoventilation and respiratory arrest in the early post-operative period.

The American Society of Anesthesiologists and the Society of Anesthesia and Sleep Medicine recommend preoperative screening of surgical patients for OSA, and treatment with continuous positive airway pressure (CPAP) during the perioperative period when significant OSA is present. Overnight polysomnography is necessary to confirm an OSA diagnosis but is expensive and often impractical. The STOP-Bang Questionnaire (Table 24.1) is a useful OSA screening tool. Pulse oximetry readings of < 95% in room air, expiratory reserve volume < 0.5 L and a serum bicarbonate concentration > 28 mmol L^{-1} each suggest OSA.

OSA risk is associated with body shape, rather than absolute BMI. Men usually exhibit central or visceral obesity ('apple shape') with abdominal, neck and airway adipose distribution, while women have a predominantly peripheral fat distribution ('pear shape') and their airways are less commonly affected. Central (male-type) obesity is significantly associated with severity of OSA.

Airway Risk Assessment

Difficult face mask ventilation is common in obese patients. Independent predictors for difficult or impossible mask ventilation are described in the mnemonic OBESE (Table 24.2). Additional factors include modified Mallampati class III–IV and neck circumference > 50 cm. Mask ventilation in the obese patient

Table 24.1 The STOP-BANG screening questionnaire for obstructive sleep apnoea. One point is scored for each positive feature; a score ≥ 5 is a significant risk.

STOP BANG	
S	Snoring. Do you snore loudly (louder than talking or heard through a closed door)?
T	Tired. Do you often feel tired, fatigued or sleepy during the daytime? Do you fall asleep in the daytime?
O	Observed. Has anyone observed you stop breathing or choking or gasping during your sleep?
P	Blood Pressure. Are you hypertensive or do you take medicine for blood pressure?
B	BMI. BMI > 35 kg m^{-2}
A	Age. Age > 50 years
N	Neck Circumference. (measured around Adam's apple) > 43 cm (17 in) for males, > 41 cm (16 in) for females
G	Gender. Male

Chung et al. (2012). *British Journal of Anaesthesia*, 108, 768–775

Table 24.2 Five independent risk factors (OBESE) for difficult mask ventilation

OBESE	
O	Obese
B	Beard
E	Edentulous
S	Snoring (OSA)
E	Elderly (> 55 years)

Holland J, Donaldson W. (2015). WFSA Tutorial 321, https://open airway.org/difficult-face-mask-ventilation-atotw-321

often requires two operators, one to hold the face mask and another to squeeze the reservoir bag.

A meta-analysis reported a threefold higher incidence of difficult intubation in obese patients. The Intubation Difficulty Score (IDS) (Table 24.3) can be used to measure airway difficulty. An IDS > 5 was reported in 15.5% of obese patients compared with 2.3% of non-obese patients. Nevertheless, the relationship between obesity and difficult intubation is more complex as 378 of the 379 obese and morbidly obese patients in the four cited studies in that review were successfully intubated with direct laryngoscopy. Direct laryngoscopy is successful in most morbidly obese patients, but risk factors for increased difficulty include male sex, Mallampati class III/IV and neck circumference > 60 cm.

Preparation for and Induction of General Anaesthesia

Position

Pulmonary mechanics are markedly altered in supine patients because the increased intra-abdominal pressure causes diaphragmatic impedance, which reduces FRC and total lung capacity. These effects impair the capacity of obese patients to tolerate apnoeic episodes. Their safe apnoea time, i.e. the time between apnoea onset and desaturation (SpO$_2$ ≤ 90%), is very short. Positioning the operating room table in a 30° reverse Trendelenburg position increases safe apnoea time.

Direct laryngoscopy is conventionally performed on a supine patient in the 'sniffing' (flextension) position with a single pillow under the head. The laryngeal view is significantly improved in obese patients when their head, shoulders and upper body are 'ramped', such that their ear level and sternal notch are aligned. This head-elevated laryngoscopy position (HELP) can

Table 24.3 Intubation Difficulty Score. IDS > 5 = moderate-major difficulty

Variable	Score	Rules
Number of attempts > 1	N1	Each additional attempt adds 1 point
Number of operators > 1	N2	Every additional operator adds 1 point
Number of alternative techniques	N3	Every alternative technique adds 1 point
Cormack Grade -1	N4	1 point for each grade above 1
Lifting forced required	N5	Add 1 point if increased
Laryngeal pressure	N6	Add 1 point if applied. Cricoid force adds no points
Vocal cord mobility	N7	Abduction = 0 points, adduction = 1 point
Total IDS = sum of scores	N1–N7	

Adnet et al. (1997). *Anesthesiology*, 87, 1290–1297.

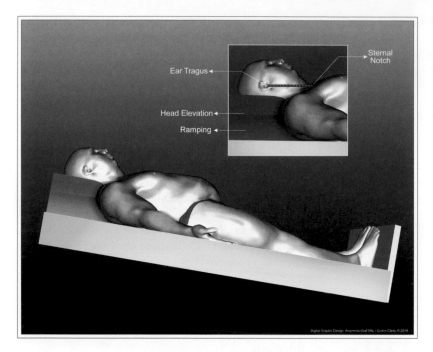

Figure 24.1 Position for tracheal intubation in the obese patient ramped position (head-elevated laryngoscopy position) with patient's ear level aligned with the sternal notch, and operating table in reverse Trendelenburg. This increases safe apnoea time and improves the view during direct laryngoscopy by aligning the oral, pharyngeal and laryngeal axes.

be achieved by placing multiple folded blankets, pre-manufactured foam pillows or inflatable pillows under the upper body, head and neck.

The combination of the HELP and reverse Trendelenburg position decreases dependent atelectasis by reducing mass-loading on the chest, increases the safe apnoea time and improves the laryngoscopic view by aligning the oral, pharyngeal and laryngeal axes (Figure 24.1) (see also Chapter 14).

Pre-oxygenation

Routine pre-oxygenation (e.g. tidal ventilation of 100% oxygen for 3 minutes or eight vital capacity breaths) increases safe apnoea time to 8–10 minutes in non-obese patients, but to only 2–3 minutes in supine obese patients.

Pre-oxygenation in the obese should be meticulous and proceed until end-tidal oxygen is > 0.9. Safe apnoea time can be increased by passive oxygenation during the apnoeic period ('apnoeic oxygenation') (see also Chapter 8). This may be provided in a number of ways including:

- Dry oxygen at 5–15 L min^{-1} via standard nasal cannula
- Dry oxygen at 10 L min^{-1} via small Ring–Adair–Elwyn (RAE) tube placed along the cheek so its distal tip sits in the buccal cavity
- High flow nasal oxygen (transnasal humidified rapid-insufflation ventilatory exchange, THRIVE)

using high flow, warmed, humidified oxygen at a rate of up to 70 L min^{-1}. This provides both apnoeic oxygenation and modest levels of CPAP (up to approximately 7.5 cmH$_2$O). High flow nasal oxygen increases safe apnoea time in obese patients and may also be used to maintain oxygenation in spontaneously breathing obese patients during awake intubation and sedation procedures.

- CPAP, which increases safe apnoea time by ≈50% in obese patients, with the optimal level being 10 cmH$_2$O.
- Non-invasive ventilation, which improves alveolar recruitment and prolongs the safe apnoea time and is commonly used for rapid sequence induction (RSI) in the critically ill (see Chapter 28).

Aspiration Risk

The incidence of perioperative pulmonary aspiration is similar between fasting obese and lean patients undergoing elective surgery. However, obese patients with severe gastro-oesophageal reflux and those with adjustable gastric bands *in situ* are at increased risk of aspiration.

A cuffed tracheal tube is the best protection against aspiration, once placed. If an RSI technique is chosen either thiopental or propofol may be suitable. Both suxamethonium and rocuronium achieve acceptable intubating conditions during RSI. However, suxamethonium-induced muscle fasciculations increase oxygen consumption and decrease safe apnoea time. Rocuronium can be rapidly antagonised with sugammadex if intubation fails, provided the drug is immediately available and prepared for use. In an obese patient the dose of sugammadex should be based on adjusted body weight: ideal body weight plus 40% of the patient's weight above this.

The role of cricoid force remains controversial (see Chapter 11). Cricoid force may:

- impede mask ventilation if excessive force is used or the force is misplaced
- in extreme cases displace the normal airway anatomy or cause airway obstruction thereby worsening both mask ventilation and intubation attempts
- relax the lower oesophageal sphincter
- interfere with supraglottic airway (SGA) placement unless it is released
- be more difficult to apply correctly in the obese patient due to difficulty identifying the correct anatomical landmarks

Therefore, if cricoid force is used in obese patients it is important that the person applying it is trained and that great attention to detail is applied in its application.

Due to the short safe apnoeic period in obese patients, mask ventilation with only low inspiratory pressure, with or without cricoid force, is recommended during induction of anaesthesia before and between any attempts to secure the airway.

Airway Techniques

Direct and Videolaryngoscopy

Prior to surgery, an airway management plan should be discussed and additional personnel should be available if required. The technique of choice in morbidly obese patients is tracheal intubation and controlled ventilation. Use of an SGA as the primary airway device should be reserved for highly selected patients undergoing elective procedures and where the patient can be positioned with head elevated and the upper airway accessible.

The decision to proceed with standard anaesthetic induction, RSI or awake intubation will depend on the patient's history and co-morbidities, as well as a thorough preoperative airway examination.

Difficulty or failure of direct laryngoscopy intubation should be promptly managed according to a difficult airway algorithm. As in all cases, the number and duration of direct laryngoscopy attempts should be limited to prevent airway trauma and progression to a 'cannot intubate, cannot oxygenate' (CICO) situation. Direct laryngoscopy aids include bougies and stylets, external laryngeal manipulation, backward, upward and rightward pressure and various laryngoscopy blades. Short laryngoscope handles are useful to avoid the interference between the large chest wall pads and placement of the laryngoscope blade in the mouth.

Both the American Society of Anesthesiologists (ASA) Guidelines for Management of the Difficult Airway and the Difficult Airway Society's 2015 guidelines advocate having a low threshold for the use of videolaryngoscopy. The literature includes studies showing that, compared with direct laryngoscopy, the GlideScope improves intubation conditions in morbidly obese patients and that both the C-MAC and GlideScope reduce intubation attempts in obese patients. Videolaryngoscopy improves the view at laryngoscopy and this may mean that successful intubation is achieved sooner, thus avoiding hypoxaemia, and that multiple attempts may be avoided. Videolaryngoscopy also reduces the lifting force required, which may avoid airway trauma and which reduces haemodynamic responses to laryngoscopy. Videolaryngoscopy enables both the operator and assistant (or supervisor) to view the airway anatomy and passage of the tracheal tube. Finally, videolaryngoscopy may be combined with flexible optical bronchoscopy to achieve intubations where visualisation is otherwise very difficult (see Chapter 19). In view of the multiple benefits of videolaryngoscopy a videolaryngoscope should always be available for management of the obese patient. It should be used when direct laryngoscopy fails, and could usefully be considered for the initial intubation attempts (Figure 24.2).

Supraglottic Airway Devices

Although a tracheal tube is recommended to be the default airway for most obese patients, an SGA may be suitable for elective procedures in overweight and moderately obese patients. SGAs retain an important role in selected elective procedures in obese patients. Their use may be associated with improved quality of recovery and reduced complications on emergence compared with intubation. There is no strong evidence to determine at which weight or for which operation a tracheal tube should be preferred over an SGA, and even expert opinion will vary in this area. The UK Society for Obesity and Bariatric Anaesthesia recommends a cut-off for default tracheal intubation to be a BMI > 35 kg m^{-2} in obese patients. Although anaesthestists with significant bariatric experience may balance risks and benefits and use an SGA in patients with a significantly higher BMI, the decision to use an SGA in an obese patient should be based on considerations of safety, rather than expediency or speed.

When an SGA is used in an obese patient it is logical to use a high performing second generation SGA with a drain port and higher sealing pressure (see Chapter 13). Such a device can be used to provide reliable controlled ventilation with positive end-expiratory pressure (PEEP) without causing gastric inflation. However, SGA use should be carefully considered and requires meticulous performance. When an SGA is used, it is useful to consider administering drugs to decrease gastric volume and increase the pH of gastric contents preoperatively.

An SGA can also function as an alternative to mask ventilation before tracheal intubation, and as a rescue device if ventilation and intubation fail. Intubation via an SGA should be performed with the assistance of a flexible optical bronchoscope with or without an airway exchanger catheter (e.g. Aintree intubation catheter).

Awake Tracheal Intubation

Awake intubation is performed whenever the anaesthetist considers it the safest method for securing the airway and should be actively considered in the obese patient (Table 24.4). Local anaesthetic techniques are the same as in non-obese patients. Sedation should only be used with caution and with careful monitoring. Short-acting or non-respiratory depressant agents including remifentanil, dexmedetomidine and ketamine may be particularly useful.

Both conventional flexible optical bronchoscopy and videolaryngoscopy may be suitable awake tracheal intubation techniques in the obese and both have comparable success rates in obese patients. Whichever is chosen the patient should be placed in the sitting or ramped position and supplementary oxygen should be administered throughout the procedure, especially when sedation is used. Any awake technique may be challenging because of airway narrowing caused by fatty tissue. First-attempt success rates above 70% and without serious

Table 24.4 Indications for performing safe awake intubation

ALIVE	
A	Accepts what is going to happen
L	Loose (relaxed and cooperative)
I	In the proper way oxygenated
V	Void of pain and secretions
E	Eager to do it again

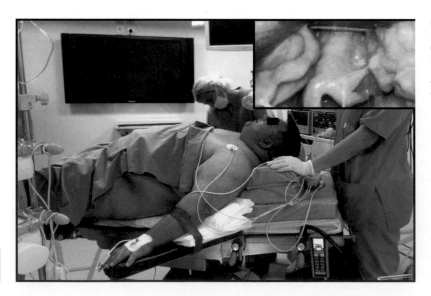

Figure 24.2 Increased difficulty. Obese patient, 35 years old, BMI 55 kg m^{-2}, with obstructive sleep apnoea, compliant with preoperative CPAP. SpO$_2$ in room air 97%, neck circumference 55 cm. Plan A: videolaryngoscopy. Insert: view obtained with the videolaryngoscope.

complications have been reported. The 4th National Audit Project (NAP4) noted reluctance by clinicians to use awake intubation but also noted that it was not always successful especially when excessive sedation led to airway obstruction. There is an increasing argument that awake videolaryngoscopy and awake flexible optical bronchoscopy should both be skills acquired by airway experts. For examples see Figures 24.3 and 24.4.

Cannot Intubate, Cannot Oxygenate and Emergency Front of Neck Airway

A CICO situation is a high-risk, low-frequency event but the consequences are severe and the risk (and speed of hypoxaemia when obstruction occurs) is significantly increased in obese patients. NAP4 reported that major airway complications occurred twice as often in obese patients and four times as often in morbidly obese patients compared with the non-obese. Obese patients – in the operating theatre and in settings outside the theatre – are at increased risk of CICO and of failure to successfully perform an emergency front of neck airway (eFONA). In NAP4 such failures were caused by decision-making delays, knowledge gaps and equipment and technical failures. An important cause of failure in the obese is inability to palpate the cricothyroid membrane (CTM) and difficulty in extending the neck due to excessive fat pads. During preoperative assessment of a patient with impalpable landmarks at high risk of a difficult intubation, good practice includes attempting to

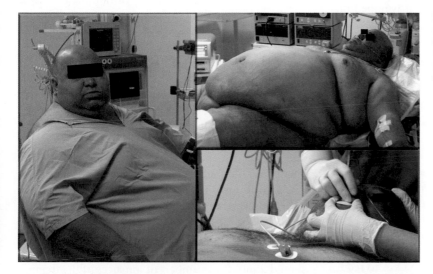

Figure 24.3 Greater difficulty. Obese patient, 48 years old, BMI 88 kg m^{-2}, with obesity hypoventilation syndrome with preoperative bilevel positive airway pressure (BIPAP) for 6 weeks. SpO$_2$ in room air 85%/91%, neck circumference 70 cm. Plan: awake flexible optical bronchoscope (FOB)-guided intubation without sedation.

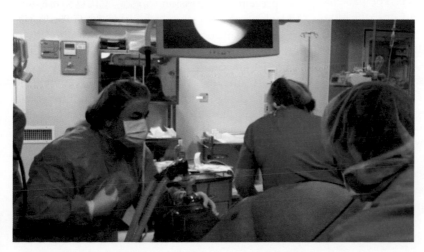

Figure 24.4 Considerable difficulty obese patient, 43 years old, BMI 63.5 kg m^{-2}, with severe obesity hypoventilation syndrome with partial compliance with bilevel positive airway pressure (BIPAP) and not cooperative for awake technique, neck circumference 62 cm. Plans: videolaryngoscopy but anticipating difficulty, difficult SGA, difficult mask ventilation. Proceed to emergency front of neck airway if above techniques fail.

identify the CTM by palpation and/or ultrasonography. Ultrasonography in the obese patient should be embraced as even training over one day can increase the success rate of CTM identification from below 50% to above 80%.

The best approach for rescue of CICO in the obese is unclear, as it is in the non-obese population (see Chapter 20). What is generally accepted is that in patients with non-palpable landmarks, a surgical technique including a large skin incision (e.g. up to 10 cm) and blunt dissection of the tissues to identify the CTM is likely to be necessary. Since CICO occurs more often and eFONA fails more often in the obese than in the non-obese it is logical to ensure airway managers are taught to manage these situations. At present there are insufficient manikins available to simulate the obese airway, particularly for eFONA. This is an active area of research and it is hoped that the issue will be redressed in the next few years.

Emergence from Anaesthesia and Post-anaesthesia Care

Development of a plan for safe extubation and emergency reintubation of the obese patient is crucial. Neuromuscular blockade should be completely reversed, and quantitative neuromuscular monitoring is needed to confirm this. Prior to tracheal extubation, the patient should be pre-oxygenated. The patient should be fully awake, cooperative and breathing with an adequate tidal volume to maintain normal end-tidal carbon dioxide and pulse oximetry levels. The patient should be ramped or sitting upright. A nasopharyngeal airway may be inserted in patients with OSA to reduce the risk of post-extubation obstruction. For patients with a difficult airway, SGA placement or extubation over an airway exchange catheter can be performed (see Chapter 21). Maintaining positive pressure with pressure support ventilation and CPAP application improves oxygenation and decreases complications, especially in patients with OSA.

Post-operative management in a level-2 or -3 high-dependency post-operative care unit should be considered for obese patients with severe OSA/OHS, with serious co-morbidities, and for patients undergoing extensive surgical procedures requiring parenteral opioids. Patients may require chest physiotherapy, incentive spirometry and supplementary oxygen including high flow nasal oxygen, CPAP or non-invasive ventilation to maintain oxygenation.

Obese patients who are suitable to recover in the post-anaesthesia care unit (PACU) should be fully monitored, receive oxygen and be in either a sitting or in a 45° head-up position. Obese patients experience frequent desaturations during the first 24 hours after surgery and opioid analgesia exacerbates this tendency. Opioid-sparing multimodal analgesia techniques should be used but are beyond the remit of this chapter. PACU management practices should be continued in the ward or until the patient completely recovers and becomes ambulatory.

Conclusions

In all obese patients, preoperative assessment to identify or exclude a potential 'difficult' airway is important. Obesity is associated with difficult mask ventilation, difficult SGA insertion, modest difficulty at laryngoscopy, increased risk of CICO and of failed eFONA. Predictors of difficult direct laryngoscopy are male sex, large neck circumference (> 60 cm), and modified Mallampati class III/IV. There is a high incidence of OSA/OHS, especially in patients with increased upper body fat distribution. OSA is associated with difficult mask ventilation and direct laryngoscopy. Airway managers need to establish skills and maintain them through practice in the different airway techniques that may be needed routinely or as rescue techniques to manage the obese airway. Obese patients have a very short safe apnoea time so tracheal intubation must be accomplished promptly. Clinicians should always have primary and backup plans including difficult airway algorithms. These should limit the number of unsuccessful attempts to prevent progression to a CICO situation. Videolaryngoscopy should be used when direct laryngoscopy fails or as a first choice when difficulty is anticipated. Help should be requested immediately from a trained anaesthetist when difficulties occur. The first attempt at tracheal intubation should be the best attempt. This should include optimal positioning and pre-oxygenation (and apnoeic oxygenation). RSI is not mandatory for every obese patient but should be considered. Gentle gas ventilation should be performed after induction and can be used with cricoid force during RSI. Before extubation, neuromuscular blockade must be completely reversed, the patient should be pre-oxygenated and sitting or ramped. Extubation should take place when the patient is fully awake. Plans for reintubation should be in place. Post-operative management includes multimodal opioid-sparing analgesia, incentive spirometry, high flow nasal oxygen, CPAP or non-invasive ventilation in the sitting position, and careful monitoring until the patient is fully recovered and mobile.

Further Reading

Brodsky JB, Lemmens HJM, Brock-Utne JG, Vierra M, Saidman LJ. (2002). Morbid obesity and tracheal intubation. *Anesthesia & Analgesi*a, **94**, 732–736.

Frerk C, Mitchell VS, McNarry AF, et al.; Difficult Airway Society intubation guidelines working group. (2015). Difficult Airway Society 2015 guidelines for management of unanticipated difficult intubation in adults. *British Journal of Anaesthesia*, **115**, 827–848.

Heinrich S, Horbach T, Stubner B, et al. (2014). Benefits of humidified high flow nasal oxygen for pre oxygenation in morbidly obese patients undergoing bariatric surgery: a randomised controlled study. *Journal of Obesity and Bariatrics*, **1**, 1–7.

Marrel J, Blanc C, Frascarolo P, Magnusson L. (2007). Videolaryngoscopy improves intubation condition in morbidly obese patients. *European Journal of Anaesthesiology*, **24**, 1045–1049.

Nicholson A, Cook TM, Smith AF, Lewis SR, Reed SS. (2013). Supraglottic airway devices versus tracheal intubation for airway management during general anaesthesia in obese patients. *Cochrane Database Systematic Reviews*, **9**, CD010105.

Nightingale CE, Margarson MP, Shearer E, at al. (2015). Peri-operative management of the obese surgical patient *Anaesthesia*, **70**, 859–876.

Maxillofacial and Dental Surgery

Hanne Abildstrøm and Brian Jenkins

Maxillofacial and dental surgery presents novel challenges to the skill of the anaesthetist, due to sharing the anatomical space with the surgeon and because of the particular conditions required for surgical success. The anaesthetist should have knowledge of the surgical terms and techniques peculiar to this field. Although elective surgery is largely routine and predictable, emergency surgery may challenge the skills of even very experienced anaesthetists. Of note, surgical procedures that start out as routine and predictable have the potential to deteriorate into life-threatening situations. To avoid poor outcomes, a knowledge of the techniques and challenges of the subject, supplemented by development of skills in the workplace, is essential. This chapter provides a brief introduction to anaesthesia for maxillofacial and dental surgery.

Dental Surgery

Dental surgery refers to minor surgery to the gums and teeth, whether dealing with extraction of teeth (exodontia), preservative treatments (fillings) or replacement (implants).

Patient Population

Patients presenting for dental surgery under general anaesthesia typically either require extensive procedures or are unable to comply safely with dental treatment under local anaesthesia. The latter patients tend to be younger children, adults with learning difficulties or patients with severe dental phobia. Extensive dental infection may also prevent local anaesthesia from working adequately and thus may require general anaesthesia.

Because of the potential complications of general anaesthesia, it is useful to discuss whether the planned procedure could be managed with sedation or other techniques. In adults, sedation using benzodiazepines or nitrous oxide administered via a nasal mask is

useful, but in children, friendly staff and surroundings and the use of distractors such as tablet computers may be enough to avoid general anaesthesia.

Recommended standards for fasting, monitoring, resuscitation equipment and personnel for general anaesthesia are applicable for dental surgery, wherever it is carried out. Historically, there have been reports of a number of deaths in otherwise healthy children and adults from airway complications, often contributed to by substandard practice.

Patients with learning difficulties often present for dental surgery, and they may pose significant challenges for the anaesthetist because of difficulties with communication, compliance and associated co-morbidities. Down syndrome patients have the potential for airway problems (see Chapter 5), but also may have congenital cardiac defects that increase the risks of general anaesthesia and also endocarditis (from poor dental hygiene). It is not unusual for patients to present for dental extraction under general anaesthesia whilst awaiting cardiac transplantation.

Anaesthesia

Post-operative nausea and vomiting is a common problem in this patient population: total intravenous anaesthesia supplemented with antiemetics is an effective way to minimise this risk. Airway management should aim to provide optimal conditions for the surgeon. Sedation in a spontaneously breathing patient without an airway device is possible, but is a compromise between providing adequate surgical conditions whilst maintaining an open and free airway. Blood, debris, saliva and foreign bodies pose a threat during the whole procedure, and the avoidance of soiling of the airway depends to a large extent on the skill, diligence and speed of the surgeons. With all but the briefest procedures, general anaesthesia with tracheal intubation or airway management with a supraglottic airway device (SGA) is strongly recommended.

The choice of airway device is often dictated by the flexibility of the dental surgeon and the procedure to be carried out. Many dental surgeons prefer complete oral access, not limited by a tracheal tube or SGA, and for some procedures they have to test occlusion, which precludes the use of an oral tracheal tube. However, for simple dental extractions an SGA gives adequate oral access, although risk of displacement and airway soiling is always present and more likely with prolonged and bloody procedures. An SGA with reinforced tubing (although more difficult to insert) is more flexible and mobile, enabling repositioning of the connecting tube without compromising the laryngeal seal.

If surgery allows, an oral tracheal tube is less traumatic than a nasotracheal tube. This may be either a preformed south-facing type fixed in the midline, or a straight standard oral tube moved from side to side at the request of the dental surgeon. Nasal tubes provide ideal oral access for the operator, but at the risk of trauma to the nasal mucosa and post-operative haemorrhage.

Nasal Intubation

Nasal intubation remains the gold-standard airway management technique for dental surgery, providing the best conditions for the dental work by providing excellent surgical access and enabling the bacterial/heat and moisture exchanger filter to be placed away from the surgical field. Ideally it should be performed with a soft PVC nasal tube to reduce the incidence of nasal trauma and complications, such as epistaxis and the abruption of conchae. Use of a small tube – e.g. 6.0–6.5 mm ID – will reduce trauma. Some precautions and techniques are useful to help avoid trauma to the nasal mucosa.

Preoperative history and examination can determine the occurrence of complications during previous surgical procedures, and also identify the best nasal airway by asking the patient to occlude one nostril followed by the other. Vasoconstrictors can be administered nasally prior to intubation to reduce the risk of bleeding and to shrink the nasal mucosa.

Laryngoscopy prior to introduction of the nasal tube will help to assess intubation difficulty and the presence of potential problems (such as large tonsils) before committing to a procedure that could cause haemorrhage and threaten the airway. The nasal tube may be railroaded over a lubricated suction catheter or bougie before introduction into the nasal cavity to help guide the larger tube past the conchae. Nasotracheal intubation is usually easy to achieve by gentle rotation of the tube and flexion/extension of the head, but often progress of the tube tip through the larynx is held up by impaction against the tracheal rings. In these circumstances, the tube can be gently rotated anticlockwise to achieve passage of the whole cuff past the laryngeal inlet. External pressure on the cricoid cartilage by an assistant or flexion of the neck to reduce the angle between the tube and the tracheal wall may also facilitate passage of the tracheal tube. If these manoeuvres fail, a Magill forceps may be used to change the angle of tube insertion into the trachea, but this risks damage to the cuff and so is only appropriate if other measures fail.

Throat Packs

It is usual to place throat packs before surgery to prevent surgical debris such as blood, surgical drill bits, fragments of bone and soft tissue from entering the oesophagus or the airway during the procedure and upon extubation. Because of the potential complications associated with the use of a throat pack, the practice of routine insertion is currently being reviewed. If a throat pack is inserted it is essential to remove it at the end of surgery, and if overlooked this can cause airway obstruction immediately following extubation or in the recovery area. Pack removal may usefully be included in the surgical checklist at the end of the procedure, but it is the responsibility of the anaesthetist to ensure that the pharynx is clear before extubation.

Emergency Dental Surgery

Infection originating from dental caries is a common condition that in most cases can be dealt with by dental extraction under local anaesthesia. However, if left unresolved it can produce severe anatomical distortion due to oedema, collection of pus and may progress to systemic infection which may be life-threatening. In these circumstances, surgical intervention under general anaesthesia is required.

Poor oral hygiene provides optimal conditions for acid-producing bacteria to dissolve dental enamel, leading to odontogenic infection. Most commonly, the infection starts in a mandibular molar from where it can spread to the alveolar bone, giving rise to a periapical abscess protruding into the oral cavity or spreading through the submandibular tissue. There can be swelling of the soft tissue in the oral cavity and the tongue. Posteriorly and inferiorly the tongue, pharynx and glottis can become inflamed with oedema, eventually resulting in an obstructed airway. Infection may also spread along the great vessels of the neck to the mediastinum, which is a serious complication with high mortality. CT imaging may reveal mediastinal gas formation with pleural and epicardial effusions. From the maxillary teeth, infection can spread superiorly to the maxillary sinuses and the infraorbital cavity. Infection can also expand intracranially and give rise to cavernous sinus thrombosis.

Ludwig's angina can arise from either a peritonsillar abscess or dental infection, with hardening and swelling (cellulitis) of the floor of the mouth and the masseter muscles, giving rise to trismus and making conventional laryngoscopy impossible. The patient may be unable to lie supine and/or may be unable to swallow saliva, which are indications of the severity of the condition. Dysphonia is a late sign that precedes complete airway obstruction. Awake flexible optical bronchoscope (FOB)-guided intubation is usually the preferred approach, but may also be complicated by poor patient cooperation and difficulty with obtaining good local anaesthesia (due to changes in tissue pH secondary to infection).

Following surgical drainage, safe extubation may not be possible until resolution of airway oedema. Ventilation in the intensive care unit for a prolonged period may be required, as may repeated surgical drainage of the infected tissues. Establishing a tracheostomy prior to transfer to intensive care may be extremely difficult in the presence of submandibular oedema, but is often a safer option than relying on a precarious oral or nasal tracheal tube which may be pulled out by increasing oral and pharyngeal oedema. Broad-spectrum antibiotics are used to control infection and steroids are often used in an attempt to reduce airway oedema. Occasionally, severe sepsis, septic shock and multi-organ failure is a complication of dental infection.

Maxillofacial Surgery

Orthognathic Surgery

Orthognathic is a word of Greek derivation that means to straighten or correct the jaws. Osteotomies of the maxilla and mandible change the shape of the facial skeleton in order to treat malocclusion and deformities of the face. The purpose is both aesthetic and functional, enabling patients to chew, masticate, and breathe freely through the nose and to speak clearly.

Most patients are in late adolescence, and typically present for surgery after 12–18 months of orthodontic presurgical treatment with braces and appliances to correct malocclusion. The orthodontic treatment is continued post-operatively. All permanent teeth have erupted and the bone structures of the face have finished growing, but orthognathic surgery is required for definitive treatment of the underlying skeletal deformity causing malocclusion. The patients are generally healthy without co-morbidities. Surgery is elective and well planned by a multidisciplinary team of surgeons and orthodontists. Dental models are worked out after virtual planning on the basis of three-dimensional CT or cone-beam CT (CBCT) imaging (Figure 25.1).

Mandibular sagittal split osteotomy (Figure 25.1) is used to correct both over- and under-bite, mandibular retro- and pro-gnathism and asymmetries. An osteotomy is performed bilaterally in the rami of the mandible, allowing for both anterior and posterior sliding of the anterior tooth-bearing segment. All cuts are made intra-orally in the middle of the bone where the marrow is present, giving a surface of slightly bleeding bone. When aligned, the fragment is fixed in its new position with titanium plates and screws.

The most common form of maxillary osteotomy is the Le Fort I osteotomy (Figure 25.1), with intra-oral vestibular incisions from the lateral part of the nose downwards, separation from the nasal septum and mobilisation of the maxilla bone structure that is still attached in its pedicle of soft tissue and blood supply from the maxillary artery and venous plexuses of the palate. The maxilla can now be moved in anterior, posterior, cranial and caudal directions, and it can be rotated before fixation in the desired position, guided by occlusion with the lower teeth via a surgical splint (wafer). For this part of the procedure inter-maxillary fixation is needed. The procedure is used for patients with upper jaw deformities.

Bimaxillary osteotomy refers to the combination of the Le Fort I and sagittal split osteotomy, allowing for extensive remodelling to achieve a correct bite with an aesthetic result and enlarged airway.

Craniofacial Surgery

A smaller group of patients for orthognathic surgery are younger children with congenital craniofacial malformations, such as Apert syndrome or Morbus Crouzon,

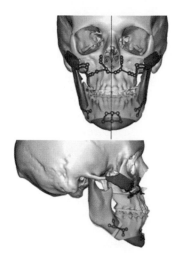
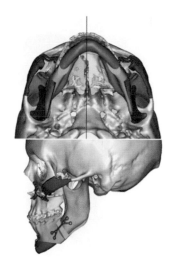

Figure 25.1 Three-dimensional planning before surgery on the basis of a CT scan. Bimaxillary osteotomy is the combination of the Le Fort I and sagittal split osteotomy, allowing for extensive remodelling of the facial bones.

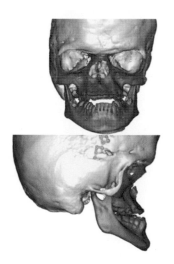
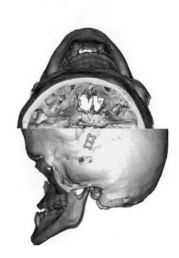

Figure 25.2 CT scan of a patient with Morbus Crouzon with hypoplasia and retrognathia of the middle face.

with hypoplasia and retrognathia of the middle face (Figure 25.2). Acquired malformations in infancy due to malignancies and trauma also need correction at an earlier age. These patients often have other malformations or co-morbidities, and may present considerable airway management challenges for the anaesthetist.

High facial osteotomies of the Le Fort II or III type are used in patients with hypoplasia of the middle face (Figure 25.3). Le Fort II and III are osteotomies of the maxilla and zygoma (where the orbital complex is included in Le Fort III), performed via an external coronal incision through the scalp where the scar will be covered by hair after healing. The scalp is raised and the maxillary osteotomies are made intra-orally.

Anaesthesia

Psychological preparation for the post-operative period is needed in young healthy patients presenting for orthognathic surgery. They can expect post-operative haematomas and oedema of facial soft tissue. It is likely that there will be post-operative nausea, which may be made worse by blood in the mouth and stomach and the requirement for opioid analgesics in the immediate post-operative period. Strong analgesics and antiemetics may be required for days, and in some cases weeks after surgery.

Nasal intubation with a north-facing tube provides excellent operating conditions, enabling the surgeon to achieve the main goal of accurate

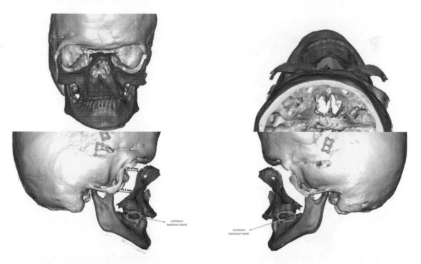

Figure 25.3 Three-dimensional planning of high facial osteotomies of the Le Fort III type in the same patient with Morbus Crouzon from Figure 25.2. The anterior sliding of the maxillary complex of approximately 2 cm corrects the hypoplasia of the middle face and results in different occlusion of the teeth.

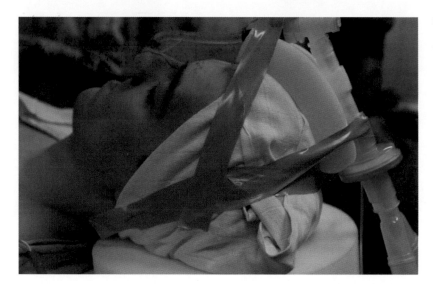

Figure 25.4 Fixation of a north-facing nasotracheal tube with padding in a patient still enabling the surgeon some mobilisation of the head.

dental occlusion. It is important to make sure that there is no pressure or traction from the nasotracheal tube on the facial structures (especially the nostrils) when the tube is secured, as this can lead to pressure necrosis during prolonged surgery. Fixation with padding should be firm, enabling mobilisation of the head and enabling the surgeon to see the whole face to help guide movement of the facial bones during the operation (Figures 25.4 and 25.5).

A throat pack is placed in the pharynx to prevent debris, blood and bone fragments from entering the airway and oesophagus, and there are similar considerations with use and removal as in dental surgery.

Emergence from anaesthesia should be quiet, gradual and stress free, aiming for an awake patient with fully recovered airway reflexes before extubation. Intermaxillary fixation is achieved with elastic rubber bands after surgery. This completely closes the mouth, although gaps in the teeth often allow pharyngeal suction with a catheter. An airway exchange device may be used if airway problems are expected, as reintubation after surgery can be difficult due to oedema and haematoma caused by the surgery (see Chapter 21). Scissors must be immediately available post-operatively to cut the elastic bands in case of emergency. If reintubation is required, extra care must be taken to avoid applying

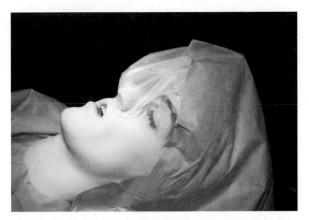

Figure 25.5 The same patient from Figure 25.4 presenting for bimaxillary surgery with surgical dressing enabling the surgeon to see the whole face during the operation.

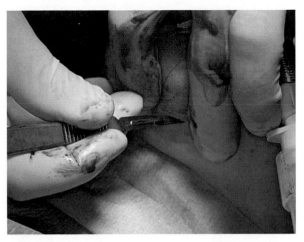

Figure 25.6 Submental tube: skin incision, one third of the distance between the chin and the mandibular angle medially to the mandibular base. (Reproduced with permission from Schopka JH, Toft P, Nørholt SE, Dahl M. (2006). Tandlaeglebadet110, 398–401.)

pressure to the newly fixated facial bones. FOB-guided intubation or use of a videolaryngoscope may help to achieve this.

In patients presenting for craniofacial surgery the airway should be expected to be difficult. In Crouzon syndrome, which is characterised by a very narrow nasal space, intubation via the nasal route is neither possible nor desirable, as the tube would be placed in the middle of the surgical field of the midface. An oral reinforced tube sutured with a perimandibular wire for security reasons is an option, but tracheostomy or a submental tracheal tube is preferred by most surgeons. Submental intubation was first described in 1986: the patient's trachea is intubated with a reinforced tube via the oral route. The surgeon creates an incision in the floor of the mouth in the submandibular region and a tunnel is created by blunt dissection (Figure 25.6). After disconnection from the ventilator the proximal end of the reinforced oral tube is pulled through this tunnel to emerge in the submandibular region and ventilation is continued (Figure 25.7). By the end of surgery, the tube is repositioned to the oral cavity with the proximal end protruding from the mouth, and the hole is sutured before extubation. There are some complications associated with the submental tube such as haemorrhage, scarring, infection, fistulae and lesions to the lingual nerve and sublingual gland.

Post-operative Haemorrhage

The bone surface where osteotomy incisions have been made in the bone marrow may continue to

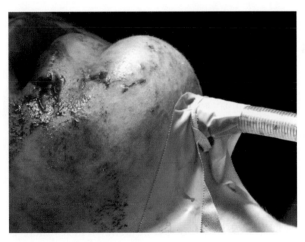

Figure 25.7 Patient intubated with a submental tube. (Reproduced with permission from Schopka JH, Toft P, Nørholt SE, Dahl M. (2006). Tandlaeglebadet110, 398–401.)

bleed in the post-operative period. A nasogastric tube may be placed before surgery to enable blood to be aspirated from the stomach. In order to reduce blood loss during surgery, a strategy of moderate hypotensive anaesthesia (maintaining a mean arterial blood pressure of 50–60 mmHg) is well tolerated in young healthy patients.

Surgical bleeding can be very difficult to control if a branch of the maxillary artery, the greater palatine artery, is cut and has retracted into the maxilla out of reach of the surgeon. This is rare, but in such situations the oral and nasal cavities may need to be packed and the patient ventilated overnight until the bleeding stops. If this does not work, angiographic embolisation may be required. Haemostatic abnormalities must always be excluded in patients with unexpected excessive bleeding. Occasionally, as blood pressure is raised at the end of surgery, bleeding from the osteotomy fracture lines may flood the mouth and nose with blood. Icepacks can be positioned round the face to promote haemostasis, but this type of bleeding usually stops after haematoma formation. After control of haemorrhage the pharynx must be thoroughly cleared of blood and clot by suction to ensure a clear airway prior to extubation.

Craniofacial surgery may be extensive and of long duration. After prolonged procedures (sometimes lasting a whole day) the patient may need ventilator support overnight. Bleeding can be substantial, and transfusion of blood products is needed to replace blood loss.

Maxillofacial Trauma

Airway

Maxillofacial trauma may present as the main problem, but is also commonly present in patients with multiple injuries depending on the trauma mechanism. Many patients will also have cervical spine fractures and injuries and/or intracranial bleeding. All trauma should be managed using an ABC algorithm, with securing the airway, adequate oxygenation and maintaining in-line stabilisation of the cervical spine as first management priorities (see Chapter 30).

In unconscious patients with a Glasgow Coma Score (GCS) < 8 and loss of airway reflexes there is urgent need to secure the airway, but this may be difficult. Blood, vomit, bone fragments, loose teeth, other foreign bodies and eventually oedema may obstruct the airway. The most experienced anaesthetist available should be in charge of the airway, but should communicate with all members of the trauma team before attempts at tracheal intubation. Initial orotracheal intubation is preferred, but this may be changed later for a nasotracheal tube for planned definitive maxillofacial surgery.

If the airway is expected to be difficult, awake FOB-guided intubation is a useful strategy in patients with sufficient spontaneous ventilation, but foreign bodies and anatomical distortion of the airway can

make this difficult. A useful alternative approach is retrograde intubation using an epidural catheter (Chapter 32), which is inserted via a cannula or a Tuohy needle through the cricothyroid or the crico-tracheal membrane and then used to guide tracheal intubation. Which technique is preferred in these circumstances depends on familiarity with equipment and techniques.

Rapid sequence induction is the gold-standard approach to anaesthetic induction, but equipment for difficult airway management should be immediately available, as should effective suction. Videolaryngoscopes are useful in cases where optimal head and neck positioning cannot be obtained, as in in-line stabilisation of the cervical spine. Should intubation fail, an oropharyngeal airway or an SGA may be used to maintain oxygenation of the patient while other more secure means of airway management are prepared. If oxygenation cannot be maintained in an un-intubated patient, an emergency front of neck airway (eFONA) must be established. In the context of maxillofacial injury this may be performed by the anaesthetist, ENT surgeon or emergency physician (see Chapter 20). FOB-guided intubation during apnoea is both difficult and time consuming, but is also a possibility. Transtracheal jet ventilation is familiar to few, but is often mentioned as an airway rescue manoeuvre: if this technique is used after airway trauma the risk of upper airway obstruction, barotrauma, pneumothorax and/or surgical emphysema is high and is likely to make a bad situation worse. Establishing an eFONA with a tube of at least 5 mm internal diameter is likely the safest approach and is recommended.

Bleeding

Fracture lines can be unilateral or bilateral and follow structural weaknesses of the facial skeleton (Figure 25.8). The face has an extensive blood supply with good collateral circulation. Disruption of large arteries such as the maxillary artery can cause heavy bleeding, but it is seldom the only cause of severe hypotension in trauma patients. In case of circulatory instability other, more obvious bleeding sites should be investigated first.

If bleeding persists from the nasal and oral cavities, packing after intubation will be sufficient for control in most cases. If not, surgical exploration and control by ligation of bleeding arteries must be considered. Arteriography with embolisation is also

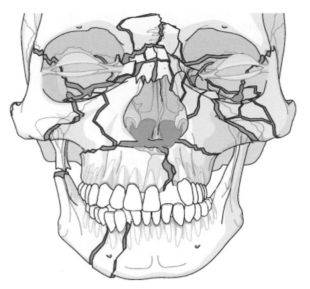

Figure 25.8 Examples of facial fractures that typically follow structural weaknesses of the facial skeleton.

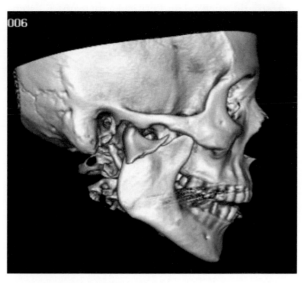

Figure 25.9 CT scan reconstruction showing a displaced mandibular condyle fracture. The head of the mandible is displaced from the temporomandibular joint.

a possibility, although there are limited options because of the abundant collateral circulation. If all else fails or in extreme circumstances the external carotid artery may need to be ligated.

Definitive Surgery

In the trauma patient life- and mobility-threatening lesions have the highest priority, and for facial trauma these are suturing of soft tissues, including the eyes. Fixation of maxillofacial fractures can be delayed until full cardiovascular stability is achieved, but should be within one week from the trauma to ensure optimal conditions for alignment and fixation. In the neuro-surgical patient, timing of surgery will need to be balanced against the ability to satisfactorily control intracranial pressure.

Before surgery, a plan for the perioperative airway management must be discussed with the surgeon. When osteosynthesis of mid-facial fractures is required, a nasotracheal tube will usually be requested, but in some instances a gap in, or lack of, dentition will leave a suitable hole for an orotracheal tube to pass without disturbing occlusion.

Coexisting skull base fracture is a relative contra-indication for nasotracheal intubation, and there are well-described cases when nasotracheal tubes have entered the intracranial space. However, if nasotracheal intubation is required, the nasal passages may be safely negotiated by using an FOB to railroad a tube into the

trachea under visual guidance. An alternative approach would be to establish surgical tracheostomy prior to surgery. This is especially recommended in patients with neurotrauma, who may have the need for assisted ventilation for a long post-operative period, or for patients who require multiple scheduled surgeries. In a patient expected to be able to return to full respiratory capacity after surgery a submental tube is recommended.

In the case of un-displaced mandibular condyle fracture, forceful manipulation of the mandible with a conventional laryngoscope could displace the head of the mandible from the temporomandibular joint (Figure 25.9). FOB-guided nasotracheal intubation may be achieved without manipulation of the jaw and may be the intubation technique requested by the surgeon. Gentle use of a videolaryngoscope may also help to reduce the risk of fracture displacement in susceptible patients.

For zygomatic fractures an oral tube may be sufficient in some cases, but often a nasal tube is preferred if correction of malocclusion is required.

Conclusion

Maxillofacial and dental surgery can present many challenges for even the most experienced of anaesthetists. The cornerstone of management is understanding what is required by the surgeon to produce good results. Good communication between the anaesthetic, surgical and critical care teams is essential to optimise patient care and maximise safety.

Further Reading

Coplans MP, Curson I. (1982). Deaths associated with dentistry. *British Dental Journal*, **153**, 357–362.

Hamaekers AE, Henderson JJ. (2011). Equipment and strategies for emergency tracheal access in the adult patient. *Anaesthesia*, **66**, 65–80.

Hernández Altemir F. (1986). The submental route for endotracheal intubation. A new technique. *J Maxillofacial Surgery*, **14**, 64–65.

Kademani D, Tiwana P. (2015). *Atlas of Oral & Maxillofacial Surgery*. St Louis: Elsevier.

Kristensen MS. (2015). Tube tip in pharynx (TTIP) ventilation: simple establishment of ventilation in case of failed mask ventilation. *Acta Anaesthesiologica Scandinavica*, **49**, 252–256.

Marlow TJ, Goltra DD, Schabel SI. (1997). Intracranial placement of a nasotracheal tube after facial fracture: a rare complication. *Journal of Emergency Medicine*, **15**, 187–191.

Shaw S Kumar C, Dodds C. (2010). *The Oxford Textbook of Anaesthesia for Oral and Maxillofacial Surgery*. Oxford: Oxford University Press.

Ear, Nose and Throat Surgery: Airway Management

Basem Abdelmalak and Anil Patel

Patients undergoing ear nose and throat (ENT, otorhinolaryngeal) surgery probably present more airway management challenges than any other branch of surgery. ENT procedures encompass a range of operations varying in duration, severity and complexity from high-volume cases such as myringotomy, simple nasal procedures and tonsillectomy through to complex resection and reconstructive surgeries for head and neck cancer. In all cases the surgical team operates close to the airway and in many within the airway, which is therefore shared with the anaesthetist. For a successful outcome these 'shared airway' procedures require close communication and cooperation between anaesthetist and surgeon, an understanding of each other's challenges, knowledge of specialist equipment, and a thorough preoperative evaluation to identify potential risk factors for poor perioperative outcomes.

Airway Safety and Maintenance

Factors affecting airway safety and maintenance during ENT surgery may be classified into eight groups.

- Patient factors. Patients may present with distorted upper airway anatomy and/or airway obstruction. Airway reactivity is more prevalent than in other surgical groups.
- Physical space factors. After surgery has begun the anaesthetist is remote from the airway, making adjustments more difficult and disruptive to the surgical procedure.
- Surgical factors. Significant lateral rotation of the head may be required for ear procedures and head extension for neck procedures. During intra-oral procedures instruments to keep the mouth open may obstruct the airway.
- Anatomical factors. Shared airway procedures involve surgery of the glottis, subglottis and trachea and require an understanding of the necessary special equipment, techniques and laser safety (when used).

- Procedure-specific factors:
  - Throat packs. Oropharyngeal and nasopharyngeal packs should be specifically recorded and accounted for at the end of the procedure. Failure to do this has led to fatal airway obstruction during or after emergence.
  - Airway soiling. For nasal and intra-oral surgery, the airway requires protection from blood and debris.
  - Coroner's clot. Direct inspection and suction clearance of blood and debris from the oro- and nasopharynx as well as the tracheobronchial tree should be undertaken at the end of the procedure to avoid a potentially deadly (Coroner's) clot in the airway.
- Recovery factors. ENT operations, particularly intra-oral, laryngeal, subglottic and tracheal procedures, have a more challenging recovery profile compared with the general surgical population with a higher incidence of coughing, laryngospasm and desaturation following tracheal extubation.

Face Mask

Historically, face mask ventilation was used for simple, short ear procedures such as myringotomy and tube (grommet) insertion. The patient retained spontaneous ventilation but this required the anaesthetist to hold the face mask and the surgeon to work around the anaesthetist's hands and the face mask. Most of these short duration procedures are now undertaken with a supraglottic airway (SGA). The quality of airway management with the SGA is superior to a face mask with better oxygenation, improved seal, less oropharyngeal air leak, better monitoring of tidal gases particularly at low flow, and with less operating room (OR) pollution. Surgical conditions are superior for ear surgery in children with an SGA compared with use of face mask because there is less movement of the surgical field.

Tracheal Tube

Tracheal tubes are commonly used in ENT surgery. Reinforced (flexible) tubes are useful for procedures where head and neck movements and positioning are anticipated for surgery. Caudad-facing oral tubes, such as the Ring–Adair–Elway (RAE) tube, are particularly suitable for surgery involving the pharynx where a gag is used. The advantages of using an oral tracheal tube are: (i) familiarity with its use, (ii) relative resistance to compression if using a wire-reinforced tube, (iii) the ability to secure and protect the *lower airway – distal to tube cuff –* from blood and debris in the oropharynx and regurgitated gastric contents, (iv) avoiding laryngospasm that may be encountered with mask or SGA ventilation, (v) allows for using higher-pressure ventilation when needed and (vi) less chance for losing the airway during surgery.

Extubation and Recovery

Tracheal extubation is usually undertaken with the patient awake; however, some anaesthetists consider 'deep' extubation as well and/or use of an SGA (often a flexible laryngeal mask airway, FLMA) as part of the extubation strategy (staged extubation).

For nasal surgery awake extubation involves removal of the tracheal tube when the patient responds to commands and makes purposeful attempts to remove the tracheal tube. The advantage of awake extubation for nasal surgery is the intrinsic airway control in an awake patient with better return of laryngeal reflexes and protection from further airway contamination by blood and secretions. The disadvantage is the higher incidence of laryngospasm, coughing, bucking, oxyhaemoglobin desaturation and increased risk of bleeding. That said, many anaesthetists who are specialised in ENT anaesthesia have developed different techniques to facilitate smooth awake extubation avoiding such complications. Some of those techniques include the incorporation of local or systemic (IV) lidocaine just before extubation, and/or a narcotic such as fentanyl, remifentanil, sufentanil, and/or alfentanil.

Deep extubation is used in an attempt to improve the recovery profile; however, for nasal surgery this leaves an unprotected airway. After surgery the nasal airway is often blocked with surgical packs and the patient is dependent on oropharyngeal airflow. In practice this may make it extremely difficult to maintain an airway in an obstructive sleep apnoea patient extubated deep lying on their side.

Considering the above considerations some anaesthetists prefer recovery with an SGA in place as they believe it provides protection of the lower airway from aspiration of blood and a superior recovery profile compared with awake or deep extubation.

Flexible Laryngeal Mask Airway (FLMA)

Amongst SGAs used for ENT surgery the FLMA has a special place and it is especially well suited to use for head and neck surgery including shared airway surgery. The ProSeal LMA has some benefits too but is not suited at all to shared airway surgery (see Chapter 13).

However, the use of any SGA including the FLMA seems to have a regional pattern; in the UK, and certain parts of the world, the FLMA is used in ear, nose and throat procedures including tonsillectomy. The cuff of the device is identical to a standard classic LMA but the flexible shaft is better suited and tolerant to head rotation, flexion and extension during surgery. The successful use of the FLMA requires the acquisition of new skills for the anaesthetist and surgeon. The FLMA requires training and experience for successful use and this is probably the main limitation. An understanding of the device, in particular sizing, insertion, placement and recognition of misplacement, is necessary.

The single greatest problem with the FLMA is placement. Unless a scrupulous technique is used (usually digital placement) that ensures that the mask portion is delivered deep into the hypopharynx and facing correctly there is risk of displacement and axial rotation. This will lead to poor device performance and poor airway protection.

During recovery the FLMA is tolerated better than a tracheal tube during emergence and can be left in place until return of protective reflexes. The improved recovery profile leads to a smoother recovery with a reduced incidence of respiratory complications including: coughing, bucking, straining, airway obstruction, laryngospasm and desaturation.

In other parts of the world, the tracheal tube is the preferred airway to use for the reasons mentioned above regarding airway protection, and the preference of some surgeons, as the tracheal tube has a lower profile in the oral cavity compared with an SGA.

FLMA: Nasal Surgery

Using an FLMA during nasal surgery requires care and attention to detail and if there is incorrect sizing or insertion, malposition, dislodgement or suboptimal recovery there is the potential for airway obstruction and blood contamination of the airway.

It seems intuitive that a tracheal tube would protect the airway more effectively than a FLMA because of the seal offered by contact of the tracheal tube cuff on the tracheal wall; however, this may not be completely true. The tracheal cuff is below the glottic and subglottic airway and blood can pass down from the nasopharynx, past a throat pack, along the outer surface of the tracheal tube to the level of the vocal cords, subglottis and upper trachea. In contrast, a correctly placed FLMA covers and protects the supraglottic and glottic airway and blood is diverted laterally to the pyriform sinus and post-cricoid region.

Direct comparisons of airway contamination by flexible optical bronchoscope (FOB) examination at the end of nasal surgery show patients managed with a FLMA are significantly less likely to have blood staining the airway (glottis and trachea) than patients managed with a tracheal tube. The FLMA effectively and satisfactorily protects the glottic and tracheobronchial airway from blood exposure during nasal and sinus surgery and may offer *better* protection of the tracheobronchial airway than a tracheal tube in many instances.

Those who are in favour of using FLMA believe that the emergence quality and overall airway protection following nasal surgery appear to be *better* for a FLMA than a tracheal tube – and it is certainly true that emergence with an SGA is better than with a tracheal tube in other settings. This must be balanced against the potential for misplacement and intraoperative problems that arise with the FLMA, especially when used by an inexperienced anaesthetist or with an inexperienced surgeon.

Whether the airway is managed by FLMA or tracheal tube, if there is considerable bleeding from nasal/sinus surgery an orogastric tube should be inserted to evacuate any blood that may have entered the stomach, before waking the patient up, to decrease the risks of post-operative nausea, vomiting and aspiration.

FLMA: Tonsillectomy

The use of a FLMA for tonsillectomy is an advanced technique and requires an experienced anaesthetist who is familiar with the insertion and maintenance of the device and a surgeon who is competent at working around a FLMA. In small children, the inexperienced should not use a FLMA for tonsillectomy.

The use of a FLMA for tonsillectomy requires close cooperation and meticulous attention to detail by both the anaesthetist and surgeon. Particularly, care is required by the surgeon on placement and opening of the mouth gag and intraoperative manipulation of the gag. Mechanical obstruction during the use of a tonsillar gag varies from 2% to 20% and for the majority of these cases the obstruction is correctable. Access to the inferior pole of the tonsil has been documented as being more difficult.

The FLMA is removed when patients open their eyes to command. The cuff should remain inflated enabling blood and secretions on the backplate to be suctioned out as the FLMA is removed from the mouth.

Potential advantages of using a FLMA for tonsillectomy are (i) the superior recovery profile with fewer episodes of bronchospasm, laryngospasm and desaturation, (ii) less aspiration of blood when compared with an uncuffed tracheal tube and (iii) better protection of the lower away from blood and secretions until awake.

The alternative to the FLMA for tonsillectomy is the use of a standard or oral RAE tracheal tube. A cuffed tracheal tube will also provide good protection of the lower airway at the end of surgery (Figures 26.1–26.3). The anaesthetist will need to make a clear decision about deep extubation or with the patient fully awake.

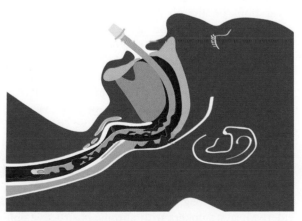

Figure 26.1 Uncuffed tube – note blood can pass tube.

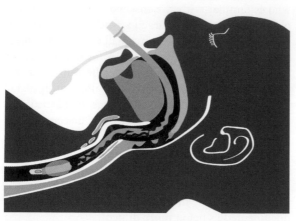

Figure 26.2 Cuffed tube – note blood can pass down to cuff.

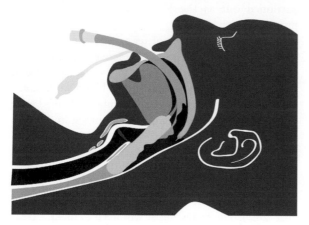

Figure 26.3 Correctly placed LMA protects laryngeal inlet from soiling.

Laryngeal Surgery

Operations on the airway are unique in that both anaesthetist and surgeon are working in the same anatomical field. The anaesthetist is concerned with oxygen delivery, removal of carbon dioxide (ventilation), maintenance of an adequate airway and the prevention of soiling of the tracheobronchial tree, while the surgeon requires an adequate view of a clear motionless operating field. Close cooperation and communication between anaesthetist and surgeon are essential for success. Patients presenting for laryngeal surgery vary from young healthy individuals, with voice changes secondary to benign vocal cord pathology (e.g. small nodules and polyps), to elderly, heavy smokers with chronic obstructive pulmonary disease and alcohol users/abusers with

Table 26.1 The ideal anaesthetic technique - goals

Simple to use
Provide complete control of the airway
No risk of aspiration
Control ventilation with adequate oxygenation
Provide smooth induction and stable maintenance of anaesthesia
Provide a clear motionless surgical field, free of secretions
No time restrictions on the surgeon
No risk of airway fire
No cardiovascular instability
Allow safe emergence with no coughing, bucking, breath-holding or laryngo/bronchospasm
Produce a pain-free, comfortable, alert patient with minimum hangover effects upon emergence

malnutrition and liver disease presenting with stridor caused by glottic carcinoma.

The Ideal Anaesthetic for Laryngeal Surgery

There is no 'ideal anaesthetic technique' (Table 26.1) for all laryngoscopy procedures. The technique chosen will be dependent on (i) the patient's general condition, (ii) the size, mobility and location of the lesion and (iii) surgical requirements including the use of a laser.

The presence of a standard polyvinyl chloride (PVC) cuffed tracheal tube, whilst providing control of the airway and preventing aspiration, may obscure a glottic lesion and is not 'laser safe'. A cuffed laser tube provides some protection against laser-induced airway fires but has a greater external diameter to internal diameter ratio and may obscure laryngeal lesions. Jet ventilation techniques require special equipment and knowledge and understanding of their limitations and do not protect the airway from soiling.

Preoperative Assessment

Causes of laryngeal pathology are listed in Table 26.2.

At the end of the preoperative assessment, the anaesthetist should have some idea of the size, mobility, vascularity and location of the lesion. Standard airway assessments to predict the ease of ventilation, visualisation of the laryngeal inlet and tracheal intubation should be performed but should factor in the airway pathology and its impact on airway management (Table 26.3).

The severity and size of lesions at the glottic level are assessed by direct or indirect laryngoscopy undertaken by ENT surgeons in an outpatient setting and a photograph of the findings is often recorded in the notes (Figures 26.4–26.7). The anaesthetist may perform their own assessment with nasendoscopy (also see Chapter 6). Information about subglottic and tracheal lesions is provided by chest radiography, CT and MRI.

Table 26.2 Causes of vocal cord pathology

Cysts
Polyps
Nodules
Sulcus
Granulomas
Papillomas
Haemangiomas
Reinke's oedema
Microweb
Post-operative scarring or stenosis
Congenital lesions
Malignant tumours
Paralysis
Fixation

Lesion size gives an indication of potential airflow obstruction. Stridor indicates a significantly narrowed airway. In the adult, stridor implies that the airway diameter is probably less than 5 mm, but the absence of stridor does not exclude a narrowed airway, especially if the lesion is chronic.

Very mobile lesions (e.g. multiple large vocal cord polyps or papillomas) may cause *partial* airway obstruction following induction of anaesthesia but *total* airway obstruction is extremely uncommon. Obstruction may change (worsen) after induction of anaesthesia because of the loss of supporting tone in the oropharynx and laryngo-hypopharynx collapsing the airway.

Supraglottic lesions, if mobile, can obstruct the airway or make visualisation of the laryngeal inlet difficult. Subglottic lesions may allow a good view of the laryngeal inlet but may cause difficulty during the passage of a tracheal tube.

Table 26.3 Preoperative assessment of laryngeal lesions

Assessment	Implication
History of endoscopic procedures	Previous difficulty, severity, vascularity and site of obstruction. Anaesthetic technique used
Hoarse voice	Non-specific symptom. Can occur without airway compromise
Voice changes	Non-specific symptom. Minor lesions can change the voice
Dysphagia	Significant and suggests supraglottic obstruction. If associated with carcinoma implies upper oesophageal extension
Altered breathing position	Significant. Patients with partially obstructing lesions will compensate by changing their body positioning to limit airway obstruction
Unable to lie flat	Significant. Suggests severe airway obstruction and patients may need to sleep upright, could also signify recurrent aspiration (e.g. after oesophagectomy with stomach pull through)
Breathing difficulty during sleep	Significant. Difficulty in breathing at night or waking up at night in a panic suggests severe airway obstruction
Inspiratory noise – stridor	Significant and indicates critical airway obstruction with over 50% reduction in airway diameter and in adults an airway diameter of less than 5 mm
Stridor on exertion	Significant. Suggests airway obstruction is becoming critical. Patients may have no stridor at rest
Stridor at rest	Significant. Critical airway obstruction is present
Inspiratory stridor	Significant. Suggests extrathoracic airway obstruction
Expiratory noise – wheeze	Significant. Suggests intrathoracic airway obstruction
Absence of stridor or wheeze	Generally reassuring BUT in exhausted adults and children there is limited chest movements and insufficient airflow to generate enough turbulent flow for stridor. These circumstances suggest life-threatening compromise. After chronic airway obstruction stridor may also decrease
Awake flexible optical laryngoscopy ('nasendoscopy')	All adult patients should have this to visualise the vocal cords. In patients with symptoms and signs of severe airway obstruction great care must be taken to avoid local anaesthetic and scope contact with the vocal cords precipitating total airway obstruction
CXR/CT/MRI scans	Can identify severity and depth of glottic, subglottic, tracheal and intrathoracic lesions

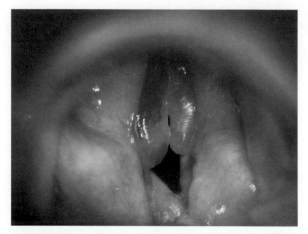

Figure 26.4 Bilateral Reinke's oedema on vocal cords.

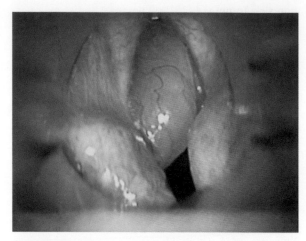

Figure 26.5 Large vocal cord cyst occluding the majority of the airway.

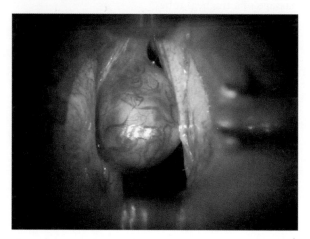

Figure 26.6 Vocal cord polyp.

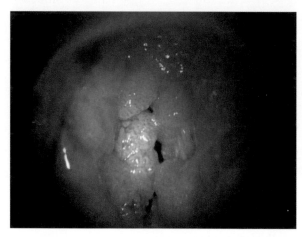

Figure 26.7 Extensive vocal cord papilloma.

Anaesthetic Techniques for Laryngoscopy

For the majority of benign vocal cord lesions and early malignant lesions, airway obstruction is not a feature. Where airway obstruction is anticipated, the anaesthetic plan will change but for non-obstructing lesions a number of anaesthetic techniques are suitable.

Anaesthetic techniques can be broadly classified into two groups: *closed* systems in which a cuffed tracheal tube is employed with protection of the lower airway and *open* systems in which no tube is used leaving the airway 'open'. Open systems use spontaneous ventilation, jet ventilation or oxygen high flow techniques.

The decision to use a closed or open technique will be dependent upon the experience of the anaesthetist

and surgeon, the equipment available, the requirements for surgical access, the size, mobility and location of the lesion and its vascularity. The technique chosen for any given procedure is not absolute and may have to change as surgical and anaesthetic requirements change. For example, an open system using jet ventilation on a lesion thought to be relatively avascular may change to a closed system employing a cuffed tracheal tube if the lesion is bleeding with the risk of soiling of the airway. Conversely a system employing a cuffed tracheal tube may have to change during surgery to an open system if the tracheal tube overlies a lesion making surgery very difficult or impossible.

Induction Technique for Laryngoscopy

An intravenous induction technique is suitable for the vast majority of benign and early malignant glottic lesions where airway obstruction is not anticipated. After intravenous induction of anaesthesia and administration of muscle relaxants appropriate to the length of surgery laryngoscopy is undertaken to visualise the larynx, establish laryngoscopy grade and local anaesthetic such as lidocaine may be administered topically. This improves cardiovascular stability, reduces airway reflexes and smooths recovery. Confirmation of pathology is important because the disease may have progressed since the last outpatient visit and the anaesthetic plan may have to change.

Closed Systems

Closed systems employ a tracheal tube with an inflatable cuff and include microlaryngeal tubes (MLT), ultra-thin tubes that need expiratory ventilatory assistance (see Chapter 18) and laser tubes (Table 26.4).

Open Systems

Open systems include spontaneous/insufflation techniques, intermittent apnoea techniques, high flow oxygen and jet ventilation techniques (Table 26.4).

Spontaneous/insufflation ventilation

Spontaneous ventilation and insufflation techniques are useful in the removal of foreign bodies, evaluation of airway dynamics (tracheomalacia) and paediatric airways. Both techniques require a spontaneously breathing patient and enable a clear view of an unobstructed glottis (Table 26.5).

Inhalational induction is commenced with sevoflurane in 100% oxygen. At a suitable depth of anaesthesia as assessed by clinical observations on the rate and depth of respiration, pupil size, eye reflexes, blood pressure and heart rate changes, laryngoscopy is undertaken and topical local anaesthetic is administered above, below and at the level of the vocal cords. Then 100% oxygen is administered by face mask with spontaneous ventilation and anaesthesia continued with inhalational (insufflation) or an intravenous anaesthetic technique (propofol infusion). At a suitable depth of anaesthesia, again assessed by clinical observations, the surgeon undertakes rigid laryngoscopy or bronchoscopy.

Insufflation of anaesthetic gases and agents can be via a number of routes:

- Small catheter introduced into the nasopharynx and placed above the laryngeal opening
- Tracheal tube cut short and placed through the nasopharynx emerging just beyond the soft palate
- Nasopharyngeal airway
- Side arm or channel of a laryngoscope or bronchoscope

Alternatively, a carefully and expertly titrated intravenous anaesthetic such as propofol or ketamine can be used to provide general anaesthesia while maintaining spontaneous ventilation.

Movements of the vocal cords are minimal or absent despite a spontaneously breathing technique provided an adequate level of anaesthesia is maintained. For satisfactory spontaneously breathing/insufflation techniques an adequate depth of anaesthesia is vital before any instrumentation of the airway takes place. If the depth of anaesthesia is too light, the vocal cords may move, the patient may cough or laryngospasm occur and if too deep, the patient may become apnoeic with cardiovascular instability. Careful observations throughout the procedure, noting movements, respiratory rate and depth, cardiovascular stability and constant observation for unobstructed breathing are vital, with the concentration of volatile anaesthetic or intravenous anaesthetic adjusted accordingly.

Intermittent apnoea

Intermittent apnoea techniques have been described for the laser resection of juvenile laryngeal papillomatosis when the presence of a tracheal tube obstructs surgery (Table 26.6). Following induction of general anaesthesia muscle relaxants are administered followed by tracheal intubation. The patient is hyperventilated with a volatile anaesthetic agent in 100% oxygen. The tracheal tube is then removed, leaving the surgeon a clear, unobstructed, immobile surgical field. After an apnoeic period of typically 2–3 minutes, surgery is stopped, the tracheal tube is reinserted and the patient hyperventilated once more. A total intravenous anaesthesia (TIVA) is an attractive technique for this.

Jet Ventilation (High-Pressure Source Ventilation)

Jet ventilation techniques involve the intermittent administration of high-pressure jets of air, oxygen or air–oxygen mixtures with entrainment of room air. In 1967 Sanders first described a jet ventilation technique using a 16-gauge jet placed down the side arm of a rigid bronchoscope relying on air entrainment to continue ventilation with an open bronchoscope.

Table 26.4 Closed and open techniques for laryngeal surgery

Closed systems

Advantages
- Protection of the lower airway
- Secured airway
- Control of ventilation
- Minimal pollution by volatile agents
- Routine technique for all anaesthetists

Disadvantages
- Limitation of exposure and surgical access
- Risk of laser airway fire when laser safe tubes are not used
- Rare risk of air entrapment and pneumothorax/hypotension with small tubes
- Risk of high inflation pressures

Open systems

Advantages
- Complete laryngeal visualisation
- Minimal risk of tube-related trauma to the glottis
- Laser safe

Disadvantages
- Unprotected lower airway
- Uncontrolled ventilation, and potential for hypoventilation
- Require specialist equipment, knowledge and experience

Table 26.5 Advantages and disadvantages of spontaneously breathing/insufflation techniques

Advantages
- Complete laryngeal visualisation
- Laser safe (no tracheal tube to act as fuel source)
- No tube-related trauma

Disadvantages
- No control over ventilation
- Loss of protective airway reflexes and the potential for airway soiling
- Theatre pollution when volatile agents are used

Table 26.6 Advantages and disadvantages of an intermittent apnoea technique

Advantages
- Immobile, unobstructed surgical field
- Laser safe (no tracheal tube to act as fuel source)

Disadvantages
- Variable levels of anaesthesia when volatile anaesthetics are used
- Interruption to surgery for reintubation
- Potential trauma through multiple reintubation
- The risk of aspiration of blood and debris with the tracheal tube removed

Sanders used intermittent jets of oxygen at 8 breaths min^{-1} and with a driving pressure of 3.5 bar (350 kPa, 2625 mmHg, 50 PSI) to entrain air and showed that the technique maintained a supranormal partial pressure of oxygen with no rise in the partial pressure of carbon dioxide.

Since 1967, modifications to Sanders' original jet ventilation technique have been made for endoscopic airway surgery. These modifications include the *site* at which the jet of gas emerges (supraglottic, subglottic,

transtracheal) and the *frequency* of jet ventilation (low frequency < 60 breaths min^{-1} or high frequency > 60 breaths min^{-1}).

In 1971 Spoerel demonstrated transtracheal jet ventilation and in 1983 Layman reported the use of transtracheal jet ventilation in 60 patients with difficult airways. In 1985, Ravussin designed a dedicated transtracheal catheter and the technique became incorporated in difficult airway algorithms in the late 1990s. Latterly the complications associated with transtracheal jet ventilation, particularly barotrauma in the emergency situation, have become apparent (see Chapter 20).

It is important to note that during low frequency jet ventilation the driving gas is at a high pressure but mode of ventilation is conventional. Traditional tidal volumes are achieved, which is the sum of the jetted 100% oxygen and entrained room air resulting from the negative pressure created by the strong linear oxygen jet. A pressure catheter placed at the trachea will record normal or below normal (negative) depending on the position of its tip within the trachea and the psi of the jetted oxygen. Expiration is by normal elastic recoil of the lungs and via the patient's native airway. Jet ventilation is therefore contraindicated where expiration cannot occur, including during total airway obstruction. The high-pressure source of the driving gas can readily raise the pressure many 100-fold and there is a risk of barotrauma if there is continuous inspiration or if expiration is not completed before inspiration (breath stacking).

High Frequency Jet Ventilation –# High frequency jet ventilation techniques typically use rates around 100–150 per minute. This enables:

1. A continuous expiratory flow of air, enhancing the removal of fragments of blood and debris from the airway

2. Reduced peak and mean airway pressures (compared with low frequency) with improved cardiovascular stability

3. Enhanced diffusion and interregional mixing (compared with low frequency) within the lungs resulting in more efficient ventilation

These advantages are of particular importance in patients with significant lung disease and obesity. High frequencies are achieved by automated high frequency jet ventilators, such as Monsoon or TwinStream ventilators, which have alarms and automatic interruption of jet flow when preset pause pressure limits have been reached (i.e. blockage of entrainment or exhalation have occurred). During ENT procedures both manual low frequency techniques (which deliver conventional ventilation) or high frequency techniques are appropriate. High frequency jet ventilation is also used as a mode of ventilation in neonatal and paediatric ICUs.

Jet Ventilation Techniques – Jet ventilation techniques are suitable for the vast majority of benign glottic pathology and early malignancy where airway obstruction is not anticipated. Ideally, the surgeon prepares to insert the rigid (suspension) laryngoscope onto which a jetting needle has been attached in preparation for supraglottic jet, before the induction of anaesthesia. A typical jet ventilation technique will include pre-oxygenation followed by intravenous induction and administration of a muscle relaxant. Mask ventilation is maintained while the muscle relaxation is taking effect, then immediately followed by suspension laryngoscopy! If for any reason, the surgeon requires longer time to prepare the rigid (suspension) laryngoscope, the airway may be maintained with an SGA. Anaesthesia is maintained with an infusion of propofol, supplemented by bolus or infusion of alfentanil or remifentanil. At the end of surgery, an SGA is reinserted and muscle relaxation reversed before emergence.

During the procedure, the adequacy of jet ventilation should be continuously assessed by observation of chest rise and fall (to ensure complete exhalation), oxygen saturation and by listening for changes to the sound during air entrainment and exhalation. The patency of the airway and any surgical obstruction can also be assessed by watching the endoscopic image on a video screen. Set-ups for supraglottic, subglottic and transtracheal jet ventilation are shown in Figure 26.8.

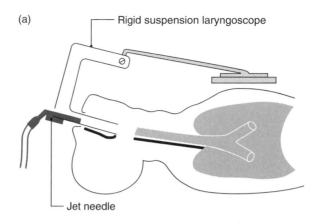

(a) Rigid suspension laryngoscope
Jet needle

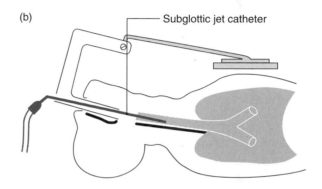

(b) Subglottic jet catheter

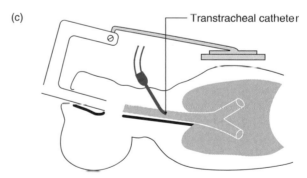

(c) Transtracheal catheter

Figure 26.8 The three sites used for jet ventilation: (a) supraglottic, (b) subglottic and (c) transtracheal.

Supraglottic Jet Ventilation – Supraglottic jet ventilation describes a technique in which a rigid suspension laryngoscope is placed by the surgeon with its tapered tip at the glottis and a jetting needle attached to the laryngoscope enables gas to emerge in the supraglottic area and ventilate the lungs. Alignment of the suspension laryngoscope with the airway is essential to success of the technique and requires careful cooperation between the surgeon and anaesthetist. It is important that the vocal cords do not move, both for ventilation and safe surgery, and so muscle relaxation should be maintained. High or low frequency ventilation can be employed. See Table 26.7.

Subglottic Jet Ventilation – During subglottic jet ventilation a small (2–3 mm diameter) catheter or specifically designed tube (Benjet, Hunsaker catheter and Tritube) is placed through the glottis and into the trachea. This enables delivery of a jet of gas directly into the trachea (see Table 26.8).

Transtracheal Jet Ventilation – Transtracheal catheter placement can be performed after general anaesthesia for elective laryngeal surgery and under local anaesthetic in patients with significant airway pathology. Compared with supraglottic and subglottic jet techniques, transtracheal techniques carry the greatest risk

Table 26.7 Advantages and disadvantages of supraglottic jet ventilation

Advantages
- Clear, unobstructed view for the surgeon
- No risk of a laser-induced airway fire

Disadvantages
- Risk of barotrauma with pneumothorax, pneumomediastinum and subcutaneous emphysema
- Gastric distension with entrained air
- Misalignment of the suspension laryngoscope or jetting needle resulting in poor ventilation
- Blood and debris or fragments being blown into the distal trachea
- Vibrations and movements of the vocal cords
- Inability to monitor end-tidal carbon dioxide concentration (in some jet systems)

Table 26.8 Advantages and disadvantages of subglottic jet ventilation

Advantages
- Greater minute ventilation at any given driving pressure (compared with supraglottic)
- Greater minute ventilation at any given frequency (compared with supraglottic)
- Minimal influence on ventilation of laryngoscope alignment to the laryngotracheal axis
- No vocal cord movements
- No time constraints for the surgeon in the placement of the rigid laryngoscope

Disadvantages
- Potential for a laser-induced airway fire (laser-resistant tubes are available, e.g. Hunsaker)
- Greater risk of barotrauma compared with supraglottic techniques

of barotrauma and a high risk of subcutaneous emphysema. Its use for benign glottic pathology should be questioned and requires careful evaluation of the potential risks and benefits. Other potential problems include: misplacement, blockage, kinking, infection, bleeding and failure to site the catheter.

New Jet Ventilation Technology – Ventrain is a relatively new manual device that enables both active inspiration and expiration through one of the narrow tubes used for subglottic or transtracheal jet ventilation. It can therefore be used for cases where complete airway obstruction (which is a contraindication for traditional jet ventilation) is present or suspected. The ventrain technology has been incorporated into an automated ventilator, the Evone, and may be used with a long narrow (2 mm ID) cuffed tracheal tube (Tritube). These techniques are discussed further in Chapter 18.

High Flow Nasal Cannula Oxygenation Ventilation

Recently Patel et al. described the use of high flow warmed and humidified nasal oxygen (high flow nasal oxygen – HFNO) delivered at 30–70 L min^{-1} for ENT surgery. This technique is able to maintain oxygenation and carbon dioxide clearance in most anaesthetised patients during spontaneous ventilation and during apnoea. During apnoea the partial pressure of carbon dioxide normally rises by approximately 0.5 kPa min^{-1} but HFNO may reduce this to < 0.1 kPa min^{-1}. This therefore can enable prolonged surgery without anaesthetic equipment in the airway (Figure 26.9).

This technique has a potentially major role to play in ENT surgery but it is important to understand its limitations. It will not overcome airway obstruction or pulmonary shunt. In obese patients while there is useful prolongation of safe apnoea time this is still considerably shorter than in non-obese patients. Due to the high concentration of oxygen throughout the upper airway there is a risk of airway fire and it is now generally accepted that HFNO should not be used with laser or diathermy. HFNO is also discussed in Chapter 8.

Head and Neck Surgery

Head and neck surgery involves the treatment of patients with diseases of the upper airway, larynx and pharynx. When airway compromise is not an issue most procedures are largely uneventful. When

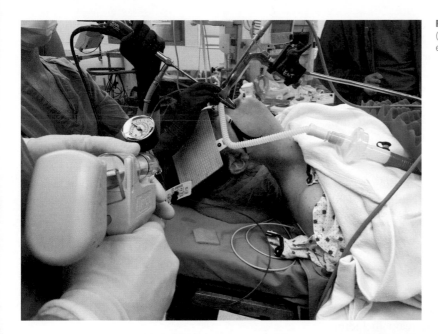

Figure 26.9 High flow nasal oxygen (HFNO) for surgery without anaesthetic equipment in the airway.

airway compromise is a feature, the anaesthetic plan needs to change according to the severity and site of obstruction.

Major head and neck procedures include laryngectomy, pharyngolaryngectomy, radical neck dissection and the resection of large thyroid or parotid lesions. A laryngectomy involves the resection of the larynx and the creation of an end-tracheal stoma, a pharyngolaryngectomy also resects structures within the pharynx including part or all of the tongue and oesophagus. A radical neck dissection resects sternomastoid, internal and external jugular veins and cervical lymph nodes.

The treatment of upper airway tumours depends on the staging (Tumour, Node, Metastasis – TNM classification) and site. The principal treatment options include chemotherapy, radiotherapy, laser endoscopic resection, transoral laser surgery, major soft tissue and organ excision, radical neck dissection and flap reconstruction, alone or in combination.

All patients with airway compromise should be considered as a potentially difficult intubation, whereas not all patients with a difficult intubation have airway compromise.

Patients with No Airway Compromise

Laryngeal pathology without symptoms or signs of airway compromise, such as early T1 and some T2 tumours, can be managed by a number of anaesthetic techniques including intravenous induction of general anaesthesia and placement of a cuffed tracheal or laser

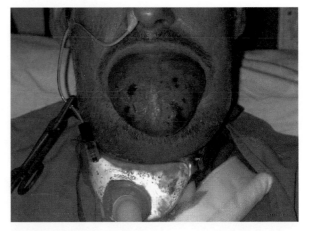

Figure 26.10 Massive tongue swelling causing airway compromise.

tube. Alternatively, a supraglottic or subglottic jet ventilation technique can be employed for biopsy and laser resection.

Patients with Airway Compromise

The recognition of a compromised or anatomically distorted upper airway is paramount in the preoperative assessment of head and neck patients. For elective procedures a detailed history, examination and investigations can be undertaken, but for more urgent procedures with severe airway compromise investigations may not be possible. Anaesthetic management will depend on the urgency of the intervention, site of the lesion, size of the lesion, level of obstruction, extension of the lesion and degree of airway compromise (Figure 26.10).

Symptoms and signs of airway compromise include respiratory distress, tachypnea, accessory muscle use, sternal retraction, tracheal tug, stridor, hypoxia, tachycardia, and exhaustion.

Level of Obstruction

Difficult airways can be divided according to the level at which a problem exists (Table 26.9 and Figures 26.11–26.15). Disease states are not confined to these anatomical areas and can pass through many levels.

Management Options

Whatever technique is chosen as the primary anaesthetic technique, a backup plan should be thought through, discussed with the airway team including the surgeon and instituted when difficulties arise (see Table 26.10).

Oral Cavity/Oropharyngeal Lesions

See Figures 26.16 and 26.17. An intravenous induction in these patients may result in airway obstruction and an inability to ventilate or oxygenate. The normal techniques to prevent this such as face mask ventilation with oral or nasal airways may not be effective. The glottis and lower airway are often normal in these patients and the principal problem around intubation is one of bypassing a large obstructing mass without traumatising it whilst maintaining a patent airway. An awake FOB-guided intubation technique is often used in this group of patients. Other anaesthetic techniques include awake transtracheal catheter placement with jet ventilation, and awake tracheostomy.

Table 26.9 Levels of airway obstruction

- Oral cavity
- Oropharynx
- Tongue base and supraglottic
- Glottic
- Subglottic and upper tracheal
- Midtracheal
- Lower tracheal and bronchial

Table 26.10 Potential management options for airway compromise

- Awake intubation by FOB or other technique
- Intravenous induction of general anaesthesia
- Inhalational induction with maintenance of spontaneous ventilation
- Inhalational induction with 'take over' of ventilation
- Asleep FOB-guided intubation
- Awake transtracheal catheter placement and jet ventilation
- Awake tracheostomy under local anaesthesia
- Asleep tracheostomy under general anaesthesia

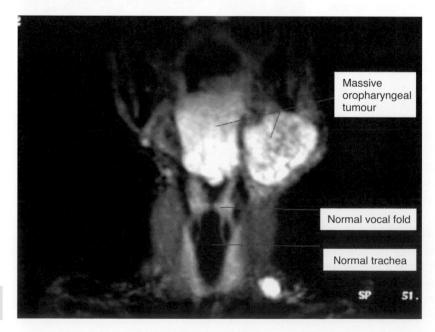

Figure 26.11 Level of obstruction: oropharyngeal tumour.

Massive oropharyngeal tumour

Normal vocal fold

Normal trachea

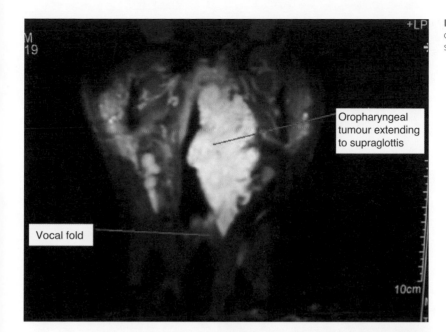

Figure 26.12 Level of obstruction: oropharyngeal tumour extending to supraglottis.

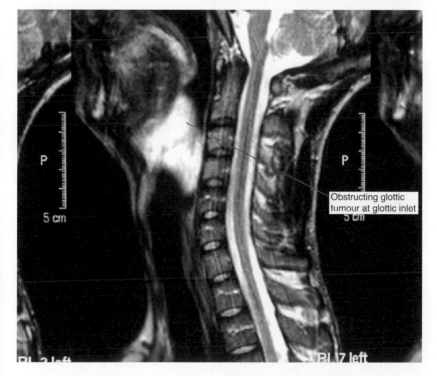

Figure 26.13 Level of obstruction: glottic inlet.

Tongue Base/Supraglottic Lesions

See Figures 26.18–26.20. Even small lesions at the tongue base and supraglottis can have significant effects on the airway because of their location at the entrance to the glottis, and their effect on the epiglottis. As a tongue base lesion expands it fills the space in the vallecula and directs the epiglottis downwards increasing airway obstruction. A large epiglottic or

235

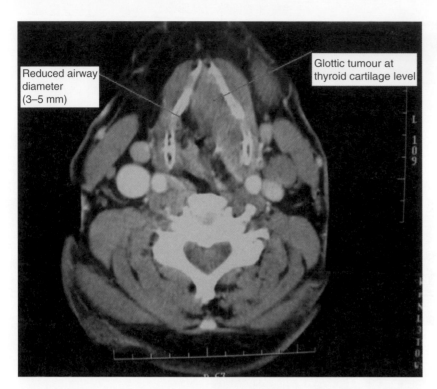

Reduced airway diameter (3–5 mm)

Glottic tumour at thyroid cartilage level

Figure 26.14 Level of obstruction: glottic tumour with grossly narrowed airway.

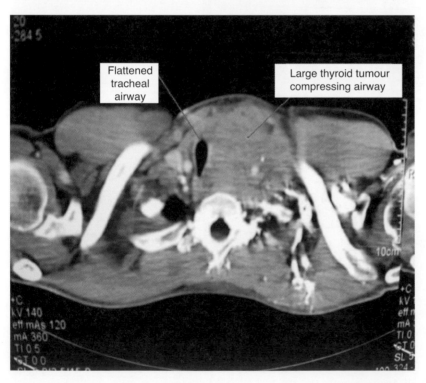

Flattened tracheal airway

Large thyroid tumour compressing airway

Figure 26.15 Level of obstruction: compressed trachea.

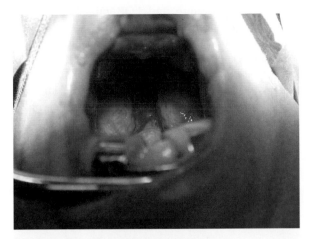

Figure 26.16 Oral cavity with large tonsils.

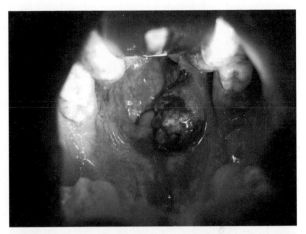

Figure 26.17 Oral cavity with right-sided tonsillar tumour.

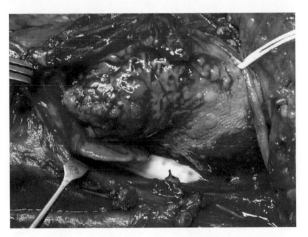

Figure 26.18 Tongue base cancer during resection. Note tracheal tube and downward displacement of the epiglottis.

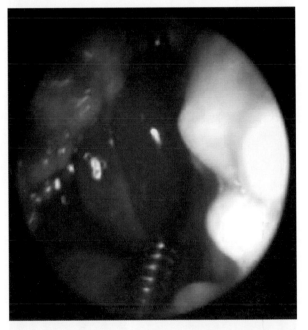

Figure 26.19 Acute epiglottitis with cherry red appearance.

vallecular cyst results in airway obstruction and compromise in a similar manner to epiglottitis. The danger of an intravenous induction in these patients is airway obstruction following the loss of supportive tone from the soft tissues. An oral or nasal airway may be ineffective in relieving the obstruction, and a strong jaw thrust which displaces the mandible and tongue base forward may create an airspace at the supraglottic inlet, but this is not guaranteed to be effective.

Standard curved blade laryngoscopy can traumatise any lesion at the tongue base and vallecula, causing bleeding and swelling with the potential for complete airway obstruction. Although straight blade laryngoscopy aims to pass below the epiglottic tip and lift the

epiglottis upwards, this can be difficult with a distorted epiglottis. Great care and attention needs to be taken during attempted laryngoscopy with these lesions.

In any patient in whom there is concern about a lesion at the tongue base or supraglottis, or in whom there is evidence of significant airway obstruction, an awake FOB-guided intubation, awake transtracheal catheter, or an awake tracheostomy with local anaesthetic should be considered.

Glottic Lesions

See Figures 26.21–26.23. Awake FOB-guided techniques are ideal for oral cavity, oropharyngeal and tongue base lesions because they *pass around* the mass, but are unsuitable for advanced obstructing laryngeal disease in which the FOB has to *pass through* the mass as this will cause complete airway occlusion. This is tolerated poorly by patients and can result in complications. Good topical anaesthesia is also difficult to achieve in this group and FOB-guided intubation through an anatomically distorted, large, vascular, friable, necrotic tumour is often technically difficult.

Some experts advocate inhalational induction techniques for the obstructed airway in which spontaneous ventilation is maintained throughout. That said, inhalational induction for advanced laryngeal tumours with airway obstruction is difficult, slow, extremely challenging and often fails.

Physiological problems include a reduction in airflow with spontaneous ventilation, an increased

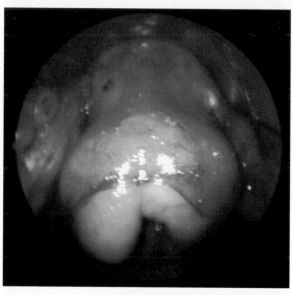

Figure 26.20 Chronic inflammatory epiglottitis.

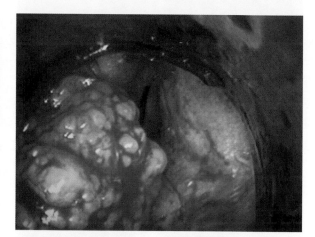

Figure 26.21 Glottic lesion, extensive carcinoma.

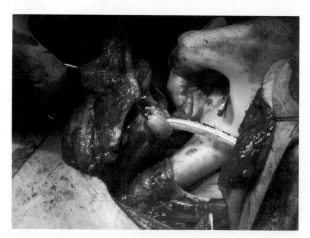

Figure 26.22 During laryngectomy showing tube through glottis and finger in upper oesophagus.

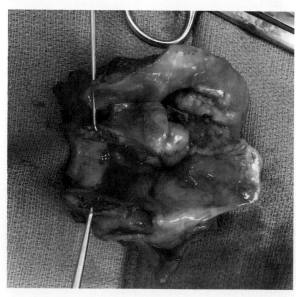

Figure 26.23 Glottic mass extending from supra- to infra-glottic regions.

collapsibility of the airway, increased work of breathing, critical instability at points of narrowing leading to further airway collapse, and a reduction in functional residual capacity. Induction is slow with apnoeic periods and episodes of obstruction are common. Patients often become more hypoxic and hypercarbic with long periods of instability, arrhythmias and apnoea.

The traditional view is that the inhalational technique is safe because if the patient obstructs, the volatile agent will no longer be taken up, and the patient will lighten up. This frequently does not happen and the technique is therefore often unreliable and at its worst unsafe.

Controversy exists as to the suitability of 'taking over' the patient's own spontaneous ventilation with bag-mask ventilation. Taking over ventilation allows a suitable depth of anaesthesia for laryngoscopy to be achieved more easily, but overrides all the claimed advantages of maintaining spontaneous ventilation. It does avoid the long periods of spontaneous ventilation waiting for an adequate depth of anaesthesia in which the patient may become unstable.

Other experts consider the inhalational technique to be too prone to difficulty and complication in this group of patients and advocate an intravenous induction and administration of a muscle relaxant to provide optimum ventilation and intubating conditions. This relies on the subsequent ability to intubate and clear backup plans if this fails. The differences in expert opinion highlight the complexity of these patients and their high-risk nature. These cases are not suitable for the anaesthetist who only has general experience and are best managed by those with significant experience in this field.

Whichever anaesthetic technique is chosen, at a suitable depth of anaesthesia laryngoscopy is undertaken and the best chance of success is usually at the first attempt when bleeding, trauma and swelling are minimal. Videolaryngoscopy will reduce forces used and optimise laryngeal view. A gum elastic bougie may be useful to negotiate the narrowed airway. Failure to intubate requires an urgent tracheostomy or cricothyroidotomy and the surgeon should be gowned and immediately ready.

Transtracheal catheter placement under local anaesthesia at a level below the distal margin of the tumour is a recognised technique for the difficult airway. The catheter is placed usually at the level of the second or third tracheal rings, avoiding the tumour and the risk of bleeding and tumour seeding. Once catheter placement has been confirmed in an awake patient by an end-tidal capnography trace, intravenous induction is started. After induction, jet ventilation through the transtracheal catheter is commenced, ideally with a high frequency ventilator with automated cut-off at a preset pause pressure limit to reduce the risk of barotrauma. If a manual jet ventilation technique is used expiration must be confirmed before initiating the next breath. An experienced anaesthetist should remain at the head end of the patient ensuring a patent and adequate upper airway by chin lift, jaw thrust, oral or nasal airway.

Subglottic and Upper Tracheal Lesions

Patients with advanced laryngotracheal stenosis may have airway diameters of 2–4 mm and airway management usually involves a supraglottic jet ventilation technique. It should be noted that mask ventilation through a stenotic trachea due to a subglottic or upper tracheal lesion is usually successful and should be attempted while the muscle relaxant is taking effect to facilitate suspension laryngoscopy/rigid bronchoscopy, and the initiation of a jet ventilation.

Tracheal resection is often used to treat a recurring short segment upper tracheal stenosis resistant to conventional therapy; the airway management would be in stages. It starts with oral tracheal tube insertion, followed by cross-field lower trachea intubation during the resection and posterior tracheal anastomosis phase (i.e. a sterile tracheal tube inserted into the lower end of the divided trachea), followed by reintubation from above under direct vision to facilitate completion of the anterior tracheal anastomosis. Utmost care should be given to a motionless extubation to avoid tracheal disruption from vigorous coughing. See Figures 26.24–26.26.

Mid and Lower Tracheal Lesions

See Figures 26.27–26.31. Tracheal obstruction can be caused by lesions arising within the trachea itself or by compression from surrounding structures or tumours. The upper airway is usually normal at laryngoscopy. Airway problems are caused by an inability to pass a tracheal tube distal to the obstruction and the fact that a front of neck airway will not resolve the problem. For mediastinal masses compressing the lower trachea, awake FOB-guided intubation should be considered, anaesthesia is then maintained with gradual increase in depth while maintaining spontaneous ventilation to the point at

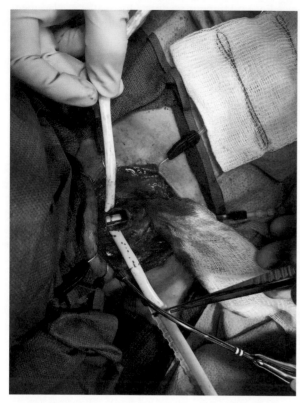

Figure 26.24 Tracheal resection, 1/3: the oro-tracheal tube is seen in the trachea.

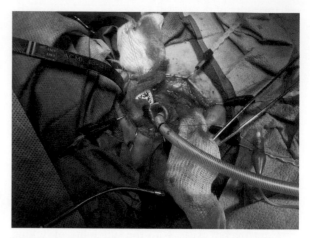

Figure 26.25 Tracheal resection, 2/3: a sterile tracheal tube inserted into the lower end of the divided trachea.

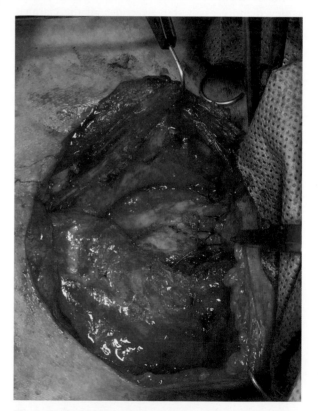

Figure 26.26 Tracheal resection, 3/3: the patient is reintubated from above to facilitate completion of the anterior tracheal anastomosis.

which insertion of a rigid bronchoscope is possible. As soon as the vocal cords are seen through the rigid bronchoscope, the tracheal tube is removed, and the trachea is intubated with the rigid bronchoscope. Subsequently the lesion is dealt with whether by a temporising measure by inserting a silicone Y stent at the carina level, or resection by the thoracic surgery team.

The Returning ENT Patient

Many patients who undergo resection of a head and neck tumour or cervical lymph node dissection with or without neck radiation, with or without reconstruction, return at a later date for follow-up for additional biopsies when tumour recurrence is suspected, or for other surgeries. Extreme caution is advised and should be exercised in evaluating and managing their airways. The altered anatomy due to resection and reconstruction as well as neck radiation are known risk factors for difficult mask ventilation and/or using the conventional direct laryngoscopy technique, thus awake FOB-guided intubation may be the preferred technique. Additionally, radiation-induced changes as well as tumour recurrence may result in trismus, making oral intubation impossible or very difficult at best,

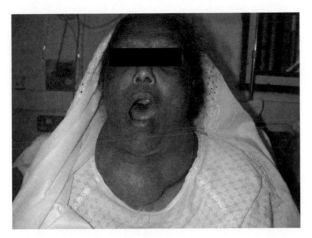

Figure 26.27 Large thyroid mass: awake FOB-guided intubation needed.

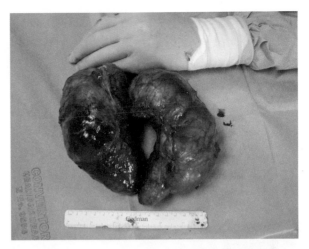

Figure 26.28 Large thyroid mass: post-resection specimen.

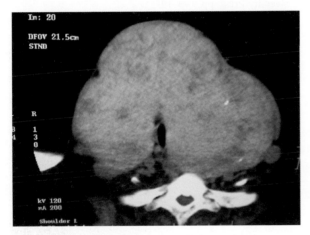

Figure 26.29 Large thyroid mass: grossly flattened trachea.

Figure 26.30 Large thyroid mass: tracheal distortion.

therefore nasal intubation may become the preferred alternative.

Bleeding and the ENT Patient

Bleeding is a common complication of ENT surgery. It may occur after simple procedures such as tonsillectomy or adenoidectomy or after more major head and neck surgery such as thyroidectomy or neck dissection. Blood may therefore be inside the airway soiling it or around the airway compressing and distorting it. It may present in the immediate aftermath of surgery or as a late complication.

It can present problems of

- Difficult airway management due to impaired vision within the airway

- Difficult airway management due to bleeding into the neck and associated oedema caused by interruption of lymphatic drainage
- Risk of aspiration of blood before or during anaesthesia (note cricoid force will not prevent aspiration of blood from bleeding in the nose, mouth or pharynx)
- Actual or potential cardiovascular collapse – including when head and neck reconstructions are compromised by bleeding

These are always high-risk cases that require a clear plan, experienced operators and good anaesthetic and surgical cooperation. The topic is discussed further in Chapter 32.

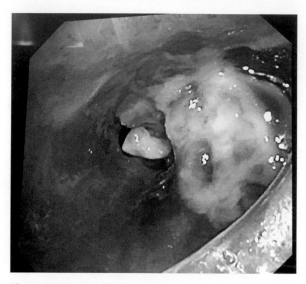

Figure 26.31 Near obstructing intratracheal tumour.

Further Reading

Abdelmalak B, Doyle J (Eds.). (2013). *Text Book of Anesthesia for Otolaryngologic Surgery*. London: Cambridge University Press. ISBN-9781107018679.

Abdelmalak B, Marcanthony N, Abdelmalak J, et al. (2010). Dexmedetomidine for anesthetic management of anterior mediastinal mass. *Journal of Anesthesia*, **24**(4), 607–610.

Abdelmalak B, Sethi S, Gildea T. (2014). Anesthesia and upper and lower airway management for advanced diagnostic and therapeutic bronchoscopy. *Advances in Anesthesia*, **32**, 71–87.

Cook TM, Woodall N, Frerk C; Fourth National Audit Project. (2011). Major complications of airway management in the UK: results of the Fourth National Audit Project of the Royal College of Anaesthetists and the Difficult Airway Society. Part 1: anaesthesia. *British Journal of Anaesthesia*, **106**, 617–631.

George J, Lorenz R, Abdelmalak B. (2017). Airway management for tracheal resection surgery. In: Doyle DJ, Abdelmalak B (Eds.), *Clinical Airway Management: An Illustrated Case-Based Approach*. London: Cambridge University Press. pp. 190–197.

Joffe AM, Aziz MF, Posner KL, et al. (2019). Management of difficult tracheal intubation: a closed claims analysis. *Anesthesiology*, **131**, 818–829.

Patel A, Nouraei SA. (2015).Transnasal Humidified Rapid-Insufflation Ventilatory Exchange (THRIVE): a physiological method of increasing apnoea time in patients with difficult airways. *Anaesthesia*, **70**, 323–329.

Chapter 27

Lung Separation

Jay B. Brodsky

Introduction

The modern practice of thoracic surgery depends on the anaesthetist's ability to collapse and selectively ventilate the lungs. Selective lung collapse facilitates surgical exposure, while anatomical isolation protects the non-operated lung from contamination. Lung isolation and selective collapse are achieved with either a bronchial blocker (BB) or a double-lumen tube (DLT).

Bronchial Blocker (BB)

Lung tissue distal to an obstructed conducting airway will collapse. Modern BBs are thin semi-rigid plastic catheters with a high-volume low-pressure balloon at their distal tip. When inflated the balloon obstructs the airway. Many BBs have an inner channel that can be opened to hasten lung deflation. The channel can be used to suction the lung and for application of continuous positive airway pressure (CPAP).

A BB is introduced under visual guidance using a flexible optical bronchoscope (FOB) alongside or through a tracheal tube (TT), tracheostomy tube or supraglottic airway, into a bronchus. The ETView VivaSight SL (Ambu, Copenhagen, Denmark) is a new TT with an integrated high-resolution imaging camera. Using a BB with this tube does not require an additional endoscope. A three-way connector allows both the BB and FOB to be advanced simultaneously without interrupting ventilation (Figure 27.1).

A variety of independent BBs are available (Figure 27.2).

The Fuji Uniblocker (Teleflex, Wayne, PA, USA) has an angulated distal tip. Digital rotation at the catheter's proximal end directs the tip into either bronchus.

The Cohen Flexitip Endobronchial Blocker (Cook Critical Care, Bloomington, IN, USA) uses a rotational wheel at the operator's end to mechanically manoeuvre the distal tip into position.

The Arndt Endobronchial Blocker (Cook Critical Care) has a wire loop in its central channel. The loop is snared over an FOB, which is then advanced into a bronchus. The loop with the BB is slid over the bronchoscope directly into the bronchus. Once in position, the FOB is removed and the wire is withdrawn into the catheter's lumen.

The EZ-Blocker (AnaesthetIQ BV, Rotterdam, the Netherlands) has a distal end that splits into two 4-cm-long extensions, each with its own balloon. The extensions are symmetrical, with one balloon dyed blue and the other yellow for identification. The EZ-Blocker is advanced into the trachea under FOB control until the **Y** engages the carina preventing further advancement. Either balloon can then be inflated as required. When correctly positioned each extension will be in a main-stem bronchus, so either lung can be collapsed. An EZ-Blocker can be placed 'blindly' if necessary.

A unique approach to bronchial blockade is the Papworth BiVent Tube (P3 Medical Limited, Bristol, UK). It is a single-cuffed DLT with a bifurcated distal end to 'blindly' engage the carina with each lumen opening into one main bronchus. A BB can be advanced down either lumen into the desired bronchus for rapid lung isolation without the need for FOB guidance.

Double-Lumen Tube (DLT)

A DLT consists of two tubes of unequal length moulded together (Figure 27.3). The shorter tube ends in the trachea and the longer tube ends in a main-stem bronchus. There is a cuff above the opening of the shorter 'tracheal lumen' and a second cuff above the distal opening on the 'bronchial lumen'. Proximally the two tubes have their own connectors to attach to a dual lumen catheter mount (Figure 27.3). Adult sizes are 41 Fr, 39 Fr, 37 Fr and 35 Fr.

Inflating only the tracheal cuff enables positive pressure ventilation to both lungs. Inflating both

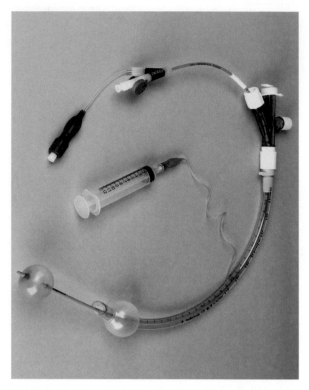

Figure 27.1 A bronchial blocker (BB) is introduced into the airway either alongside or within the lumen of a standard tracheal tube or supraglottic airway. A special three-port connector allows advancement of both the BB and a paediatric flexible optical bronchoscope (FOB) without interfering with ventilation. The FOB allows direct visualisation of BB placement.

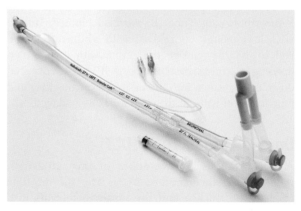

Figure 27.3 Double-lumen tubes (DLTs) consist of two tubes of unequal length moulded together. The shorter tube ends in the trachea and the longer tube in a main bronchus. There is a proximal cuff on the tracheal portion and a distal cuff on the bronchial lumen. Inflating the tracheal cuff allows positive pressure ventilation to both lungs. When both the bronchial and tracheal cuffs are inflated, the lungs can be ventilated together or separately. Selectively clamping the lumen to either lung at a connector at the proximal end of the DLT enables separation and collapse of that lung, while ventilation continues through the unclamped lumen to the other lung.

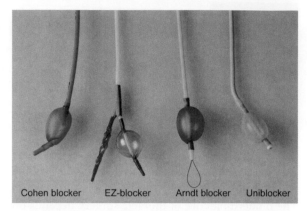

| Cohen blocker | EZ-blocker | Arndt blocker | Uniblocker |

Figure 27.2 Several different independent bronchial blockers are shown.

cuffs enables both lungs to be ventilated separately: clamping one of the lumens of the catheter mount will stop ventilation to that lung, while ventilation can continue to the other lung. If the catheter mount tubing to the non-ventilated lung is then detached that lung will collapse.

DLTs are constructed of clear plastic, which enables observation of condensation, blood or purulent material coming from the lungs. Suction catheters or a paediatric FOB can be passed down either lumen. The bronchial cuff is usually dyed blue for easy visual identification.

Human airway anatomy is asymmetric. The left main bronchus is longer (average 5.4 cm males, 5.0 cm females) than the right main bronchus (average 2.3 cm males, 2.1 cm females). In as many as 10% of adults the right upper-lobe bronchus originates at the carina or even in the trachea. DLTs are designed for intubation of either the left or the right bronchus. Either tube can be used to isolate either lung, but a left DLT is usually preferred. A left DLT has a greater 'margin of safety' since there is less chance of it obstructing the ipsilateral upper-lobe bronchus. Right DLTs have an additional slot in the bronchial lumen wall to reduce the risk of obstructing the upper-lobe orifice. Right DLTs are used when placement of a left DLT is impractical or unsafe.

Selecting a DLT based on height and gender has a poor correlation with actual airway size. The width of the left bronchus and/or trachea can be measured from the patient's chest radiograph or CT scan. Left main bronchial width can be accurately estimated from tracheal width using the formula:

Left Bronchial Width$_{mm}$ = (0.68) Tracheal Width$_{mm}$.

If the dimensions of the DLT and left bronchus are known an appropriate size left DLT can be chosen for that patient.

A large DLT is preferred for several reasons:

- There is less resistance to airflow during one-lung ventilation through a larger lumen and less chance of developing auto-PEEP (positive end-expiratory pressure) and air trapping in patients with chronic obstructive pulmonary disease.
- A larger lumen more easily accommodates an FOB or suction catheter.
- Larger DLTs cannot be advanced as far into the airway as smaller tubes, reducing the chance of malpositioning.
- The bronchial cuff of a large DLT requires less air to seal the bronchus, which in turn may reduce the risk of trauma from overinflation.

A DLT can be placed by clinical examination and auscultation, followed by bronchoscopy to confirm or adjust position. Alternatively, a DLT can be directly guided into the intended bronchus using an FOB. The VivaSight DL DLT (Ambu, Copenhagen, Denmark) has an integrated high-resolution camera which enables faster insertion and initial positioning and reduces or eliminates the need for an FOB. It provides continuous visual monitoring throughout the procedure, so malposition and dislocation are easily detected by real-time high-resolution video images transmitted to a monitor.

Familiarity with the clinical signs for DLT placement is important since a clean, functioning FOB may not always be available. An FOB may also be too large for smaller DLTs, and blood or mucus in the airway can interfere with the ability to identify the carina or the blue bronchial cuff.

Since a left DLT is used most often, the steps for left DLT placement are described.

Following successful laryngoscopy, the blue bronchial cuff is passed just past the vocal cords. Before advancing the tube further the stylet in the bronchial lumen is withdrawn. The DLT is then rotated 90°–120° anticlockwise until its tip is directed towards the left and advanced down the airway. The former recommendation was to advance a DLT until moderate resistance was encountered. With thin plastic DLTs this practice will often result in the tube being inserted too deeply. For both men and women, the depth of placement for a left DLT is highly correlated with height, and can be expressed by the formula:

Depth L–DLT$_{cm}$ = 12 + (0.1) Height$_{cm}$.

Once in the bronchus both cuffs are inflated. If an appropriate size (large) left DLT has been selected, the bronchial cuff should require < 3 mL air to seal the airway. If > 3 mL is needed the bronchial cuff is most likely partially in the trachea. An exception is the patient with an extremely large airway, since the bronchial cuff of even the largest 41 Fr DLT may require > 3 mL. The volume of air in the bronchial cuff and the tension of that cuff's pilot balloon should be noted.

Both lungs are ventilated. A capnograph will demonstrate an appropriate waveform and end-tidal carbon dioxide. Water vapour should be visible in both lumens and bilateral breath sounds and chest wall excursions should occur. Condensation in only one lumen (with both cuffs inflated) usually means that the bronchial lumen of a left DLT has inadvertently entered the right bronchus.

Next clamp the tracheal (right) lumen, while ventilating the left (bronchial) lung. Breath sounds should be heard only over the left lung. If breath sounds are present only over the right lung the left DLT is in the right bronchus. In this event both cuffs should be deflated and the tube withdrawn until its tip is above the carina. After bending and turning the patient's head and neck towards the right shoulder with the chin pointed to the left, the DLT should be re-rotated to the left and re-advanced. This manoeuvre will direct the DLT into the left bronchus. If unsuccessful, an FOB down the bronchial lumen can be used as a stylet to advance the DLT into the left bronchus.

Next clamp the bronchial lumen and ventilate only the right lung noting peak inspiratory pressure (PIP); then clamp the tracheal lumen and ventilate only the left lung noting PIP. In the absence of a pleural effusion, large intrathoracic or pulmonary mass, or previous pulmonary resection, this sequential ventilation of each lung should produce almost identical PIPs and end-tidal carbon dioxide waveforms.

If ventilation of only the left lung produces a significantly higher PIP than with identical tidal volume ventilation to the right lung, the tube is probably too deep and obstructing the left upper-lobe bronchus. The DLT should be withdrawn in 0.5 cm increments. If ventilation through the tracheal lumen to the right lung produces higher PIPs than ventilation to the left, the inflated bronchial cuff is probably herniating above the carina partially obstructing ventilation to the right lung. The DLT should be advanced in 0.5 cm increments.

An FOB down the tracheal lumen should always be used to confirm DLT position. The right main bronchus should be fully visible with a rim of the blue bronchial cuff just below the carina in the left main bronchus. If more than the edge of the bronchial cuff is present the DLT should be advanced further into the bronchus. If the bronchial cuff is not seen, the DLT is too deep and should be slowly withdrawn under FOB guidance until just a rim of blue is visible. The FOB should then be introduced down the bronchial lumen to demonstrate a patent non-obstructed left upper-lobe bronchus.

Bronchoscopy with the patient supine confirms that the correct bronchus has been intubated. After turning the patient laterally tube position must be rechecked as many DLTs require repositioning. The tension of the bronchial cuff's pilot balloon should be palpated. If the bronchial cuff is no longer completely within the bronchus its pilot balloon will no longer be as tense as when the patient was supine. Do not add more air. Rather, both the bronchial and tracheal cuffs should be deflated and the tube advanced 0.5–1.0 cm deeper into the airway. After re-inflating the bronchial cuff with the same volume of air that was initially used its pilot balloon should once again be as tense as before. Bronchoscopy should then be repeated to reconfirm correct placement.

When lung isolation or selective ventilation is not needed the bronchial cuff should be deflated. It is best to avoid nitrous oxide in the anaesthetic technique as this will expand the bronchial cuff and increase the risk of DLT displacement or airway injury. If nitrous oxide is used the bronchial cuff should be deflated periodically to the original inflation volume.

Choice of Bronchial Blocker and Double-Lumen Tube

For most thoracic procedures either a DLT or BB can be used and both are equally safe and effective. The choice depends on the requirements of the specific case, the patient's airway and most importantly the preferences and experiences of the anaesthetist. There are situations when there may be an advantage to using one technique rather than the other (Box 27.1).

A DLT enables safe collapse and re-inflation of the operated lung during a procedure. Sequential inflation/deflation with a BB greatly increases the risk of balloon displacement. If the BB's balloon is no longer in correct position it will fail to isolate the operative lung, which may then re-expand and interfere with surgery. Intraoperative BB movement occurs much more frequently than DLT displacement, especially when changing the patient's position from supine to lateral and/or from surgical manipulation of the operated lung.

A DLT can be positioned in less time than a BB and complete lung deflation is more rapid. This may be a benefit for very short procedures. Although it takes longer for the lung to initially collapse with a BB, once the lung is fully deflated there are no differences between techniques.

A collapsed, operated lung should be suctioned prior to re-expansion in order to avoid contamination of the dependent airway. A DLT facilitates suction of the operated lung at any time without interrupting ventilation to the non-operated lung. Adequate suctioning of the operative lung is difficult or impossible through the narrow channel of a BB. When a BB's balloon is deflated, either during the procedure or at the completion of surgery, the contralateral healthy airway is potentially exposed to contamination from the operated lung.

A DLT enables fibrescopic examination of the operated lung during surgery. The VivaSight DLT enables continuous monitoring. Intraoperative visual examination is not possible through a BB. CPAP is easily applied to the collapsed lung through a DLT during one-lung ventilation (OLV).

A BB cannot be used if the main bronchus on the side of surgery is obstructed or if the procedure involves the main bronchus. A BB cannot be used to collapse a right lung if the upper-lobe bronchus originates at the carina or in the trachea. In these situations, a DLT can be placed on the contralateral side.

Selective lobar collapse is not possible with a DLT but can be accomplished with a BB. This can be an advantage in patients with limited respiratory reserve, especially those who have had a previous pulmonary resection of the same or contralateral lung. A BB is indicated for lung isolation in young children since the smallest DLTs (26–28 Fr) may still be too large for children less than 8 years old.

Expense may be a factor in choosing one device over another. Actual cost will vary with supplier and

Box 27.1 Advantages and disadvantages – double-lumen tube vs. bronchial blocker

Favours double-lumen tube (DLT)

- Quicker and easier to place
- 'Blind' placement possible (if FOB is not available)
- More rapid lung deflation
- Intraoperative tube displacement less frequent
- Enables FOB examination of operated lung during surgery
- CPAP easily applied to treat hypoxaemia
- Enables suctioning before re-inflation of operative lung
- Operative lung can be re-expanded and collapsed as needed
- One DLT can be used for bilateral sequential surgery during same procedure
- Can be used for operations on contralateral lung if main bronchus on operated side obstructed
- Provides complete anatomical lung isolation
  - Used for bronchopulmonary lavage
- Facilitates 'split lung' ventilation in ICU

Favours bronchial blocker (BB)

- Placed through or alongside a TT or supraglottic airway
  - Patients with difficult airway when DLT difficult or impossible to use
  - Can be placed through oral, nasal or tracheostomy tube, or supraglottic airway
  - Patients with *in-situ* TT when tube exchange dangerous
  - Patients requiring post-operative ventilation
- Multi-port adaptor enables ventilation during placement
- Less potential for serious airway trauma
- Allows selective lobar isolation
- Can be used in children too small for a DLT

institution, but BBs are much more expensive than DLTs. Therefore, unless there is a clear-cut clinical advantage, from a cost perspective a DLT may be a better choice.

Difficult Cases

Intubation with a DLT is more difficult than with a single-lumen TT. Bronchial blockade is therefore recommended for patients with difficult airways in whom placement of a DLT can be challenging or impossible. Once the airway is secured (by oral, nasal, tracheostomy tube or supraglottic airway), then bronchial blockade is always possible. Patients who arrive at the operating room with a TT, either from the ICU or emergency room, may be at risk for tube exchange. A BB through an *in situ* TT avoids that risk. If post-operative ventilation is anticipated, or

when exchanging tubes at the completion of surgery is dangerous, a BB is a good choice.

At the beginning of the procedure if there is difficulty placing a DLT, the patient's airway can be intubated with a TT which can then be exchanged for a DLT over an airway exchange catheter (AEC). Similarly, at the end of surgery, especially where airway management has been difficult and post-operative ventilation is planned, exchange of a DLT to a standard TT can be readily achieved with an AEC. Guidelines for safe use of an AEC are in Box 27.2.

Complications

A BB's balloon must be deflated and withdrawn before that bronchus is stapled during pulmonary resection. If not, the catheter can be sheared or even incorporated into the staple line.

Box 27.2 Guidelines for use of an airway exchange catheter (AEC)

- Select an AEC > 70 cm length when using with a DLT
- Choose an AEC with a large outer diameter relative to the bronchial lumen's inner diameter (i.e. 'tight fit')
- Lubricate the AEC
- Test the fit between the AEC and the tube before attempting tube exchange
- Pre-oxygenate fully
- Insert the AEC. Note the depth markings on both the AEC and *in situ* tube; never insert the AEC deeper than 25 cm into the airway (beyond the teeth)
- Never advance the AEC against resistance
- Once the AEC is in position remove the DLT without advancing the AEC
- Place the new TT on the AEC
- Use a laryngoscope to lift supraglottic tissue to facilitate tube passage of the new TT through the glottis
- If passage is obstructed, rotate the tube 90° anticlockwise to avoid arytenoid or vocal cord impingement
- Have a rescue intubation plan ready to manage failed exchange
- Oxygenation via the AEC is very rarely needed and should be avoided unless absolutely necessary because of the risk of barotrauma if the AEC becomes wedged in the lung

---

Box 27.3 Risk factors for airway rupture with a double-lumen tube

- Trauma during insertion
- Too large a tube
- Tube advanced down bronchus with stylet in bronchial lumen
- Overinflation of tracheal and/or bronchial cuff
  - Too rapid inflation
  - Too large a volume
  - Use of nitrous oxide during procedure
- Asymmetric cuff distention pushing distal tip into airway wall
- Movement of tube with cuffs inflated
- Pre-existing airway pathology
  - Congenital airway wall abnormalities
  - Airway wall weakness
    - Tumour infiltration
    - Infection
    - Steroids
- Airway distortion from mediastinal lymph node tumours

Minor tracheobronchial trauma (sore throat, hoarseness) is more common with a DLT. Tracheobronchial rupture is a rare but potentially lethal complication of DLTs (Box 27.3).

A malpositioned DLT or BB will present either as failure to collapse the lung or as obstruction to ventilation. If the inflated cuff or balloon is displaced into the trachea it must be immediately deflated to re-establish ventilation to both lungs. If the lung on the operated side fails to collapse FOB examination is required to ensure the DLT or BB is completely sealing the bronchus.

Conclusion

The 'best' technique for lung separation has been debated for years. There are situations when there is an advantage to one technique or the other, so every anaesthetist must be familiar with both BBs and DLTs.

Further Reading

Benumof JL, Partridge BL, Salvatierra C, et al. (1987). Margin of safety in positioning modern double-lumen endotracheal tubes. *Anesthesiology*, **67**, 729–738.

Brodsky JB. (2009). Lung separation and the difficult airway. *British Journal of Anaesthesia*, **103**(Suppl 1), i66–i75.

Brodsky JB. (2015). Con: a bronchial blocker is not a substitute for a double-lumen endobronchial tube. *Journal of Cardiothoracic and Vascular Anesthesia*, **29**, 237–239.

Brodsky JB, Lemmens HJ. (2003). Left double-lumen tubes: clinical experience with 1,170 patients. *Journal of Cardiothoracic and Vascular Anesthesia*, **17**, 289–298.

Fitzmaurice BG, Brodsky JB. (1999). Airway rupture with double-lumen tubes. *Journal of Cardiothoracic and Vascular Anesthesia*, **13**, 322–329.

Narayanaswamy M, McRae K, Slinger P, et al. (2009). Choosing a lung isolation device for thoracic surgery: a randomized trial of three bronchial blockers versus double-lumen tubes. *Anesthesia & Analgesia*, **108**, 1097–1101.

Schuepbach R, Grande B, Camen G, et al. (2015). Intubation with VivaSight or conventional left-sided double-lumen tubes: a randomized trial. *Canadian Journal of Anaesthesia*, **62**, 762–769.

Airway Management in the Critically Ill

Andy Higgs and Audrey De Jong

Introduction

Airway interventions are the procedures most commonly associated with mortality and serious morbidity in the intensive care unit (ICU). Approximately 6% of ICU patients have either a known difficult airway or features indicating anatomical difficulty. Physiological abnormalities such as pre-existing hypoxia and haemodynamic instability add to the degree of difficulty because they shorten the safe apnoea time and cognitively overload the operator. Added to this, ICU is rarely designed for airway management in the same way as the operating theatre is, creating logistical challenges to airway management. Thus, intubation in ICU will often include anatomical difficulty, physiological difficulty and logistical difficulty.

Anticipating difficult intubation is particularly important: complications are higher in difficult intubation than non-difficult intubation (51% vs. 36% for severe life-threatening complications such as hypoxaemia and cardiovascular collapse). De Jong reported that intubation-related cardiac arrest occurred in 2.7% of ICU patients (1000-fold higher than in elective surgery) and 28-day mortality was increased 3-fold when cardiac arrest occurred (hazard ratio 3.9 (95% CI 2.4–6.3), $p < 0.0001$, after adjustment for confounding variables). Five independent risk factors predictive of intubation-related cardiac arrest were hypoxaemia, haemodynamic failure, absence of pre-oxygenation (all modifiable before intubation), body mass index (BMI) > 25 kg m^{-2} and age > 75 years.

Difficult intubation occurs in about 10% (range: 1–23%), but ICU intubation is still commonly managed in a relatively primitive manner. NAP4 reported that airway-related death and brain damage may be 50- to 60-fold more common than operating room practice. Jaber and colleagues demonstrated that using didactic ICU intubation bundles improves outcome. Elements of such a bundle are described in this chapter.

Reducing the Risks in the ICU by Using an Intubation Bundle Approach

In 2018, several UK organisations (the Difficult Airway Society (DAS), Intensive Care Society and the Faculty of Intensive Care with endorsement from the Royal College of Anaesthetists) created a UK national guideline for tracheal intubation in the critically ill adult. This establishes an *intubation bundle*, which retains the standard algorithmic structure of Plans A–D seen in the DAS guidelines, albeit with a unified Plan B/C, similar to the 'Vortex' approach.

Human Factors

More than individual technique or innovative devices, human factors may be the single most important modifiable element in ICU intubation: an average of 4.5 human factor elements per case were seen in reports of major airway complications reported to NAP4 (see also Chapter 36). The nature of modern critical care means that the team assembled to achieve intubation may never have performed this task together before. This can lead to rigidly vertical or chaotic communication, to poorly planned and executed actions and, when difficulty arises, to increasingly urgent and technically challenging cognitive tasks falling on a single team member, who receives limited support from others.

To avoid this, the intubation team leader must ensure the intubation plan is explained to all team members prior to induction and empower them to speak up or raise concerns. This is 'sharing the mental model': not only must the whole team know how the operator intends to secure the airway, but crucially, what will be needed should difficulty arise – the 'plan for failure'. The team leader verbalising an appropriate intubation checklist in which the team prepares the patient, themselves, the equipment and also agrees on the plan for managing difficulty is an extremely powerful tool (Figure 28.1). This occurs concurrently with pre-oxygenation. Such proactive leadership engenders active followership in other team members.

Team performance is optimised using real-world simulation together in their own unit, following an agreed algorithm and using equipment with which they are trained. The intubation trolley should be identical to that used elsewhere in the hospital to avoid presenting operators with unfamiliar devices. The algorithm should be displayed clearly whenever intubation is performed (Figure 28.2). Shift handovers should detail potential airway difficulties and specific plans tailored to that resident team's skill set should be made. Regular whole-team no-blame discussion of critical incidents and near misses is an efficient means of improving practice.

Assessment

Predicting difficult intubation enables the team to prepare optimally. A tool predicting difficult intubation, the MACOCHA score, was developed and externally validated in a prospective multicentre French study and is shown in Table 28.1.

A cut-off of ≥ 3 predicts difficulty. This score has a negative predictive value of 98% and sensitivity of 73%. Importantly, Mallampati class can be assessed in a cooperative *supine* patient. Such prediction tools are only useful if they lead to a change in approach (see below) and none are wholly sensitive and specific, so preparing for unanticipated difficulty is crucial.

Use the 'laryngeal handshake' to identify the cricothyroid membrane (CTM). If this is

Table 28.1 MACOCHA score calculation worksheet

	Points
Factors related to patient	
Mallampati class III or IV	5
Obstructive Sleep **A**pnoea Syndrome	2
Reduced mobility of **C**ervical spine	1
Limited mouth **O**pening < 3 cm	1
Factors related to pathology	
Coma	1
Severe **H**ypoxaemia (< 80%)	1
Factor related to operator	
Non **A**nesthesiologist	1
Total	**12**

Score 0 to 12: 0 = easy; 12 = very difficult. Cut-off indicating difficult intubation = ≥3

From De Jong et al. (2013), with permission.

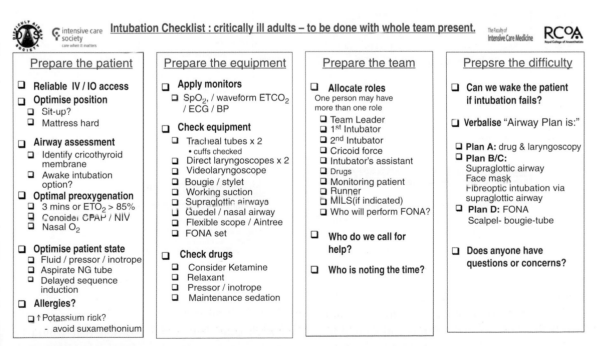

Figure 28.1 ICU Intubation Checklist. (Reprinted with permission of the Difficult Airway Society. Copyright © 2017 Difficult Airway Society. Higgs et al. (2018).)

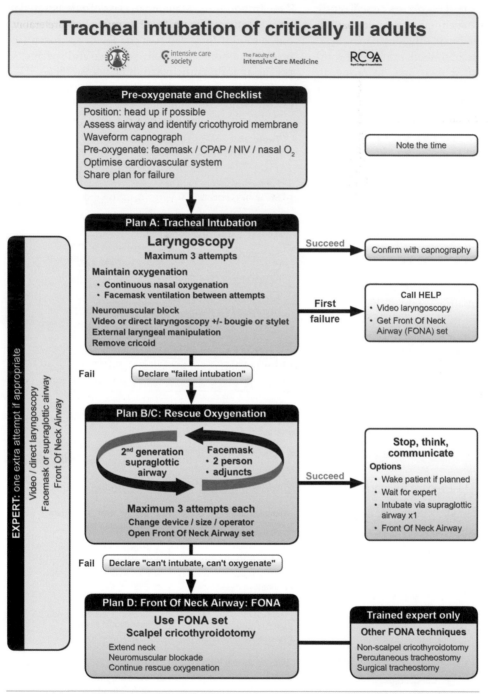

Tracheal intubation of critically ill adults

intensive care society   The Faculty of **Intensive Care Medicine**   RCoA Royal College of Anaesthetists

Pre-oxygenate and Checklist

Position: head up if possible
Assess airway and identify cricothyroid membrane
Waveform capnograph
Pre-oxygenate: facemask / CPAP / NIV / nasal O_2
Optimise cardiovascular system
Share plan for failure

Note the time

Plan A: Tracheal Intubation

Laryngoscopy
Maximum 3 attempts

Maintain oxygenation
- **Continuous nasal oxygenation**
- **Facemask ventilation between attempts**

Neuromuscular block
Video or direct laryngoscopy +/- bougie or stylet
External laryngeal manipulation
Remove cricoid

Succeed → Confirm with capnography

First failure → **Call HELP**
- Video laryngoscopy
- Get Front Of Neck Airway (FONA) set

Fail → Declare "failed intubation"

EXPERT: one extra attempt if appropriate
Video / direct laryngoscopy
Facemask or supraglottic airway
Front Of Neck Airway

Plan B/C: Rescue Oxygenation

2nd generation supraglottic airway ⟷ **Facemask**
- 2 person
- adjuncts

Maximum 3 attempts each
Change device / size / operator
Open Front Of Neck Airway set

Succeed → **Stop, think, communicate**
Options
- Wake patient if planned
- Wait for expert
- Intubate via supraglottic airway x1
- Front Of Neck Airway

Fail → Declare "can't intubate, can't oxygenate"

Plan D: Front Of Neck Airway: FONA

Use FONA set
Scalpel cricothyroidotomy

Extend neck
Neuromuscular blockade
Continue rescue oxygenation

Trained expert only
Other FONA techniques
Non-scalpel cricothyroidotomy
Percutaneous tracheostomy
Surgical tracheostomy

This flowchart forms part of the DAS, ICS, FICM, RCoA Guideline for tracheal intubation in critically ill adults and should be used in conjunction with the text.

Figure 28.2 Algorithm for tracheal intubation in critically ill adults. (Reprinted with permission of the Difficult Airway Society. Copyright © 2017 Difficult Airway Society. Higgs et al. (2018).)

impalpable but time permits, ultrasound should be used to locate the CTM, or as a minimum to mark the midline. This should be done with the head and neck extended in the position that would be used during an emergency front of neck airway (eFONA) procedure.

Haemodynamic assessment is also necessary; pre-intubation optimisation may prevent peri-intubation collapse.

Airway Plan A

This refers to the phase of preparation (including pre-oxygenation and haemodynamic optimisation), modified rapid sequence induction (RSI), peroxygenation (oxygenation throughout intubation attempts), laryngoscopy and intubation. Decide before induction whether awakening the patient is indicated if intubation fails; most ICU patients require intubation because of neurological, respiratory or cardiovascular failure and so attempting to awaken the patient is usually inappropriate.

Sit the patient 25–30° head-up (use reverse-Trendelenberg tilt if spinal instability is suspected). This maximises functional residual capacity (FRC) and may reduce passive regurgitation of gastric contents. Together with extending the head on the flexed neck, this permits optimal access to the airway. Ramp obese patients (see Chapter 24).

To help avoid cardiovascular collapse, administer a fluid load (500 mL balanced crystalloid) in the absence of cardiogenic pulmonary oedema and start vasopressors early if the blood pressure is low.

Pre-oxygenation

Critically ill patients with respiratory failure have significant intrapulmonary shunt with a reduced FRC, which limits the effectiveness of all pre-oxygenation techniques. Pre-oxygenation recruitment manoeuvre may improve pre-oxygenation effectiveness.

Pre-induction non-invasive ventilation (NIV) or continuous positive airway pressure (CPAP) can recruit and stabilise alveolar lung units available for gas exchange: 'opening the lung' with the pressure support and 'keeping the lung open' with positive end-expiratory pressure (PEEP). The UK guideline follows this approach, such that if NIV is already being used it should be continued. If not, a Waters circuit with an adjustable valve and anaesthetic face mask should be used to provide CPAP/assisted breaths for 3 minutes or until the end-tidal oxygen is > 85%.

However, NIV/CPAP must be removed during laryngoscopy and intubation: this creates an apnoeic period during which profound desaturation may occur. Oxygenation at this time should be by face mask ventilation between intubation attempts, together with 'apnoeic

oxygenation' via nasal cannulae. The latter includes standard dry oxygen at up to 15 L min^{-1}, or preferably, warmed and humidified high flow nasal oxygen (HFNO) at up to 60 L min^{-1}. To date, the evidence for apnoeic oxygenation being beneficial in ICU intubations is conflicting, most likely because its efficacy depends on upper airway patency during laryngoscopy and intubation, the FiO_2, oxygen flow rate, patient position and the extent and cause of any pre-existing hypoxaemia. There is little or no evidence of harm.

Optimising alveolar recruitment stabilisation by combining NIV or CPAP with apnoeic oxygenation may be better than NIV alone in hypoxaemic patients, but is only possible when the HFNO tubing does not prevent a good face mask seal being achieved, because this causes PEEP to be lost. The corollary is that if the face mask seal is good, concomitant HFNO may generate high airway pressures in a sealed breathing system, with the risk of barotrauma.

Aspiration Risk

Most critically ill patients are at risk of aspiration of pulmonary contents because of urgency of intubation or gastric stasis. A modified RSI is recommended. This implies IV induction, rapid-onset neuromuscular blockade, cricoid force applied by a trained assistant and face mask ventilation between intubation attempts. Nasogastric tubes should be left in place and aspirated before induction. Cricoid force is recommended but remains controversial (see Chapter 11): it should certainly be reduced, or removed fully, if there is difficult laryngoscopy, difficulty inserting the tracheal tube, difficult face mask ventilation, the need to insert a supraglottic airway (SGA) during airway rescue, or active vomiting.

Obesity

Obese patients are at especially high risk during ICU airway management. The pathophysiology of obesity includes reduced FRC (particularly with central, android fat disposition), greater oxygen consumption (1.5 times higher), greater risk of aspiration, increased work of breathing and heightened cardiovascular risk (including right ventricular strain, which may be revealed at intubation). Obstructive sleep apnoea (OSA) syndrome (diagnosed or not) is an unambiguous marker of potentially complicated airway management. Obesity increases the risk of difficulty with almost all airway interventions, but the main reason obesity increases risk during ICU intubation is the propensity for abrupt, profound and often refractory desaturation at induction: the shortened safe apnoea time may cause hypoxaemia, cardiovascular collapse and cardiac arrest.

These findings are not purely theoretical. A French study of obese patients intubated in ICU reported difficult intubation in 16% of obese subjects and notably increased risk of complications. Compared with intubation of the obese patient in the operating room, obese patients in ICU were 21-fold more likely to experience complications including severe hypoxia, oesophageal intubation, cardiovascular collapse, cardiac arrest and death. Advanced airway management strategies were used infrequently in the ICU, but commonly in the operating room. Similarly, in NAP4 half of reports from ICU described obese patients and these patients were at increased risk of death or brain damage compared with non-obese patients (twofold higher if BMI > 30 kg m^{-2} and fourfold higher if BMI > 40 kg m^{-2}).

Serious consideration should be given to securing the airway awake if possible. Where general anaesthesia is used this should include a ramped position, thorough pre-oxygenation with CPAP/NIV, apnoeic oxygenation, ventilation with CPAP between intubation attempts, laryngoscopy prioritising prompt first-pass success, airway rescue using a second generation SGA which provides a higher seal pressure to ventilate poorly compliant chest walls and protection against aspiration. The CTM is often impalpable but most often identifiable with ultrasonography. eFONA using a vertical incision through skin and subcutaneous tissue with a second, horizontal, incision through the CTM is usually best.

Airway (tracheal tube or tracheostomy) displacement is far more common in obese individuals and this was prominent in NAP4.

Drug Choice

Induction drug choice depends on the clinical situation; reduced doses are usually indicated. Ketamine is commonly used in ICU intubations because it provides optimal haemodynamic stability and bronchodilation. Etomidate provides cardiovascular stability but induces adrenal suppression. Thiopentone and propofol can cause catastrophic hypotension.

Neuromuscular blocking agents reduce complications of intubation and failed airway management. Rocuronium is as effective as suxamethonium and avoids hyperkalaemia in those at risk (critical illness-

related immobility, neuromuscular diseases and burns of > 24 hours). Suxamethonium is short-acting and may partially wear off during prolonged intubation attempts, complicating matters further. Sugammadex reverses rocuronium, but even complete reversal of neuromuscular blockade alone may not restore airway patency and adequate spontaneous respiration after the administration of hypnotics and multiple intubation attempts.

Laryngoscopy

Optimal laryngoscopy should minimise the number of attempts and avoid trauma to the airway. The presence of two operators is strongly advised in the critically ill patient. During difficult airway management, situation awareness is often lost and prolonged periods of time pass during repeated efforts to intubate the trachea. To avoid this, note the time at induction and limit intubation to *three* attempts. A fourth attempt should be restricted to a suitably experienced 'expert' if this is thought appropriate (Figure 28.2).

When intubation is expected to be uncomplicated (MACOCHA score 1–2, without other features of difficulty), either direct or videolaryngoscopy may be used. When difficulty is suspected (MACOCHA ≥ 3 or other features), videolaryngoscopy is preferable. All operators must be trained to use the videolaryngoscope available in their unit. A videolaryngoscope screen visible to all is advantageous: it facilitates optimal cricoid force, external laryngeal manipulation, teaching and team-working.

A potential disadvantage of videolaryngoscopy with a hyperangulated blade is that it can prolong straightforward intubations, which may worsen outcome. The obvious solution to this is to use a videolaryngoscope with a MacIntosh-shaped blade: if the view is good, there is no delay. If difficulty is encountered, a hyperangulated blade such as the C-MAC D-Blade or GlideScope is then indicated. Hyperangulated blades necessitate use of the screen and the use of an angled stylet or bougie (see Chapter 17).

Systematic reviews of videolaryngoscopy in the critically ill have reported conflicting findings. A 2014 systematic review reported that videolaryngoscopy was beneficial in that it improved process (reducing difficult intubations, grade 3–4 laryngeal views, oesophageal intubation and improving first-attempt success) without improving outcomes (severe hypoxaemia, severe cardiovascular collapse, airway injury). Other meta-analyses have been less positive. Overall many studies of videolaryngoscopy in the critically ill are of poor design, too small, involve inappropriate operators or exclude patients of interest, with the result that the study results are heterogeneous and difficult to summarise. The largest study was the 2016 MACMAN study of 371 patients, which reported that a McGrath Macintosh VL did not improve first-pass success rates. A post hoc analysis identified higher rates of severe life-threatening complications with videolaryngoscopy. Study limitations included using very inexperienced intubators, who lacked clinical experience in videolaryngoscopy, and avoiding use of a bougie or stylet. It is likely that these limitations led to prolonged intubation attempts, which might have been avoided by suitably experienced intubators.

While many operators are strongly supportive of videolaryngoscopy in the critically ill, the overall quality of evidence supporting or refuting benefit remains poor. Training and education are essential to improve safety during tracheal intubation, whether using videolaryngoscopy or not. Videolaryngoscopy undoubtedly improves laryngeal view but passing the tracheal tube requires a different technique to direct laryngoscopy and mastering this requires training. Videolaryngoscopes should not be used without appropriate training as this likely causes harm.

After the first failed intubation attempt, ensure help has been summoned and that, if not already done, the FONA set is immediately accessible at the bedside.

Confirmation of Intubation

Successful intubation is confirmed by *waveform* capnography. Universal adoption of this monitor was described as the single most important change which could reduce airway-related mortality and morbidity in the NAP4 report. Importantly, a discernible waveform is seen even during cardiac arrest, providing effective CPR is in progress (see Figure 28.3). Absence of a recognisable waveform trace should always be regarded as indicative of oesophageal intubation until proven otherwise.

Other causes of a flat trace such as the ventilator not being turned on or connected or a blocked circuit should also be considered, but oesophageal intubation *must* be excluded. Clinical signs such as chest wall movement or misting are highly insensitive in critically ill patients and should not be relied upon.

Post-intubation Management

Provided the patient is haemodynamically stable, a recruitment manoeuvre (CPAP 30–40 cmH$_2$O for 30–40 seconds, FiO$_2$ 100%) can be performed. This technique is associated with a higher P_aO_2 at both 5 minutes and 30 minutes after intubation (Table 28.2).

It is beyond the remit of this chapter, but it is notable that most complications of airway management in the critically ill occur after intubation. Tracheal tube displacement and tracheostomy tube displacement are particular problems. Accidental airway tube displacement will occur in all ICUs and occurs most often in the obese, during sedation holds and after minor procedures such as changes in patient position, tracheal tube suction or nasogastric tube aspiration. Continuous display of waveform capnography is crucial to detect displacement and monitor airway integrity. It is a standard of care. Every ICU should anticipate that airway displacements will occur and have plans (monitoring, equipment, personnel and training) in place to ensure these events are promptly recognised and managed (see also Chapter 29).

Extubation is a particularly high-risk period as up to 20% of patients who are extubated on ICU will require reintubation in the next 24 hours, often as an emergency. Where there has been difficulty at intubation or reintubation is anticipated to be difficult for other reasons the greatest caution should be taken. The DAS guidelines for tracheal extubation are readily applicable to critically ill patients (see Chapter 21).

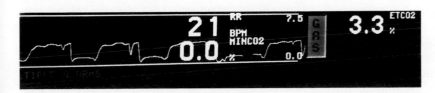

Figure 28.3 Capnography (end-tidal carbon dioxide (ETCO$_2$)) trace during cardiac arrest with CPR. Note the low amplitude, recognisable waveform CO$_2$ trace.

Table 28.2 A post-intubation care bundle (Montpellier, France)

POST-INTUBATION

1. Immediate confirmation of tube placement by waveform capnography
2. Noradrenaline if MAP < 60–70 mmHg or diastolic blood pressure < 35 mmHg
3. Initiate long-term sedation
4. Initial 'protective ventilation': tidal volume 6–8 mL kg^{-1}, FiO$_2$ to maintain target SpO$_2$, PEEP as per FiO$_2$ ARDSnet table, respiratory rate between 10 and 20 cycles/min, plateau pressure < 30 cmH$_2$O
5. Recruitment manoeuvre: CPAP 40 cmH$_2$O for 30–40 s, FiO$_2$ 100% (if no cardiovascular instability)
6. Maintain cuff pressure 25–30 cmH$_2$O
7. Closed tracheal suction if indicated
8. Arterial blood gas
9. Chest X-ray to check tube position in relation to carina and identify complications of intubation
10. Note length of tube (at facial landmark, e.g. lips or teeth) on ICU chart

CPAP, continuous positive airway pressure; MAP, mean arterial pressure; PEEP, positive end-expiratory pressure.

Adapted from Jaber et al. (2010).

Failed Intubation

After three failed attempts – or a single optimal attempt – declare: '*This is a failed intubation, move to Plan B/C: Airway Rescue*' (Figure 28.2).

Plan B/C: Airway Rescue after Failed Intubation

The traditional intubation sequence follows Plan A with Plan B then Plan C and finally Plan D. This helps to rationalise the process but is a linear representation of interventions which often proceed in parallel. After failed laryngoscopy in ICU, airway rescue commences most commonly as an alternating cycle of attempted oxygenation using an SGA or a face mask. This is analogous to the Vortex approach and this concept is incorporated into the UK algorithm.

Second generation SGAs, such as ProSeal LMA and i-gel, are preferable as they have higher seal pressures (enabling use of higher airway pressures and PEEP needed with poorly compliant lungs) and a drain tube, which provides some protection against aspiration of gastric contents (see Chapter 13).

After one failed attempt using either an SGA or face mask, open the FONA set, to prime the team for the possibility of eFONA.

Successful placement of an SGA (recognisable capnograph trace and stable or improving oxygen saturation) presents the opportunity to 'Stop, think and communicate' (Figure 28.2). Options at this point are:

- Awaken the patient. If this was planned prior to induction and the airway has not been traumatised.
- Wait for the *prompt* attendance of a more experienced operator (an expert, whose skills are discernibly superior to the current team).
- A single attempt to intubate via the SGA (e.g. with an Aintree intubation catheter) (see Chapter 13).
- Proceed to eFONA. Indicated when awakening the patient is impractical and appropriate intubation techniques have failed.

Failed SGA oxygenation leaves only one remaining method of oxygenation 'from above': face mask ventilation. If this is successful (recognisable capnograph trace and stable or improving oxygenation), the options are similar: wake the patient if indicated, await an expert if they can attend promptly or proceed to eFONA.

If both SGA and face mask oxygenation fails, declare '*This is a "cannot intubate, cannot oxygenate" situation. We will proceed to emergency front of neck airway.*'

Plan D: Emergency Front of Neck Airway (eFONA)

The most important aspect of successful eFONA is to avoid delay in performing it. The most likely successful approach is the scalpel-bougie-tube technique through the CTM (Figure 28.4).

Scalpel-bougie-tube cricothyroidotomy is a core skill for all ICU airway operators. It is associated with high success rates and uses equipment found in all

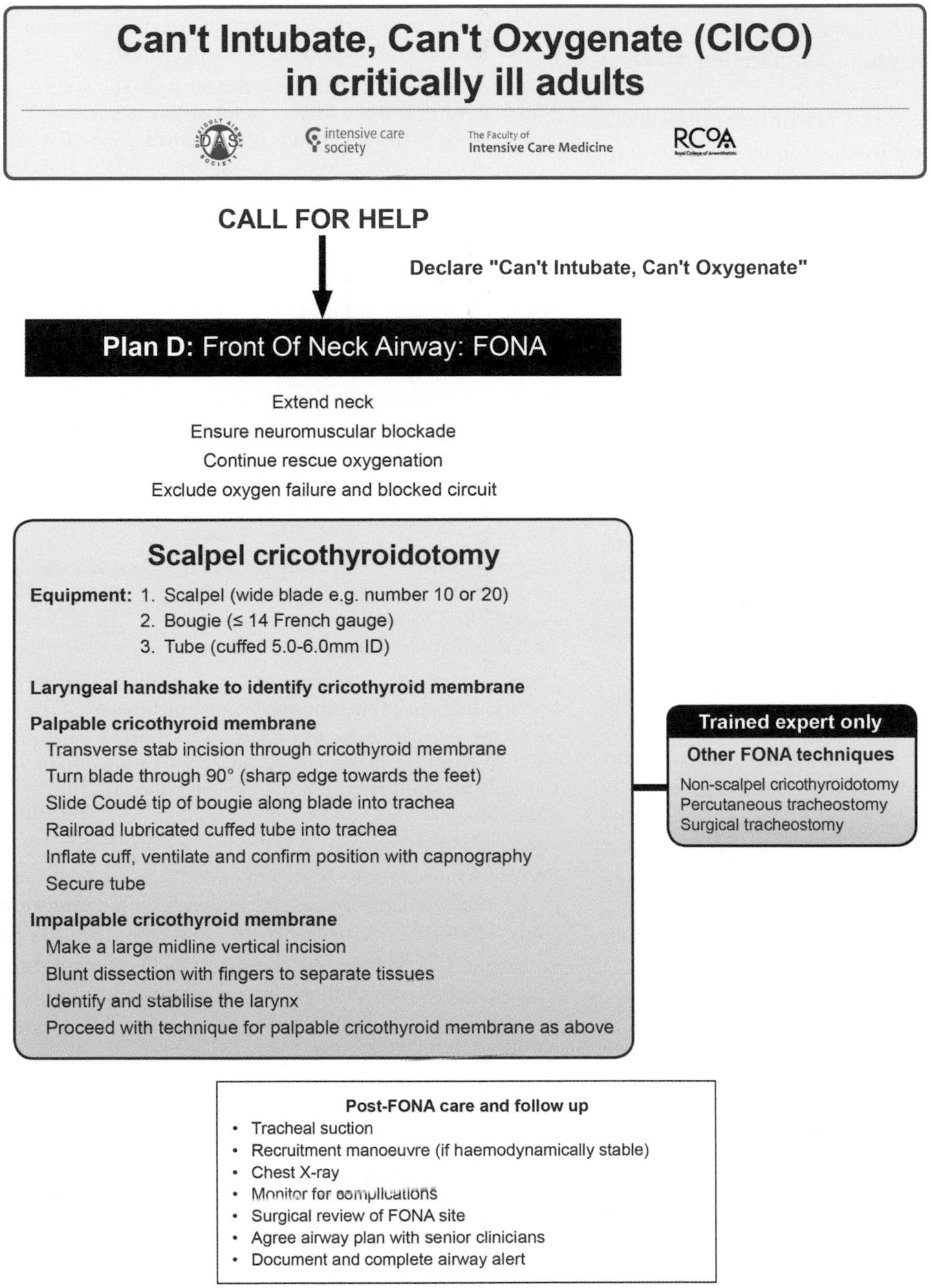

Figure 28.4 'Can't Intubate, Can't Oxygenate' in critically ill adults. (Reprinted with permission of the Difficult Airway Society. Copyright © 2017 Difficult Airway Society. Higgs et al. (2018).)

ICUs. It is recognised, however, that many intensivists have a skill set which enables appropriately trained experts to use non-scalpel techniques such as percutaneous tracheostomy. These techniques are inevitably slower than scalpel cricothyroidotomy, but are potentially very useful when cricothyroidotomy fails, when the CTM is inaccessible or soon after a tracheostomy has been decannulated. Evidence indicates that so-called 'jet ventilation' techniques through narrow cannulae are fraught with danger; they are associated with failure and extremely high complication rates (see Chapter 20).

After eFONA is achieved, a recruitment manœuvre is indicated as above and tracheal toilet. Prompt conversion to a more definitive airway such as a surgical tracheostomy should be performed.

Summary

NAP4 indicated that the incidence of death and brain damage in ICU airway management is 50- to 60-fold more common than in theatre-based anaesthetic practice. Human factors play an even greater role in improving airway safety in critically ill patients than in other forms of airway management. Use of an intubation checklist, designed for the critically ill patient, including the plan for failure and shared with the whole intubation team, is invaluable. The MACOCHA assessment score predicts difficult intubation in the critically ill patient. Pre-oxygenation of critically ill patients requires CPAP or NIV, with or without nasal oxygen. A modified RSI is recommended, as is peroxygenation with intermittent face mask ventilation and nasal oxygen. Early recourse to videolaryngoscopy by an individual trained in its use is recommended. Second generation SGAs are suitable for airway rescue. Plans B/C airway rescue are best regarded as a continuum, a philosophy in keeping with the Vortex approach. All intensivists should be trained in the scalpel-bougie-tube eFONA technique and this is the default rescue technique.

Further Reading

Baillard C, Fosse JP, Sebbane M, et al. (2006). Noninvasive ventilation improves preoxygenation before intubation of hypoxic patients. *American Journal of Respiratory and Critical Care Medicine*, **174**, 171–177.

Chrimes N. (2016). The Vortex: a universal 'high-acuity implementation tool' for emergency airway management. *British Journal of Anaesthesia*, **117**(Suppl 1), i20–i27.

Cook TM, Woodall N, Harper J, Benger J. (2011). Fourth National Audit Project. Major complications of airway management in the UK: results of the Fourth National Audit Project of the Royal College of Anaesthetists and the Difficult Airway Society. Part 2: intensive care and emergency departments. *British Journal of Anaesthesia*, **106**, 632–642.

De Jong A, Molinari N, Pouzeratte Y, et al. (2015). Difficult intubation in obese patients: incidence, risk factors, and complications in the operating theatre and in intensive care units. *British Journal of Anaesthesia*, **114**, 297–306.

De Jong A, Molinari N, Terzi N, et al. (2013). Early identification of patients at risk for difficult intubation in the intensive care unit: development and validation of the MACOCHA score in a multicenter cohort study. *American Journal of Respiratory and Critical Care Medicine*, **187**, 832–839.

Higgs A. (2018). Airway management in intensive care medicine. In: Hagberg CA, Artime CA, Aziz MF (Eds.), *Hagberg and Benumof's Airway Management*. 4th ed. Philadelphia: Elsevier. pp. 754–780.

Higgs A, McGrath B, Goddard C, et al.; Difficult Airway Society; Intensive Care Society; Faculty of Intensive Care Medicine; Royal College of Anaesthetists. (2018). Guidelines for the management of tracheal intubation in the critically ill adult. *British Journal of Anaesthesia*, **120**, 323–352.

Jaber S, Jung B, Corne P, et al. (2010). An intervention to decrease complications related to endotracheal intubation in the intensive care unit: a prospective, multiple-center study. *Intensive Care Medicine*, **36**, 248–255.

Lascarrou, J. B., J. Boisrame-Helms, A. Bailly, et al. (2017). Video laryngoscopy vs direct laryngoscopy on successful first-pass orotracheal intubation among ICU patients: a randomized clinical trial. *JAMA*, **317**, 483–493.

Mosier JM, Hypes CD, Sakles JC. (2017). Understanding preoxygenation and apneic oxygenation during intubation in the critically ill. *Intensive Care Medicine*, **43**, 226–228.

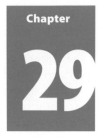

The Patient with a Tracheostomy

Brendan McGrath and Sheila Nainan Myatra

History

A tracheostomy is an artificial opening made into the trachea through the anterior neck (Figure 29.1). This may be temporary or permanent. A tracheostomy tube is usually inserted, enabling gas to enter the trachea and lungs directly, bypassing the nose, pharynx and larynx.

Tracheostomy is one of the earliest described surgical procedures, probably dating to the sixteenth century. Historically it was undertaken to relieve obstruction to the upper airway caused by trauma or tumour. In countries with advanced critical care services the majority of tracheostomies are now performed percutaneously by intensivists rather than by surgeons, with the commonest indication being to facilitate prolonged ventilation.

Indications

Indications for temporary and permanent tracheostomy are:

- to secure and maintain a patent (clear) airway in actual or potential upper airway obstruction

- to secure and maintain a safe airway in patients with injuries or surgery to the face, head or neck
- to facilitate weaning from artificial ventilation
- to facilitate long-term artificial ventilation
- to facilitate tracheal suctioning where there is poor cough effort with sputum retention
- to protect (partially) the airway of patients at high risk of aspiration

There is no convincing data that can guide clinicians as to the timing of tracheostomy. Prolonged use of a translaryngeal tracheal tube can damage the larynx and the upper airway and requires prolonged sedation. Balancing these risks against the risks of tracheostomy (procedural and post-placement) can be difficult.

Types of Tracheostomy

Tracheostomy may be temporary (short/long term) or permanent and may be formed electively or in an emergency. They may also be classified by their method of initial insertion.

(a)

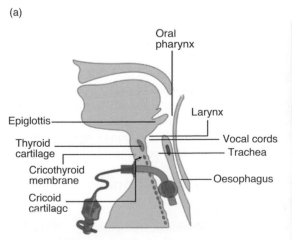

(b)

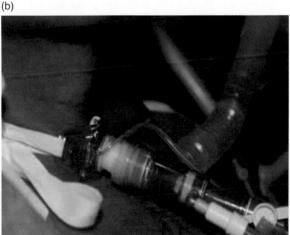

Figure 29.1 (a and b) Tracheostomy tube in the anterior neck.

259

Temporary tracheostomies are often used in patients with a temporary need for:

- bypass of upper airway obstruction
- 'tracheobronchial toilet'
- 'protection' against aspiration in patients with disordered pharyngolaryngeal neurological control mechanisms (e.g. head injuries or neurological diseases)

Certain maxillofacial or ENT surgical procedures require a temporary tracheostomy to facilitate the procedure.

It should be noted that while cuffs provide some protection against aspiration this is not complete, especially with low-pressure PVC cuffs, which have microfolds through which aspiration may occur. Silicone cuffs which have fewer folds may provide better protection.

Long-term/permanent tracheostomies are used when the underlying condition is chronic, permanent or progressive, including carcinoma of the naso-oropharynx or larynx, chronic respiratory support or long-term airway protection.

Surgical Tracheostomy

Surgical tracheostomies are usually undertaken in an operating theatre where conditions are sterile and lighting is good, although this is also possible in the emergency department or intensive care unit (ICU). General anaesthesia is commonly used, although tracheostomy under local anaesthesia is possible. Anaesthesia for tracheostomy requires careful consideration of airway management once sedative agents are administered.

In the anterior neck, midway between the cricoid cartilage and the sternal notch, a 2–3 cm long horizontal incision is made. The skin and platysma are dissected and the strap muscles retracted laterally, exposing the thyroid isthmus, which is either mobilised or divided. Following haemostasis, a cricoid hook or lateral stay sutures are used to expose the trachea and a small opening or 'window' is made in the trachea. A Björk flap may be created, where a part of the tracheal cartilage is incised, folded and sutured to maintain stoma patency. The tracheostomy tube is inserted through the stoma and may be sutured to the skin and/or secured with cloth ties or a holder.

Airway Management for Surgical Tracheostomy

Airway management for surgical tracheostomy will depend on the setting. In all settings communication between anaesthetic and surgical teams is paramount and national audits have shown that airway management may be difficult and associated with complications.

In an elective setting it is likely the trachea is already intubated. The tracheal tube will need to be withdrawn to enable passage of the tracheostomy tube. There is a risk of damaging the tracheal tube cuff during the surgery which may be overcome by inserting the tracheal tube deeply (cuff below surgery) or withdrawing it partially (cuff and distal tube above surgery). Both have limitations.

In the emergency setting and when the patient is not already intubated airway management may be much more complex. Where feasible, nasendoscopy before the procedure may assist in planning a safe approach. If general anaesthesia is safe tracheal intubation is usual, though a supraglottic airway (SGA) may occasionally be used and this may also be the case when a surgical airway is performed after an SGA is used for airway rescue and followed by surgical tracheostomy.

The most challenging situation is awake tracheostomy in the awake patient with airway obstruction. Efforts to assist oxygenation may require heliox or high flow nasal oxygenation. The optimal position required for surgery (fully supine and the neck fully extended) is often poorly tolerated and requires explanation: surgical compromise may be needed. Sedation may be unavoidable to ensure safety in the delirious patient but should be avoided wherever possible in a critical airway. Resisting sedation/anaesthesia and reassuring the patient may actually be the anaesthetist's greatest challenge during high-risk awake tracheostomy.

Once the tracheostomy is inserted its position in the airway should be immediately confirmed with capnography. Airway suction to remove secretions, blood and debris is good practice. Endoscopy via the tracheostomy tube is useful to assess adequacy of tube placement. The distal lumen of the correctly positioned tube will be parallel to the tracheal wall – and at endoscopy the entire trachea will be visible (full moon view). If positioning is suboptimal endoscopy may only reveal a limited view of the trachea (half-moon or crescent moon) and this requires correction by repositioning or a different choice of tracheostomy tube.

Percutaneous Dilatational Tracheostomy

Percutaneous dilatational tracheostomy (PDT) has become the technique of choice in ICU as it is a relatively quick bedside procedure, can be performed by a non-surgeon and does not require transfer of the critically ill patient to theatre. It involves a modified Seldinger technique of four steps:

- needle insertion into the trachea
- guidewire insertion through the needle
- conversion to a larger stoma through some form of dilation
- insertion of the tracheostomy tube over the guidewire

Bleeding during the procedure is generally controlled by the tamponading effect of the tube in the dilated tract.

Several different dilatational techniques are described. Originally, serial dilatation using sequentially larger dilators was used, but single-step dilation with a curved tapering dilator is now the most commonly used technique (Ciaglia technique, Figure 29.2). In the Griggs technique forceps are introduced over a guidewire and then extended to dilate the stoma with the tracheostomy tube then placed between them. The Fantoni technique involves needle puncture of the trachea and passage of a retrograde guidewire through the vocal cords, followed by railroading a combined dilator and tracheostomy tube over the guidewire into the larynx and out through the anterior tracheal wall. The tracheostomy tube is then separated from the dilator and rotated 180° to face the carina. The PercuTwist technique involves rotating a screw-like dilator over a guidewire to dilate the stoma. Dilation using a high-pressure balloon has also been described.

A meta-analysis of studies comparing at least two PDT techniques included 1130 patients and reported broad equivalence between techniques and devices, except the Fantoni technique, which was associated with more significant complications. The single-step dilation technique was associated with fewer failures than Griggs, PercuTwist or balloon dilation techniques.

Indications and Contraindications for PDT

Indications for PDT are similar to those for surgical tracheostomy. Most are performed in ICU to facilitate weaning from mechanical ventilation, tracheal toilet or airway protection. It is an elective procedure and in emergency settings a surgical technique is generally preferred.

Contraindications include children, infection at the insertion site or an unstable cervical spine injury.

Distorted airway anatomy, previous tracheostomy, neck surgery or radiation, obesity (body mass index (BMI) > 30 kg m^{-2}), bleeding diatheses, high positive end-expiratory pressure (PEEP) (≥ 10 cmH$_2$O) or FiO$_2$ ($\geq 70\%$) and haemodynamic instability are relative contraindications to PDT. If a patient has notably abnormal clotting or a large vessel near the puncture site many will choose surgical tracheostomy and direct haemostasis; however, an experienced operator may still undertake PDT. The availability (and method of contact) of an airway surgeon should be established prior to commencing PDT.

Airway Management during PDT

Airway management during PDT requires an individual suitably experienced in airway management and anaesthesia. The patient should be anaesthetised and paralysed with the airway secured, as minor movements or coughing may lead to needle misplacement and injury. Perforation of the posterior tracheal wall is a particular risk.

The patients should be ventilated with an FiO$_2$ of 100%. A tracheal tube must be withdrawn so that its tip does not lie in proximity to the tracheal puncture site and so that its cuff is not damaged by needle or guidewire insertion. Before manipulating the airway, position the patient with the neck extended, shoulders elevated and the bed at 30° head-up (to reduce venous pressure) for maximum exposure of the neck. Following oral and tracheal suction, the tracheal tube is withdrawn (or replaced) and the cuff positioned to just at/above the vocal cords. Conventional or videolaryngoscopy may be used, although the view may be worsened due to positioning.

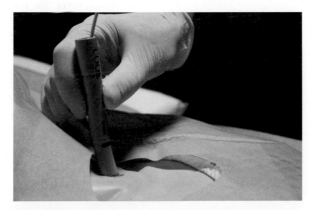

Figure 29.2 Percutaneous tracheostomy insertion into a model using the Seldinger technique and a single curved tapered dilator.

Alternatively, an existing tracheal tube may be exchanged for an SGA prior to PDT. This requires an experienced skilled operator and optimal positioning of the SGA. A second generation SGA with a high airway seal and through which airway endoscopy is readily achieved should be chosen. Endoscopy facilitates full vision of the trachea to guide needle insertion. As with conventional anaesthesia, SGAs are not suitable for all, especially the obese and those with high airway pressures.

Whichever technique is chosen, oxygenation, ventilation and anaesthesia must be maintained throughout the procedure. Following airway device displacement, inability to perform PDT, or serious bleeding, the airway manager should be prepared to reintubate the patient. Only after confirming proper placement of the tracheostomy tube using capnography should the tracheal tube be removed.

Ultrasound Prior to Surgical Tracheostomy or PDT

Bedside ultrasound screening may enable optimal needle location by identifying the tracheal rings, thyroid isthmus and pretracheal vascular structures. It enables measuring the distance from the skin to the trachea and avoidance of overlying blood vessels and is especially useful in patients who are morbidly obese or have difficult neck anatomy in whom the trachea may be impalpable and may not be in the midline (See Chapter 7).

Flexible Bronchoscopy during PDT

Flexible bronchoscopy during PDT enables passage of the needle, guidewire, dilator and tracheostomy tube to be observed and checking of tube tip position following insertion. The bronchoscope should remain within the airway device to avoid damage during needle insertion. It may not be possible to identify the level of the tracheal puncture unless an SGA is used or the tracheal tube is withdrawn significantly, as the tracheal tube within the trachea obscures the upper tracheal rings. Ventilation may be compromised by bronchoscope use and appropriate adjustments to ventilator setting should be made.

Care after PDT

The PDT tract will typically take 7–10 days to mature, compared with 2–4 days for a surgical tracheostomy. Proper fixation of the tracheostomy tube is particularly important after PDT as tube displacement in the first few days after stoma formation means the recently dilated tissues can 'spring' into their original positions, making reinsertion difficult or impossible (Figure 29.3).

Percutaneous versus Surgical Tracheostomy

During PDT there is less dissection and cutting than with a surgical tracheostomy and this may cause less tissue trauma and bleeding. However, a meta-analysis of 22 studies comparing techniques found no differences in mortality or intraoperative or post-operative bleeding, though PDT was quicker and led to less infection.

(a)

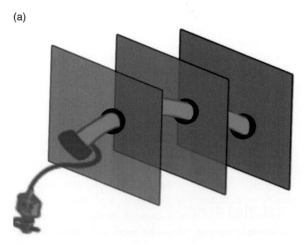

(b)

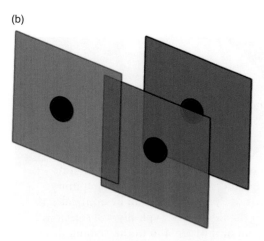

Figure 29.3 If a percutaneously inserted tracheostomy (a) becomes displaced, the recently dilated tissues can 'spring' into their original positions (b), making reinsertion difficult.

After the first week or so, there is little practical difference between the tracheostomy stoma. Better follow-up of tracheostomies may reveal subtle differences in the future.

Physiological Changes for the Patient with a Tracheostomy

Airway anatomy and physiology are altered following tracheostomy. Some physiological changes are advantageous whilst others necessitate extra vigilance.

- Upper airway anatomical dead space can be reduced by up to 50%.
- Dead space takes no part in gas exchange and adds to the work of breathing. This can be advantageous when weaning patients from mechanical ventilation.
- The natural warming, humidification and filtering of air by the upper airway is lost.
- Secretions will become thick and dried and can easily obstruct a stoma or tube.
- The patient's ability to speak is removed.
- Limited or absent vocalisation causes distress and anxiety. Vocalisation strategies such as above-cuff vocalisation or early cuff deflation may be tolerated and one-way speaking valves can help. Non-verbal communication is important and speech and language therapists, attentive nursing staff and communication boards are useful.
- Sense of taste and smell can be lost.
- This can reduce appetite and general well-being of the patient – easily overlooked when managing 'medical' problems.
- The ability to swallow is adversely affected.
- Initially, most will have a nasogastric or gastrostomy tube and feeding regimen established. The cuff of the tracheostomy or the tube itself interferes with the swallowing mechanics of the larynx. These muscles can waste if not used (during prolonged ventilation) and require careful rehabilitation and assessment.
- Altered body image.
- This is an important factor as it can have a major psychological impact, mitigated by careful explanation and support. After a temporary tracheostomy scarring should be minimal and speech should return. Typically, the stoma will close and heal within 4–6 weeks, though this is variable.

Types of Tracheostomy Tubes

Cuffed Tubes

The soft, inflatable distal cuff seals the airway, to facilitate positive pressure ventilation or to minimise aspiration of oral or gastric secretions. Cuffs are not an absolute barrier to (micro)aspiration (Figure 29.4). If the tracheostomy tube lumen is occluded or blocked the patient will not be able to breathe around the tube.

Uncuffed Tubes

Uncuffed tubes allow gas to escape around and above the tracheostomy tube, facilitating vocalisation. If the patient requires a degree of ventilatory support, a mode or type of ventilator that will allow for this 'escape' of gas must be used. Patients must have an effective cough and gag reflex to reduce aspiration risks, although the continual translaryngeal expiratory gas flow may help expel secretions and rehabilitate the larynx (Figure 29.5).

'Minitrach' tubes are uncuffed and typically 4 mm internal diameter. They are designed to enable airway toilet (suction) and are not suitable as a ventilatory device but can deliver supplementary oxygen. The manufacturers do not recommend their use for emergency front of neck airway (eFONA). They are prone to blocking and have limited role outside the carefully monitored setting of ICU.

Double Cannula Tubes

Double cannula tubes have an outer tube (or cannula) to keep the airway patent and an inner, removable 'liner' to facilitate cleaning of secretions. Some inner cannulae are disposable; others must be cleaned and reinserted. They are often favoured in patients who are fully weaned from ventilation and in whom airway blockage from secretions is a risk. Secretions are easily managed by removal of the inner and replacement by a new or cleaned inner. Whilst safer outside the specialist environment, they reduce the diameter of the tube, increasing resistance, and so may not be favoured during mechanical ventilation, when closed-circuit humidification and regular suctioning reduce blockage risks.

Fenestrated Tubes

Fenestrated tubes usually are part of a double cannula tube – with the outer tube having an opening or

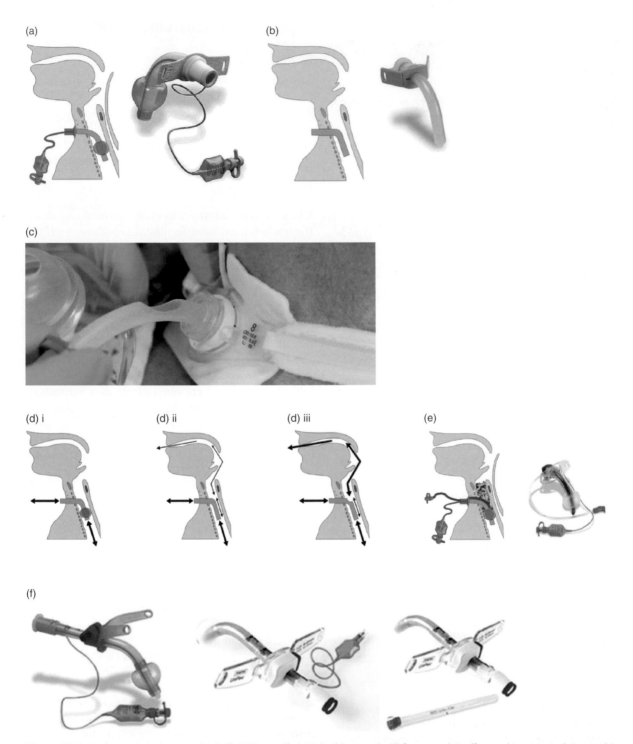

Figure 29.4 Tracheostomy tube types. (a) Cuffed, (b) uncuffed, (c) double cannula, (d) fenestrated: i cuff up and inner cannula inserted (no airflow via upper airways), ii cuff down and inner cannula inserted (some airflow), iii cuff down and inner cannula removed (most airflow), (e) subglottic suction, (f) adjustable flanged.

(a)

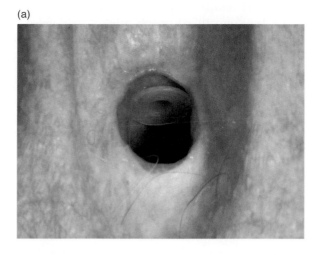

(b)

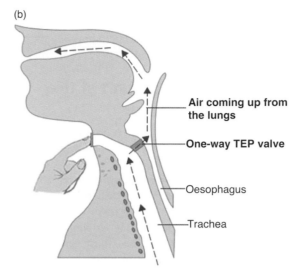

Air coming up from the lungs

One-way TEP valve

Oesophagus

Trachea

Figure 29.5 (a and b) Laryngectomy stoma with Tracheo-(o)Esophageal Puncture (TEP) valve.

openings. During exhalation, gas may pass through the patient's oral/nasal pharynx as well as the tracheal opening, facilitating vocalisation and coughing. When this function is not needed a non-fenestrated inner cannula blocks the fenestrations, with the tube then functioning as non-fenestrated.

Tubes with Subglottic Suction

A narrow tube runs along the outside of the tracheostomy tube terminating just above the cuff. This enables suction to clear secretions from above the cuff/below the glottis – subglottic suction. Subglottic suction may reduce the incidence of ventilator-associated pneumonia.

If a low flow of gas is applied retrogradely to the suction tube this can exit via the upper airway and enable 'above-cuff vocalisation'. This can help normalising laryngeal function, vocalisation and swallowing after critical illness.

Adjustable Flange Tracheostomy Tubes (Figure 29.4f)

Obese patients with a tracheostomy are at significantly increased risk of problems compared with the non-obese, including displacement. Adjustable flange tracheostomy tubes enable the length of the intratracheal portion to be adjusted and are particularly suitable for obese patients. Particular indications include:

- large neck girth/obesity
- oedema, particularly burns
- actual or anticipated oedema after surgical procedures (including tracheostomy itself)

Problems with Tracheostomies

Tracheostomy patients have significant co-morbidities and high in-hospital mortality (around 20%). When a clinical incident occurs relating to a tracheostomy, the chance of patient harm is ≈60–70%, depending on patient location.

Incidents may be classified as:

- procedural (e.g. airway loss; damage of adjacent structures; bleeding)
- blockage or displacement after placement
- equipment (lack of equipment or inappropriate use)
- competency (skills and knowledge)
- infrastructure (staffing and location)
- late complications (e.g. tracheomalacia; stenosis; infection of stoma)

The majority of these incidents are due to the same recurring themes, many of which may be prevented by prospective quality improvement strategies.

The Patient Perspective

The patient, and to some extent their family, will often have a different view of the problems a tracheostomy can bring, with a lack of vocalisation and difficulty in swallowing solids or liquids often being the most important issues. Addressing these concerns with the multidisciplinary team can help improve the quality of care.

Emergency Management of the Tracheostomy Patient

Patients with tracheostomies are uniquely vulnerable to airway problems, which may rapidly become life-threatening. Deterioration can be rapid if the patient is critically ill, ventilator-dependent or has an altered or abnormal upper airway. Many tracheostomy problems are predictable and commonly involve warning signs ('red flags') prior to a problem developing (Table 29.1).

The UK National Tracheostomy Safety Project (NTSP) developed guidance for the management of such emergencies in 2012. The resulting algorithms guide responders to address the commonest and most easily rectifiable problems in a sequential way (Figure 29.6). Removal of a confirmed blocked or displaced tube is encouraged, breaking down barriers and giving 'permission' to junior staff to undertake potentially lifesaving interventions that were previously considered a specialist skill.

Key principles of the guideline are:

1. Algorithms are paired with bedhead signs, indicating whether the patient has a tracheostomy or laryngectomy, and identifying specific airway issues.
2. Waveform capnography has a prominent role at an early stage in emergency management.
3. Oxygenation of the patient is prioritised.

Table 29.1 Tracheostomy red flags

Any physiological change, including agitation, can be caused by an obstructed or partially obstructed airway and airway problems should be excluded.

1. Absence or change of capnograph waveform with ventilation
2. Absence or change of chest wall movement with ventilation
3. Increasing airway pressure
4. Reducing tidal volume
5. Inability to pass a suction catheter
6. Obvious air leak
7. Vocalisation with a cuffed tube in place and inflated
8. Apparent deflation, or need for regular re-inflation, of the pilot balloon
9. Discrepancy between actual and recorded tube insertion depth
10. Surgical emphysema

4. Trials of ventilation via a potentially displaced tracheostomy tube to assess patency are avoided.
5. Suction is only attempted after removing a potentially blocked inner tube.
6. Oxygen is applied to both potential airways.
7. Simple methods to oxygenate and ventilate via the stoma are described, such as using a paediatric face mask or SGA applied to the skin.
8. A blocked or displaced tracheostomy tube is removed as soon as this problem is identified, not as a 'last resort'.

Whilst these algorithms are designed to be universal, local or patient-specific circumstances should be taken into account. For example, an ICU patient with a recently formed tracheostomy for weaning from ventilation may be far more easily managed via the patent upper airway than via a new PDT stoma. Bleeding from the stoma commonly represents suction-related trauma but may herald an arterial bleed. Hyperinflation of the tube cuff, aggressive resuscitation and prompt surgical intervention are warranted, although mortality rates from tracheo-innominate fistulae remain high.

Decannulation

Decannulation may be performed for temporary tracheostomies, once the primary condition for which the tracheostomy was performed has resolved. The upper airway must be patent and laryngeopharyngeal function adequate enough to 'protect' the airway following decannulation (flexible optical bronchoscopic evaluation may be required). The patient should have an adequate cough to clear secretions without invasive suctioning and should no longer be dependent on mechanical ventilation. Some centres will 'downsize' the tracheostomy tube (replacement with a smaller size) promoting translaryngeal airflow, speech and laryngeal function before decannulation.

Paediatric Tracheostomy

In-depth discussion of paediatric tracheostomy is beyond the remit of this chapter.

The indications for paediatric tracheostomy are similar to those for adults but there are key differences to consider in routine and emergency care of children with a tracheostomy. Tracheostomy may be required from the first few moments of life, for airway abnormalities or long-term ventilation, with the majority

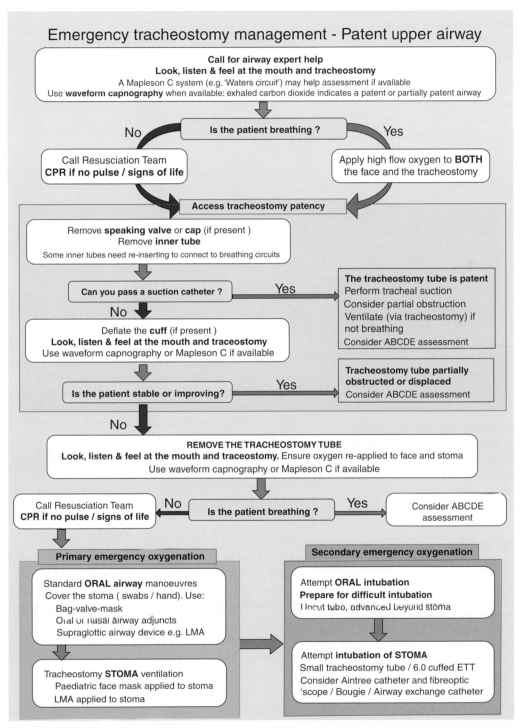

Figure 29.6 The NTSP algorithm for management of an airway emergency in a patient with a tracheostomy. (From National Tracheostomy Safety Project.)

performed in children < 4 years old: many are permanent or at least long term with significant lifestyle changes for the child and their parents or carers.

The tracheostomy is typically a surgical procedure, although percutaneous techniques are described. Uncuffed tubes without an inner cannula (which would reduce the inner diameter excessively) are used routinely. Neonatal tubes may be very short with high risk of displacement. Cuffed tubes are occasionally required to manage high ventilation pressures or aspiration risk.

Emergency guidelines developed by the NTSP are directed at multidisciplinary responders who may not be airway or tracheostomy experts, recognising that paediatric patients with a tracheostomy are more likely to be managed in the community than adults. Children with tracheostomies often have multiple other medical needs and may present for unrelated medical care.

The principles of providing emergency oxygenation and limiting the number of unnecessary airway interventions are retained from the adult guidelines, but key differences include:

- Bespoke paediatric bedhead signs reflecting paediatric tracheostomy indications and pathologies
- Recognition of (almost) exclusively surgical tracheostomies with stay sutures and maturation sutures available to aid emergency management
- Initial management includes up to three attempts at emergency tracheostomy tube changes
- Use of suction catheters to guide reinsertion

Laryngectomy Stoma

A laryngeal stoma is importantly different than a tracheostomy. Key differences are described in Table 29.2.

A total laryngectomy – usually for cancer – involves the removal of the larynx, including vocal cords. The trachea is transected and sutured to the neck skin creating a permanent stoma through which the patient breathes (Figure 29.5). These patients are often referred to as 'neck breathers', though the term 'neck-only breathers' might be even better in distinguishing them from others with tracheostomies. The upper airways are no longer connected to the trachea and thus oxygenation or ventilation via face mask, SGA or intubation is *impossible*. It is essential that the presence of a laryngectomy stoma is clearly

Table 29.2 Key differences between a laryngectomy stoma and tracheostomy

Laryngectomy stoma	Tracheostomy
Permanent procedure	May be temporary or permanent
No communication between the lungs and upper airway	The larynx is present and thus there is still a potential connection between the upper airway and the lungs
Does not typically require any tube to keep the stoma patent	A tracheostomy tube when inserted stents the tracheostomy open facilitating gas exchange and will readily close without a supportive stenting mechanism
Aspiration of gastric contents is not a concern	Aspiration of gastric contents remains possible

identified – MedicAlert bracelets, medical records or a bedhead sign are all useful – especially for potential responders to an airway emergency.

Despite removal of the larynx, 'vocalisation' is possible following laryngectomy if a tracheo-oesophageal puncture (TEP) prosthesis with a one-way valve is inserted, at the time of the laryngectomy or later. By occluding the stoma during exhalation, gas is directed via the oesophagus and pharynx, and with practice this enables quiet speech (Figure 29.5). These valves do not require removal during airway management, but may get displaced, rotated or occluded and should be reviewed following instrumentation of the trachea.

Routine Care for a Laryngectomy Stoma

A working knowledge of the basic management and equipment used in patients with a laryngectomy stoma can avoid complications and improve a patient's comfort and safety. The basic equipment required for routine care includes:

- suction device
- humidification device
- personal mirror
- soft laryngectomy tube/tracheostomy tube

Though most laryngectomy stomas do not require a tube to keep them patent, some patients may use a laryngectomy tube to assist with hygiene.

Gentle suctioning directed with a small personal mirror is performed to remove excess mucus or crusting near the stoma opening and for airway clearance.

(a) (b)

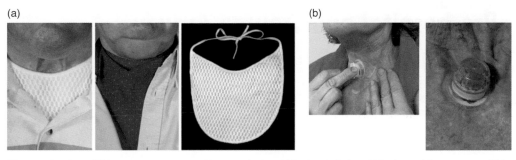

Figure 29.7 (a and b) Laryngectomy stoma with covers for humidification, including: (a) Buchanan bibs, cravats and (b) adhesive stoma covers.

Routine humidification – provided by small heat and moisture exchange (HME) devices or covers (Figure 29.7) – is required to prevent thick mucus plugs from forming. Saline nebulisers or active, warm humidification may be required if the patient becomes unwell, dehydrated or develops a respiratory infection.

Approach to Complications and Emergencies with a Laryngectomy Stoma

Dyspnoea
- Partial or complete tracheal blockage by retained secretions, mucus plugs or a foreign body can cause dyspnoea. Apply humidified oxygen to the stoma, ask the patient to cough, attempt suction with a flexible suction catheter and consider instilled saline. If the suction catheter passes easily, consider non-airway causes of dyspnoea. An otolaryngologist should evaluate the patient urgently if the condition does not improve. Oxygenation and ventilation via laryngectomy stoma can be achieved using a paediatric face mask or SGA device placed over the stoma, creating a seal. Intubation of the stoma may be required: a standard or shortened (e.g. Montandon) tracheal tube or tracheostomy tube should be directly inserted into the stoma. The remaining trachea is short and airway devices should be placed such that the balloon is nearly visible under the skin.

Pharyngocutaneous fistula
- This is most common in the first few weeks after a laryngectomy due to breakdown of the mucosal lining resulting in salivary leakage to surrounding tissue. Initial clinical signs are neck erythema, facial and neck oedema and tenderness. Early recognition is essential to prevent wound complications and potential breakdown of nearby vessels.

Bleeding
- Bleeding is an airway emergency and may result in airway compromise. All bleeding needs prompt assessment by an otolaryngologist. Causes include poor humidification, suction trauma, local or respiratory tract infection, or disease recurrence with resulting fistula formation or blood vessel erosion. Carotid artery or jugular vein 'blowouts' can result in a life-threatening emergency. In an emergency, secure the airway with a cuffed tube. Hyperinflation of the cuff or manual compression of the vessel can help to tamponade bleeding points. Bleeding may be temporarily reduced or stopped by applying finger pressure to the root of the neck in the sternal notch (see also Chapter 32). Haemodynamic and respiratory support should be started simultaneously, while preparing for surgical intervention.

Further Reading

Al-Shathri Z, Susanto I. (2018). Percutaneous tracheostomy. *Seminars in Respiratory Critical Care Medicine*, **39**, 720–730.

Bontempo LJ, Manning SL. (2019). Tracheostomy emergencies. *Emergency Medicine Clinics of North America*, **37**, 109–119.

Doherty C, Neal R, English C, et al.; Paediatric Working Party of the National Tracheostomy Safety Project. (2018). Multidisciplinary guidelines for the management of paediatric tracheostomy emergencies. *Anaesthesia*, **73**, 1400–1417.

Lerner AD, Yarmus L. (2018). Percutaneous dilational tracheostomy. *Clinics in Chest Medicine*, **39**, 211–222.

McGrath BA, Bates L, Atkinson D, Moore JA; National Tracheostomy Safety Project. (2012). Multidisciplinary guidelines for the management of tracheostomy and laryngectomy airway emergencies. *Anaesthesia*, **67**, 1025–1041.

Chapter 30

Pre-hospital and Trauma Airway Management

Leif Rognås and David Lockey

Introduction

The pathophysiology of the critically unwell or injured patient is the same in the pre-hospital setting as it is in the emergency department or intensive care unit. The requirement for high quality airway management is not dependent on the patient location.

The concepts described in other chapters are almost all applicable to pre-hospital patients. What then is different in the pre-hospital environment?

- Pre-hospital clinicians see patients at an earlier point after injury or onset of serious illness and the signs and symptoms may therefore be less developed or more difficult to detect.
- Although pre-hospital access to electronic patient charts are available in some areas, most pre-hospital clinicians have only limited information about a patient's past medical history.
- The emergency medical system (EMS) in many areas is multi-tiered, but the availability of backup is often limited, and may be a considerable distance away.
- The amount of equipment available on scene is limited.
- Patients in need of pre-hospital airway management in general, and pre-hospital advanced airway management (PHAAM) in particular, make up only a small percentage of the pre-hospital workload making airway management skill retention a challenge for some practitioners.

Tailored Care

Many pre-hospital services have structured standard operating procedures (SOPs) which dictate how anaesthesia and airway management is conducted. This contributes to predictable, high quality care.

However, this does not mean that 'one size has to fit all' and pre-hospital airway management can be tailored to patients, providers and the system delivering care.

Tailored Care: Patient Level

Before advanced airway intervention an informal risk–benefit assessment is made taking into account the condition and characteristics of the individual patient and the features of the pre-hospital situation in which they are. Typical features which may change management might include: the size and age of a patient, the presence of severe co-morbidities, airway abnormalities, access to the patient, a hazardous environment and the proximity to hospital.

Tailored Care: Clinician Level

Even with the development of pre-hospital training programmes and standardisation of advanced pre-hospital provider roles there is considerable variation in the experience and competences of providers, both between different professional groups and within them. Pre-hospital doctors may be trainee emergency physicians with the minimum anaesthetic training or consultant anaesthetists with many years of experience. Similarly, paramedics may have practised for many years at an advanced level or may have limited advanced airway skills. It is rare for pre-hospital practitioners to deliver anaesthesia frequently enough to remain competent without some in-hospital anaesthesia practice. The experience of the attending pre-hospital team may influence the decision to anaesthetise on scene.

Tailored Care: System Level

An EMS delivering PHAAM can tailor its activity by dictating what level of airway management is provided, for which patients and by what level of provider. Providers may be doctors, paramedics or nurses. The level of training and skill retention can be stipulated. The clinical governance of advanced airway management commonly lies with the ambulance service, an air ambulance or a hosting hospital. The EMS also has to consider the case mix and frequency of specific airway problems and how the evidence base for airway management should be applied to the population served. To provide the highest level of patient safety, the pre-hospital airway management offered by one EMS/helicopter emergency medical service (HEMS) may not be identical to that offered by another.

Human Factors

Using the combined knowledge of the entire team, empowering all team members to speak up when necessary and having a shared mental model is vital (see Chapter 36). In addition, we recommend the following in order to facilitate cognitive offloading and improve patient safety:

- Airway management should be performed in a well-lit place with shelter and as close to 360° patient access as possible. Many services prefer to do this outside; but occasionally this may not be possible due to weather or other external factors.
- A standardised equipment set-up should be used in every case (standard 'kit dump').
- A standardised, well-rehearsed, pre-procedure checklist that has been tailored to the service guides preparation and delivery of pre-hospital anaesthesia. Having an unnecessarily long or impractical checklist reduces compliance and leads to checklist fatigue. Figures 30.1 and 30.2 show different tailored pre-rapid sequence intubation (RSI) checklists for two different doctor–paramedic staffed HEMS.
- Regular simulations (or 'moulages') tailored to the needs of both the individual clinicians being 'moulaged' and the service should be used to practise the different components of airway management.

An in-hospital airway management expert does not necessarily translate to a pre-hospital airway management expert. The psychomotor skills of bag-valve-mask (BVM) ventilation, placing a supraglottic airway device (SGA) or tracheal intubation are transferable; the knowledge of where, when and how to use these skills in a less predictable environment may not be.

Data Collection

Pre-hospital services should record core data on airway intervention including timelines, success rates and complications. This enables service improvement and the identification of equipment, training and skill problems that require attention. Data may also be used to design and adapt service SOPs and be used by clinicians to inform decision making on-scene.

The Anatomically vs. Physiologically Difficult Airway

Anaesthetists often concentrate on the issues of difficult BVM ventilation, SGA placement and tracheal intubation. The difficulties of the anatomically difficult airway are also a routine consideration. These subjects are described in many other chapters.

The concept of a 'physiologically' difficult airway is more recent. The physiologically difficult airway has been described as one in which severe physiological derangements place the patient at increased risk for desaturation or cardiovascular collapse and death during intubation and the transition to positive pressure ventilation (see also Chapter 28).

In pre-hospital airway management this is as important as anatomical considerations. A significant proportion of patients have increased risks of desaturation or cardiovascular collapse during anaesthesia and airway management. Managing physiological considerations is essential in pre-hospital and trauma airway management to prevent potentially catastrophic hypotension, cardiac arrest or hypoxic brain injury.

Additional factors contributing to pre-hospital airway management difficulty include *logistic difficulty* (attributable to location, environment and equipment) and *educational difficulty* (lack of knowledge, training or preparation by the operator). A well-organised pre-hospital system should eliminate or minimise the impact of these.

The Practicalities of Pre-hospital Airway Management

The fundamental principle of good pre-hospital airway management is that it should be performed to the same standard and with the same level of patient safety as when performed in the emergency department or the intensive care unit. There are published recommendations on standards that should be achieved when delivering pre-hospital anaesthesia and advanced airway management from the UK, Scandinavia and the USA. All have a great deal in common.

Have a Plan

It is vital to have and to communicate both a plan and a backup plan. The plan should state intended techniques for addressing any problems which develop during the management of both anatomically and physiologically difficult airways after induction of anaesthesia.

STANDARD PRE-RSI CHECKLIST		
	⬇ START OF CHECKLIST ⬇	Expected Response
SET UP	Anticipated difficult?...	....................................Yes/No
	Position optimal?..	....Check
	C-spine control?..	..........................Yes/Not required
	Cricoid required?...	....................................Yes/No
	Roles allocated?..	Intub1 =........ Intub 2 =.......... MILS=............. Cricoid=............
	Nasal oxgen?...	....................................Yes/No
	Oxygen?...	...................2 cylinders, full & on
	Suction?...	Working, check
	Pre oxygenation with full assembly?.........................	....Check
	IV access x2..	....Check
Monitoring	ECG...	...............................Rate/Rhythm
	Sats..	....%
	BP value & Interval...	..................x/ymmHg, set to 2min, adult/paeds/neonate
	Capnography connected...	....Check
Airway	Laryngoscope (blade/size), (Spare/size)..........................	1st [blade], 2nd [blade]
	Bougie (size)...	....Check
	TT	..........1st [Size], 2nd [Size]
	Syringe..	....Check
Drugs	Induction...	.................[Drug(s)], [Dose, mg,mls]
	Rocuronium...	............................[Dose, mg/mls]
	Maintenance available?...	...............[Intended agent] Check
Drills	Plan B...	....Check
	Plan C...	....Check
	Thoracostomies required?.......................................	Yes/No.....[Side]
END OF CHECKLIST - PROCEED TO GIVE DRUGS		

Figure 30.1 (a) Pre-RSI check list from the Emergency Medical Retrieval and Transfer Service, Wales.

Basic Pre-hospital Airway Management

The term 'basic' may be misleading because basic manoeuvres can be both technically and cognitively challenging.

Positioning

- This may be the difference between success and failure. Getting it wrong can make all that follows very difficult.

- Top tip #1: never ask a patient in respiratory distress to lie flat.

- Top tip #2: almost all airway manoeuvres can be performed with the patient either sitting up or lying on their side. If a supine position is necessary to place an SGA or tracheal tube it is usually possible to wait until everything else is prepared (including induction drugs given) before placing them flat on their back.

IMMEDIATE INTUBATION CHECKLIST		
START OF CHECKLIST		Expected Response
Position optimal ?..		...............................check
Oxygen Cylinders x 2, on & flowing..		...............................check
[BVM] or [Water's Circuit] connected.......................		...............................check
End tidal CO2 connected....................................		...............................check
Suction unit working and positioned.......................		...............................check
Laryngoscope ready and working..........................		...............................check
Tube ready..		.......................size [x] check
Bougie ready...		...............................check
Induction drugs..		[drug 1], [drug 2], [drug 3] check
Vascular access..		[location where drugs to be given]
END OF CHECKLIST - PROCED TO GIVE DRUGS		

Figure 30.1 (b) immediate intubation checklist from the Emergency Medical Retrieval and Transfer Service, Wales.

Airway opening
- Both the 'head tilt–chin lift' and the 'jaw thrust' manoeuvres may be used. Jaw thrust is an effective manoeuvre and should be perfected by all pre-hospital clinicians.
- The use of suction is often required; we recommend the use of rigid, large-bore suction catheters (i.e. Yankauer or DuCanto).
- Airway adjuncts are used as indicated; the nasopharyngeal airway is better tolerated than the oropharyngeal airway in the semi-conscious patient.

BVM ventilation (see Chapter 12)
- This is often the fastest way of providing both oxygenation and ventilation in a patient with insufficient spontaneous ventilation. It is a core anaesthetic skill but when performed by other practitioners it requires training and ongoing experience to master.
- Effective pre-hospital BVM ventilation can be facilitated by:
  - using continuous waveform capnography to evaluate the effectiveness of ventilation
  - a two-handed technique using the thenar eminence grip ('V-grip') which allows a combination of an efficient jaw thrust and a tight mask seal
  - Two nasopharyngeal airways and an oropharyngeal airway can be inserted if required

Pre-hospital Advanced Airway Management (PHAAM)

The placement of an SGA, a tracheal tube or a surgical airway constitutes advanced airway management.

PHAAM in cardiac arrest patients
Detailed discussion of this topic is beyond the scope of this chapter and is discussed in Chapter 31. Principles are that
- High quality chest compressions and early defibrillation have priority
- For non-experts, the use of BVM or an SGA is preferable to tracheal intubation
- Tracheal intubation should not interrupt chest compressions for more than 10 seconds

POST RSI CHECKLIST				
	START OF CHECKLIST	Expected response		
➡	End Tidal Trace and target..	...[Good] waveform, [x] kPa		
	Oxygen saturation...	.....................Sats are [x]		
	Breath Sounds...	...............[bilateral] check		
➡	ETT Length and secured...	.........Secured, length is [x]		
➡	Thoracostomy(s) required......................................	.... check [side]		
➡	Access adequate and secured................................	.............................check		
➡	Blood needed?..	.....................[plan] check		
➡	Vasopressor needed?..	.....................[plan] check		
➡	On-going anaesthetic plan is [x]................................	.....................[plan] check		
➡	Temperature probe reading.....................................	..............[x]degrees check		
➡	Splints required?...	.....................[plan] check		
	END OF CHECKLIST			

Figure 30.1 (c) post RSI checklist from the Emergency Medical Retrieval and Transfer Service, Wales.

Pre-RSI checklist
Danish Air Ambulance

"SO BAD"

Suction	Working	Check
Oxygen	>100 bar + backup cylinder	Check
BVM	Working	Check
Airway rescue plan	Verbalised, equipment ready	Check
Drugs	Verbalised, equipment ready	Check

Figure 30.2 Pre-RSI check list from the Danish Air Ambulance.

PHAAM in non-cardiac arrest patients

In the majority of systems, tracheal intubation is the preferred modality if the patient needs PHAAM and an appropriately trained team is available.

Pre-hospital tracheal intubation in the non-cardiac arrest patient requires pre-hospital emergency anaesthesia.

Indications for pre-hospital emergency anaesthesia and tracheal intubation include:

- Impending or actual hypoxia
- Impending or actual acute hypercapnia or ventilatory failure
- Threatened or actual loss of airway patency
- Severe agitation associated with head injury
- Reduced level of consciousness
- Humanitarian indications

Expert clinicians may choose to perform pre-hospital emergency anaesthesia and tracheal intubation for other reasons (i.e. anticipated clinical course) based on an individual risk–benefit analysis.

Preparation should focus on optimising the first intubation attempt and minimising the risk of complications. Complication rates associated with first-pass success (FPS) have been reported to be 10–12% compared with 40% when FPS is not achieved.

Oxygenation

Pre-oxygenation

- In the patient who is spontaneously breathing (with sufficient minute volumes) we suggest pre-oxygenation with one of
    - A tight-fitting non-rebreather mask with oxygen reservoir in combination with nasal oxygen to maximise FiO_2
    - A Mapleson C (Waters type) circuit providing both high FiO_2 and the possibility for adding positive end-expiratory pressure
    - Continuous positive airway pressure (CPAP) or non-invasive ventilation (NIV) using an advanced transport ventilator and a tight-fitting face mask
- In patients with insufficient spontaneous ventilation, pre-oxygenation can be provided with one of
    - BVM ventilation
    - a Mapleson C circuit
    - non-invasive ventilation

In the agitated or combative patient, careful sedation (i.e. with ketamine) may be necessary in order to be able to provide effective pre-oxygenation. Induction of emergency anaesthesia without pre-oxygenation should be avoided.

Peroxygenation

Serious consideration should also be given to delivering gentle, low frequency, low tidal-volume BVM ventilation in the apnoeic period before laryngoscopy is performed.

Apnoeic oxygenation (high oxygen flow through nasal cannulae) may prevent desaturation and hypoxia during laryngoscopy.

Drug Choice

Although most anaesthetic drugs can be used safely in the pre-hospital environment most systems encourage standardisation and a limited choice of agents. Ketamine is commonly used and is a safe anaesthetic drug of choice in most pre-hospital settings. Opiates are usually administered with the induction agent but

increase the risk of post-induction hypotension if doses are too high. The most frequently administered neuromuscular blocking agent is rocuronium. Suxamethonium use is rapidly declining.

Tracheal Intubation

Laryngoscopy

There is evidence that the routine use of videolaryngoscopy by experienced and well-trained clinicians is associated with higher FPS rates in pre-hospital tracheal intubation when compared with direct laryngoscopy. However, there is currently insufficient evidence to recommend videolaryngoscopy as a standard in every HEMS/EMS and the choice of primary device has to be tailored to the individual service. It is, however, recommended that a videolaryngoscope with both a standard and hyperangulated blade is available as a primary or rescue device when pre-hospital emergency anaesthesia and tracheal intubation is performed and that team members are well trained in the use of the chosen device(s).

The use of a hyperangulated videolaryngoscope in combination with the standard bougies seen in some EMS and HEMS can be problematic. Hyperangulated videolaryngoscopes are made to 'look around corners' and most bougies are made to guide the tube in a straight line or a slight curve. The use of a hyperangulated videolaryngoscope requires a mouldable stylet (see Chapters 15 and 17).

Confirmation of Intubation

The only acceptable confirmation of tube position is continuous waveform capnography. No trace = wrong place (see Chapter 3).

Post-intubation Management

A protocolised approach to post-intubation management can free up hands as well as mental capacity while minimising the risk of adverse events:

- Make sure that the tracheal tube is properly secured
- Always have a self-inflating bag, a mask and a syringe (for cuff inflation) within reach
- Use an automated ventilator whenever practicable
- Avoid unnecessarily high FiO_2
- Provide lung-protective ventilation to all patients
- Have pre-drawn vasopressors available

275

- Choose long-acting, cardiovascular stable drugs for continuous sedation and analgesia
- Have more than one vascular access point

Failed Intubation

The 'Vortex approach' is a good framework for failed intubation in the pre-hospital setting (see Chapter 36). Every EMS/HEMS providing PHAAM should carry a second generation SGA, a videolaryngoscope and the equipment necessary to achieve an emergency front of neck airway (eFONA).

The following are also recommended:

- Have a predefined and well-practised failed intubation drill. Many services use a '30-second drill' to make sure that an optimal intubation attempt is performed within a short time period.
- Before commencing with PHAAM, always agree on how an eFONA will be achieved if needed.
- Practise the conduct of an eFONA on a regular basis.
- Think very carefully before removing or changing a well (or just decent) functioning SGA that has been placed as a rescue device.

Aspiration Risk Management

Due care should be taken to reduce the risk of aspiration. The following is a practical approach:

- Patients with blood or gastric content in their upper airways who are able to clear this themselves must be allowed to do so and to choose their own positioning until anaesthetic induction drugs (if performing an RSI) have rendered them unresponsive.
- Consider placing the unconscious patients in a lateral position in order to facilitate passive clearance of the airways during preparation for advanced airway management.
- During airway management, at least one functioning suction unit must be ready and at hand at all times.
- There is little consensus regarding the use of cricoid force during RSI. If cricoid force is applied, it must be done by a sufficiently briefed assistant and be released if laryngoscopy proves difficult. Cricoid force can be successfully used to manipulate the upper airway to improve laryngoscopic view.

- Fear of aspiration must never take priority over oxygenation.

Airway Management in Trauma Patients including Cervical Spine Protection

A detailed description of all the different presentations of airway management in trauma patients is beyond the scope of this chapter. For this we refer to the Further Reading.

Some key points when managing trauma patients include:

- Controlling catastrophic external haemorrhage takes priority over airway management.
- Deliver the basics well – oxygenation, basic airway manoeuvres, intravenous/intraosseous access, keeping the patient warm.
- Perform a full rapid primary survey whenever possible.
- Be aware of on-scene time (or time to theatre if in the emergency department).
- Positioning is key; let blood and other bodily fluids drain from the airway. Where advanced airway management is not available on scene the unconscious trauma patient can be placed in the 'lateral trauma position' to provide the best chance of a patent airway with passive drainage of blood and gastric content.
- Have backup suction ready.
- If the cervical spine of blunt trauma patients cannot be cleared using local protocol, care must be taken to limit any movement of the cervical spine during airway management:
  - The indications for semi-rigid cervical collars have recently changed in some countries but are still standard practice in many services. Anaesthetised trauma patients are likely to be effectively immobilised with blocks and tape in a neutral position.
  - The collar must be removed and manual in-line stabilisation (MILS) applied during laryngoscopy.
  - It is important that the clinician providing the MILS is properly briefed and positioned in a way that does not hinder laryngoscopy.
  - Videolaryngoscopy may be preferable for intubation of patients with suspected cervical spine injury.

- Both the induction of anaesthesia and positive ventilation will negatively influence cardiac output and blood pressure in the circulatory unstable patient.
- If at all possible, always resuscitate before induction of anaesthesia. Consider less invasive airway manoeuvres while resuscitating.
- In awake shocked patients consider delaying induction of anaesthesia until blood products and surgical intervention are available.
- Choose induction agents and opiate dosage carefully.
- Be ready to perform bilateral finger thoracostomies if the trauma patient deteriorates and pneumothorax cannot be ruled out after the initiation of positive pressure ventilation.
- Pay particular attention to pre-and post-induction end-tidal carbon dioxide in head-injured patients. Normoventilation is key unless there is evidence of imminent coning.
- In stable patients with maxillofacial or direct airway trauma, consider delaying advanced airway management. An awake technique performed by an expert in the operating theatre may be the safest option.

Summary

Pre-hospital airway management should be performed to the same standards as would be expected in the emergency department. Tailoring pre-hospital airway management in terms of clinical care delivered to the patient, skills of the clinician and the infrastructure of the EMS is recommended. Having a standardised, well-rehearsed approach, using aids to reduce cognitive load, articulating a clear airway management plan and having a structured way of handling airway management difficulties is considered essential. Excellent pre-oxygenation, peroxygenation, FPS and post-intubation care are required to maximise patient safety. Backup equipment in the form of a second generation SGA, a videolaryngoscope with both standard and hyperangulated blades and equipment for an eFONA should be available when advanced pre-hospital airway management is provided. An awareness of potential anatomical difficulties combined with careful management of physiological derangement is necessary to deliver safe, high quality care.

Further Reading

Ångerman S, Kirves H, Nurmi J. (2018). A before-and-after observational study of a protocol for use of the C-MAC videolaryngoscope with a Frova introducer in pre-hospital rapid sequence intubation. *Anaesthesia*, 73, 348–355.

Crewdson K, Fragoso-Iniguez M, Lockey DJ. (2019). Requirement for urgent tracheal intubation after traumatic injury: a retrospective analysis of 11,010 patients in the Trauma Audit Research Network database. *Anaesthesia*, 74, 1158–1164.

Gellerfors M, Fevang E, Bäckman A, et al. (2018). Pre-hospital advanced airway management by anaesthetist and nurse anaesthetist critical care teams: a prospective observational study of 2028 pre-hospital tracheal intubations. *British Journal of Anaesthesia*, 120, 1103–1109.

Kovacs G, Sowers N. (2018). Airway management in trauma. *Emergency Medicine Clinics of North America*, 36, 61–84.

Lockey D, Crewdson K, Davies G, et al. (2017). AAGBI: Safer pre-hospital anaesthesia 2017: Association of Anaesthetists of Great Britain and Ireland. *Anaesthesia*, 72, 379–390.

Rehn M, Hyldmo PK, Magnusson V, et al. (2016). Scandinavian SSAI clinical practice guideline on pre-hospital airway management. *Acta Anaesthesiologica Scandinavica*, 60, 852–864.

Airway Management during CPR

Jerry P. Nolan and Jasmeet Soar

Objectives of Airway Management during Cardiac Arrest

The priorities of airway management during cardio-pulmonary resuscitation (CPR) are to minimise interruptions in chest compressions, to optimise blood flow and oxygen delivery to vital organs and to minimise delays in defibrillation if the initial rhythm is shockable. Thus, during the initial treatment of cardiac arrest, unusually, the circulation takes priority over the airway. Maintaining a patent airway will enable ventilation and oxygenation of the lungs, which becomes increasingly important after the first 3–4 minutes of sudden primary cardiac arrest (i.e. of cardiac cause). Early oxygenation and ventilation are important after asphyxial cardiac arrest although existing resuscitation guidelines recommend the same sequence of actions regardless of cause.

Stepwise Approach to Airway Management during Cardiac Arrest

Airway management during cardiac arrest is undertaken by a range of individuals with widely varying skills, from laypeople to highly skilled anaesthetists. On witnessing an out-of-hospital cardiac arrest (OHCA) and calling the emergency medical services (EMS), untrained bystanders are usually instructed by the dispatcher to provide compression-only CPR. Bystanders trained in CPR may attempt a chin lift manoeuvre to restore airway patency and attempt mouth-to-mouth rescue breathing. An EMS technician will be trained to use an oropharyngeal airway (OPA) and bag-mask device, while a paramedic is likely to be trained to use a supraglottic airway (SGA) and, in many cases, a tracheal tube. Thus, during resuscitation following OHCA, there is often a progression in complexity of airway management, from no intervention (compression-only CPR), mouth-to-mouth, and bag-mask ventilation, through

to SGA devices and tracheal intubation. The best airway management technique is likely to vary with patient factors, the cause of cardiac arrest, the stage of resuscitation and the skills of the attending rescuers. The ideal airway management strategy during CPR remains unclear and this typical stepwise approach makes it complicated to study (Figure 31.1).

The situation is not dissimilar following in-hospital cardiac arrest (IHCA). Depending on the location in hospital, the first responders are unlikely to have advanced airway skills and there is frequently a short period of compression-only CPR while resuscitation equipment is obtained. In the United Kingdom (UK), resuscitation teams will often not include a doctor trained in intubation and the resuscitation team may use an OPA and bag-mask and/or an SGA. Intubation is more likely if the resuscitation attempt is prolonged, if the airway cannot be maintained with an SGA, or after return of spontaneous circulation (ROSC) has been achieved.

Bag-Mask Ventilation

Oxygenating and ventilating the lungs with a self-inflating bag and face mask is considered to be basic airway management. Two breaths are given after every 30 chest compressions. Many studies show EMS personnel can ventilate the lungs of anaesthetised patients using a bag-mask, but few studies show if this is successfully achieved during CPR. Many OHCA observational studies show better outcomes when a bag-mask is used compared with advanced airway management (with an SGA or tracheal tube). A meta-analysis of 17 observational studies included nearly 400,000 patients and reported that use of an advanced airway was associated with reduced long-term survival (odds ratio (OR) 0.49 (95% confidence interval (CI) 0.37–0.65)). These results are clearly biased by confounders such as the fact that those who achieve ROSC very rapidly may not then need an advanced airway ('resuscitation time bias'). Even

Stepwise approach to airway management

Figure 31.1 The stepwise approach to airway management during cardiopulmonary resuscitation.

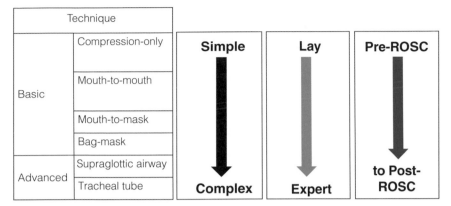

though many observational studies use statistical techniques, such as propensity analysis, in an attempt to eliminate confounders, it is possible that unaccounted for factors remain responsible for the better outcome associated with basic compared with advanced airway management.

Tracheal Intubation

Once the trachea has been intubated, chest compressions can continue uninterrupted while the lungs are ventilated at 10 breaths min^{-1} – even if inspiration coincides with a chest compression, lung inflation will still be achieved and gastric inflation prevented. Regurgitation is common after cardiac arrest and tracheal intubation will prevent subsequent aspiration of gastric contents. However, in OHCA studies two thirds of those cardiac arrest victims who regurgitate do so before arrival of EMS personnel.

Limitations of tracheal intubation during resuscitation are that the procedure may interrupt chest compressions; with less experienced intubators this may be for long periods. A United States study of 100 pre-hospital paramedic intubations documented median intubation-related interruptions to CPR of 110 (Inter-quartile range (IQR) 54–198) seconds, exceeding 3 minutes in a quarter of cases. Current European guidelines recommend compression pauses for < 5 seconds for tracheal tube insertion.

Several studies have documented rates of unrecognised oesophageal intubation after OHCA of 2–6%. Tracheal intubation would have to offer very significant advantages over other forms of airway management to offset this complication. Use of waveform

capnography during advanced life support, regardless of location, is now mandated by international guidelines and should reduce the risk of unrecognised oesophageal intubation; it also has several other functions during CPR (Figure 31.2).

The skill of intubation is difficult to establish and maintain. A systematic review of 13 studies concluded that at least 50 intubations were needed by an individual to reach a success rate of at least 90% within one or two intubation attempts. However, most intubations were in elective patients; intubation during CPR is likely to be more difficult. Skill maintenance may be difficult; for example, most paramedics in the UK perform just one or no intubations each year.

There are few data on airway management during in-hospital resuscitation. In a time-dependent propensity analysis of the American Heart Association in-hospital cardiac arrest registry, initiation of tracheal intubation within any given minute during the first 15 minutes of resuscitation, compared with no intubation, was associated with decreased survival to hospital discharge. Similar data exist for children with in-hospital cardiac arrest. Possible mechanisms for the worse outcome include prolonged interruptions in chest compressions, delays in more important interventions (i.e. defibrillation or drug administration), unrecognised oesophageal or bronchial intubation; inadequate ventilation and oxygenation during prolonged intubation attempts, and hyperventilation after intubation. Although propensity analysis should have eliminated all known confounders there is still a possibility that factors other than intubation accounted for the reduced survival.

279

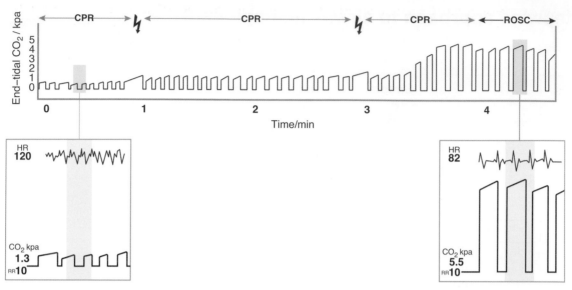

Figure 31.2 Waveform capnography showing changes in the end-tidal carbon dioxide during CPR and after ROSC. The patient's trachea is intubated at zero minutes, ventilated at 10 breaths min^{-1} and chest compressions are given (indicated by CPR) at about two per second. A minute after tracheal intubation, there is a pause in chest compressions and ventilation followed by a defibrillation attempt, and chest compressions and ventilation then continue. Higher quality chest compressions lead to an increased end-tidal carbon dioxide value. There is a further defibrillation attempt after two minutes of chest compressions. There are then further chest compressions and ventilation. There is a significant increase in the end-tidal carbon dioxide value during chest compressions and the patient starts moving and eye opening. Chest compressions are stopped briefly, the monitor shows sinus rhythm and there is a pulse indicating ROSC. Ventilation continues at 10 breaths min^{-1}. CPR – cardiopulmonary resuscitation; ROSC – return of spontaneous circulation; HR – heart rate; RR – respiratory rate. (Reproduced with permission from the European Resuscitation Council from Soar J, Nolan JP, Bottiger BW, et al. (2015). European Resuscitation Council Guidelines for Resuscitation 2015: Section 3. Adult advanced life support. Resuscitation, 95, 100–147.)

Videolaryngoscopy during Cardiopulmonary Resuscitation

In one of the few studies comparing videolaryngoscopy (VL) with direct laryngoscopy for intubation by experienced clinicians during CPR, VL (using a GlideScope) was associated with significantly fewer episodes of prolonged (> 10 seconds) interruptions in chest compressions; the intubation success rate was not significantly different. It is likely that use of VL enables a better view of the larynx during chest compressions.

Supraglottic Airways

Supraglottic airways are easier to insert than tracheal tubes. This makes it easier to acquire and maintain skills and observational studies show shorter interruptions in chest compressions when inserting an SGA compared with tracheal intubation. The SGAs studied most commonly during CPR are the classic laryngeal mask airway (cLMA), the Combitube, the laryngeal tube (LT) and the i-gel. Theoretically, SGAs do not protect the lungs from aspiration as reliably as

a tracheal tube, but two recent randomised clinical trials (RCTs) comparing the LT or the i-gel with tracheal intubation in OHCA (see below) showed no difference in pulmonary aspiration rates between these airway management strategies. Until recently, most studies have been observational and therefore likely to be confounded. A meta-analysis of 10 observational studies that included 76,000 patients managed with either tracheal intubation or an SGA during CPR reported an association between tracheal intubation and an increased rate of neurologically intact survival (OR 1.33, CI 1.09–1.61). Animal studies suggest that the cuffs of some SGAs compress the carotid artery and the reduced cerebral blood flow might account for worse outcomes during CPR; however, studies using computerised tomography scans indicate that SGAs are unlikely to compress the carotid artery in humans.

Randomised Clinical Trials of Airway Management during Cardiac Arrest

Three RCTs of airway management in cardiac arrest were published in 2018 – all in OHCA. In the Cardiac

Arrest Airway Management (CAAM) trial, patients were randomised to early tracheal intubation or bag-mask ventilation with tracheal intubation delayed until ROSC was achieved. Airway management was undertaken by EMS physicians in France and Belgium. There was no difference between the two groups in favourable neurological outcome at 28 days (the primary outcome). Difficult airway management, airway failure and regurgitation of gastric contents were all more common in the bag-mask group, and 14% of this group required 'rescue intubation'. The study intubation success rate was 97.9%. In the United States the Pragmatic Airway Resuscitation Trial (PART) was cluster-randomised by participating EMS agency and compared tracheal intubation by paramedics with LT insertion by paramedics and emergency medical technicians (EMTs). Seventy-two-hour survival was 18.3% in the LT group versus 15.4% in the tracheal intubation group (adjusted difference, 2.9% (95% CI, 0.2–5.6%); $p =0.04$); however, the success rate for tracheal intubation was just 51%. In the UK AIRWAYS-2 study, paramedics were randomised to airway management with the i-gel or tracheal intubation. There was no difference in neurologically favourable outcome at hospital discharge: 6.4% in the i-gel group versus 6.8% in the tracheal intubation group (adjusted risk difference, −0.6% (95% CI, −1.6% to 0.4%)). Among those patients in whom an advanced airway was inserted, the outcome was significantly better in those receiving an i-gel. The intubation success rate was 69.8%. Each of these RCTs was undertaken in EMS systems with many different characteristics, which limits the generalisability of the results. These studies suggest that tracheal intubation should only be used in settings where there is a high tracheal intubation success rate (e.g. first-pass success over 80%, overall success over 95%).

Conclusion

It is likely that the optimal airway management strategy during cardiac arrest will vary between systems and different types of rescuer. Ultimately, a stepwise approach may be optimal – until ROSC is achieved, start with a basic technique and change to a more advanced technique only if attempts to ventilate the lungs fail. Once ROSC is achieved those patients remaining comatose will ultimately require tracheal intubation, but this can be delayed until skilled personnel are available to undertake the procedure.

Summary

The optimal airway management strategy during cardiac arrest is uncertain. Many cardiac arrest patients are treated with multiple airway devices and this stepwise approach to airway management is difficult to study in controlled trials. Tracheal intubation should only be used in those settings with a high intubation success rate. All airway techniques should minimise interruptions to CPR and not delay defibrillation.

Further Reading

Anderson LW, Granfeldt A, Callaway C, et al. (2017). Association between tracheal intubation during adult in-hospital cardiac arrest and survival. *JAMA*, **317**, 494–506.

Benger JR, Kirby K, Black S, et al. (2018). Effect of a strategy of a supraglottic airway device vs tracheal intubation during out-of-hospital cardiac arrest on functional outcome: the AIRWAYS-2 randomized clinical trial. *JAMA*, **320**, 779–791.

Granfeldt A, Avis SR, Nicholson TC, et al. (2019). Advanced airway management during adult cardiac arrest: a systematic review. *Resuscitation*, **139**, 133–143.

Jabre P, Penaloza A, Pinero D, et al. (2018). Effect of bag-mask ventilation vs endotracheal intubation during cardiopulmonary resuscitation on neurological outcome after out-of-hospital cardiorespiratory arrest. A randomized clinical trial. *JAMA*, **319**, 779–787.

Newell C, Grier S, Soar J. (2018). Airway and ventilation management during cardiopulmonary resuscitation and after successful resuscitation. *Critical Care*, **22**, 190.

Soar J, Maconochie I, Wyckoff MH, et al (2019). 2019 International consensus on cardiopulmonary resuscitation and emergency cardiovascular care science with treatment recommendations. *Resuscitation*, **143**, 95–150.

Wang HE, Schmicker RH, Daya MR, et al. (2018). Effect of a strategy of initial laryngeal tube insertion versus endotracheal intubation on 72-hour survival in adults with out-of-hospital cardiac arrest. A randomized clinical trial. *JAMA*, **320**, 769–778.

The Bloody and Bleeding Airway

Michael Seltz Kristensen and Barry McGuire

Introduction

Bleeding in the upper airway is potentially catastrophic and is an important cause of airway-related death, even in young and otherwise healthy individuals. Severe bleeding in the airway is an emergency life-threatening situation. Conventional airway management strategies may be impossible.

The estimated lifetime incidence of epistaxis is approximately 60%; post-tonsillectomy haemorrhage occurs in 6–15% of tonsillectomy cases; and bleeding following surgery for malignancy in the upper airway is one of the leading causes of requirement of an emergency front of neck airway. Cornerstone techniques commonly employed to secure the airway, such as direct/videolaryngoscopy and flexible optical laryngoscopy, may be ineffective due to soiling of the hypopharynx – and the equipment – with blood. Supraglottic airway devices (SGAs) may be employed but are typically of limited efficacy due to the increased risk of aspiration and their potential interference with surgical access to the bleeding site in the hypopharynx, glottis and trachea. The clinician is thus forced to use other techniques and modify their approach to airway management, particularly if bleeding is profuse and/or conventional intubation and airway rescue techniques are predicted to be difficult.

Etiology and Problems of Managing a Bleeding Airway

The potential causes of bleeding in the airway include spontaneous/idiopathic; bleeding tumour/malignancy/vascular malformation; coagulopathy; trauma to the face or neck; post-surgery; iatrogenic – often due to airway management; and cocaine abuse.

Managing the bleeding airway is challenging both technically and non-technically. The following all contribute to make the bleeding airway challenging: all techniques used to manage these situations are likely to be difficult and may fail; videolaryngoscopes

and flexible optical bronchoscopes (FOBs) may be ineffective in the bleeding airway; SGAs are often not suitable as definitive airways because of risk of aspiration of blood from the stomach and interference with surgical access; denitrogenation is less efficient and high flow nasal oxygenation may fail; need for urgent intervention; obstructed vision because blood can render any technique that relies on visualisation (including direct laryngoscopy) impossible; there is a need for concomitant suctioning; blood clot can mimic tissue/pathology; the patient often cannot lie flat; hypovolaemia with impending or established circulatory collapse; aspiration risk due to blood in the stomach; 'waking up the patient' following failed airway management is rarely an option; the patient may re-bleed upon extubation and clinical care teams may become overwhelmed by stress.

Initial Management

Key points include:

- Limit the bleeding
- Upright patient positioning
- Suctioning and oxygen
- Initiate fluid/blood resuscitation and cross-match
- Airway evaluation (see Figure 32.1).

Limit the Bleeding

If possible, reduce or stop the bleeding before securing the airway. This may make subsequent airway management easier or even unnecessary. In post-tonsillectomy/adenoidectomy or other oral/pharyngeal bleeding situations, transoral compression of the bleeding vessel can be performed with a clamped swab or an index finger. Timely embolisation of the relevant artery may be considered. Epistaxis can be treated with intranasal packs soaked with a topical haemostatic agent, such as adrenaline (epinephrine) or thrombin. Administration of tranexamic acid should be considered.

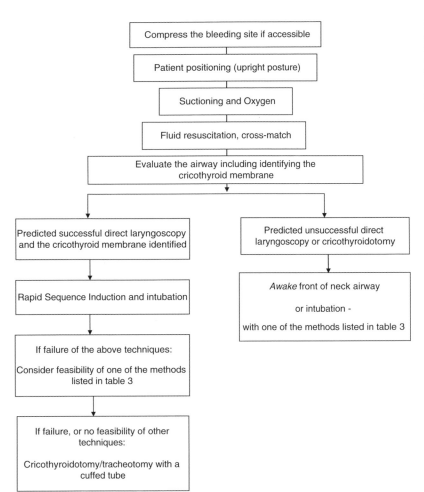

Figure 32.1 Flow chart condensing the steps for managing the bleeding *upper* airway, above the vocal cords. (Reprinted with permission from: Springer Nature. *Canadian Journal of Anaesthesia.* Managing and securing the bleeding upper airway: a narrative review. Kristensen MS, McGuire B. 2020; 67: 128–140.)

Oxygenation

Proactive oxygenation throughout airway management is essential and bi-nasal oxygen delivery prior to, and during, intubation is beneficial. This should be supplemented by face mask-delivered oxygen if possible, although this may be poorly tolerated and is relatively contraindicated in facial trauma, particularly in base of skull fractures where it increases the risk of intracranial infection. Transnasal humidified rapid-insufflation ventilatory exchange (THRIVE) should be used with extreme caution when there is bleeding and is relatively contraindicated as blood may be forced distally into the trachea. Moderate flow rates (8–20 L min^{-1}) may therefore be advisable instead of high flow rates.

Fluid/Blood Resuscitation and Correction of Coagulopathy

With severe bleeding, the patient may be hypovolaemic and large-bore intravenous access and targeted volume resuscitation should be initiated. Any coagulopathy needs to be actively managed.

Airway Management

A bleeding site in the upper airway (above the vocal cords) is a relatively common situation. Of the many possible ways of managing the airway, only those that result in the placement of a cuffed tube in the trachea fulfil the desired goals of (i) securing a conduit for oxygenation and ventilation, (ii) protecting against further aspiration of blood

283

into the lungs and (iii) providing surgical access to the source of bleeding.

A cuffed tracheal tube can be inserted via the oral or nasal route, cricothyroid membrane (CTM) or tracheal stoma. The choice will be influenced by the bleeding site and the preferred approach for safe airway management. SGAs as a means of securing the airway should be considered only as temporary solutions as they do not definitively isolate the lungs from blood in the upper airway. It is preferable to insert a cuffed tracheal tube either following rapid sequence induction (RSI) or while the patient remains awake. An RSI should only be performed if the pre-anaesthetic airway evaluation does not suggest difficulty with direct laryngoscopy and confirms that the CTM is identifiable, and thus accessible should laryngoscopy fail. A stepwise approach to managing the bleeding upper airway is summarised in Figure 32.1.

Airway Evaluation

Preoperative airway evaluation is mandatory to help inform whether an awake technique, rather than an RSI, would be a safer approach. The focus is on (i) predicting if direct laryngoscopy is likely to be successful (see Chapter 5), (ii) predicting if a front of neck airway (FONA) is likely to be successful, including identification of the CTM. However, even with a reassuring airway assessment, predicting easy direct laryngoscopy, this evaluation will occasionally mislead and therefore preparation must also include provision for a possible cricothyroidotomy or tracheostomy.

Difficult cricothyroidotomy is more likely in cases of female gender, age < 8 years, thick/obese neck, overlying pathology (inflammation, induration, radiation, tumour), a displaced airway or a fixed cervical spine flexion deformity.

Identification of the Cricothyroid Membrane

The potential need for a FONA, either pre-emptively or as part of airway rescue, is substantial in the management of the bleeding airway. The chosen route will depend on the skills and experience of the clinician. For elective FONA in the awake patient, there is less time pressure than in the emergency situation, and thus either a cricothyroidotomy or a tracheotomy may be performed. While the patient is being stabilised, and prepared for definitive airway management, the CTM and trachea should be identified and marked.

In patients who are obese or with neck pathology both conventional palpation and the 'laryngeal handshake' technique have a high chance of failure to identify the CTM. In such cases, identification of the CTM and trachea may be achieved quickly and reliably using ultrasonography (see Chapter 7), facilitating both pre-emptive and rescue cricothyroidotomy, tracheostomy or even awake retrograde intubation. Once identified, the position of the CTM should be marked with the patient's head and neck in the same position that the clinician would use to access the CTM.

Rapid Sequence Induction

If the airway evaluation reassures that intubation under direct laryngoscopy is likely to be successful, and that the CTM and trachea are identifiable, then an RSI is indicated. The patient may be hypovolaemic and induction with ketamine should be considered. The patient often needs to be sitting, or even leaning forward, until unconsciousness is achieved and can subsequently be placed in a sniffing, semi-lateral or head-down position depending on circumstance and preference. An assistant solely dedicated to managing haemodynamic changes and fluid resuscitation may be necessary.

Two direct laryngoscopes should be available in case one fails and ideally one of these should be a videolaryngoscope with a Macintosh-shaped blade; this can be used as a direct laryngoscope if blood obscures the video function or as a videolaryngoscope if the blood soiling is less than expected and the direct view is unexpectedly difficult.

Two rigid, large-bore Yankauer-type suction catheters attached to separate suction sources (use of a shared suction source will reduce the suction force achieved) should be available, as well as Magill forceps to retrieve clots deeper in the oropharynx. When the best view of the larynx is achieved, the suction catheter can be wedged to the left side of the laryngoscope, in the upper oesophagus, or in the hypopharynx below the glottis to prevent re-flooding of the airway during intubation. A malleable bougie or introducer may be useful if the larynx is partially covered with blood, as visibility of the epiglottis, and not the larynx, may be sufficient to enable intubation with the aid of one of these devices.

Following intubation, correct tracheal placement must be confirmed with waveform capnography, as the risk of inadvertent oesophageal intubation is greatly increased in the bleeding airway. Inspection with a FOB to confirm correct tracheal placement is an alternative. It is advisable to suction down the

Table 32.1 Airway techniques that do not rely on visualisation of the glottis and may be considered when the upper airway is severely soiled with blood. Significant bleeding airway situations are challenging to manage and may necessitate the use of techniques less familiar to the treating physician. These should ideally be performed by individuals who have experience with these techniques and have rehearsed the bleeding airway situation.

Technique	Indication	Comments
Supraglottic airway devices	For failed ventilation and/or as a conduit for intubation, in the awake or in the unconscious patient	Only suitable for bleeding above the larynx. Requires adequate mouth opening. Limited protection against aspiration. Mainly temporising technique until intubation is achieved
Retrograde intubation	An awake approach is recommended but can be applied in the unconscious patient	May be used in patients with critical cervical spine lesions. Can additionally be applied with an SGA in place or combined with a light-guided intubation
Light-guided intubation, using either a lightwand or an FOB as light-guide	Awake, following induction, or unconscious	High success rate in predicted difficult intubation in spontaneous breathing, or anaesthetised patients. Can be combined with retrograde intubation
Blind nasal intubation	Must be guided by breath sounds Awake patients or in those with preserved spontaneous ventilation	High success rate in spontaneous breathing patients with neck trauma in those skilled in technique, but now less recommended
Cricothyroidotomy	Pre-emptive or rescue. Awake, following induction, or unconscious	Patient may be unable to lie flat (but semi-recumbent may be an option)
Tracheostomy	Pre-emptive or rescue, Awake, following induction, or unconscious	
Ultrasound-guided intubation	Visualisation obscured by blood. Awake, following induction, or unconscious	Requires separate operator. Has been recommended for the bleeding airway, but only limited clinical use reported in the literature
Oral digital intubation	Difficult technique; demands adequate mouth opening	Rarely tolerable for the awake patient
Cardiopulmonary bypass/extra corporeal membrane oxygenation	Has been used for massive haemoptysis and tracheal granuloma cases	Does not protect from aspiration; may not be available for emergency use. Anticoagulation requirement may complicate haemostasis

Reprinted with permission from: Springer Nature. *Canadian Journal of Anaesthesia*. Managing and securing the bleeding upper airway: a narrative review. Kristensen MS, McGuire B. 2020; 67: 128–140.

tracheal tube prior to commencing assisted ventilation to limit blood contamination of the distal airways.

What to Do If the Airway Examination Suggests Risk of Failure of Direct Laryngoscopy

The approaches recommended in airway management algorithms almost exclusively depend on visualisation of the glottis and so may be inadequate when employed in the bleeding airway, particularly when the bleeding is profuse. Table 32.1 summarises methods for securing the airway that are less affected by the presence of blood. These include: FOB-guided intubation via an SGA, retrograde intubation, blind oral and blind nasal intubation, lightwand-guided intubation, ultrasound-guided intubation, cricothyroidotomy and tracheotomy. Finally, cardiopulmonary bypass or extracorporeal membrane oxygenation (ECMO) may be employed for bridging in desperate situations.

These methods may be employed in an *awake* patient when techniques for visualising the glottis (typically FOB or videolaryngoscopy) are anticipated to fail or have already failed in the awake patient. These methods may also be considered in the unconscious or anaesthetised patient, if clinically appropriate, when techniques dependent on visualisation have failed due to excessive bleeding. Otherwise, FONA will be the technique of choice for airway rescue.

Awake Approach

An awake approach to securing the airway is prudent if the airway assessment suggests that intubation after induction of general anaesthesia may fail and/or that the rescue technique, usually cricothyroidotomy, may prove to be difficult or impossible. The awake approach can be via either tracheal intubation or FONA. A sitting position may be helpful along with applying pressure to the bleeding site with forceps loaded with gauze rolls. If the bleeding is limited, then awake tracheal intubation with FOB or videolaryngoscopy can be attempted, but the operator must be prepared for the possibility of failure. For intubation over an FOB the adjunct of a blinking infrared light emitting device (InfraRed Red Intubation System, 'IRRIS') placed over the cricothyroid membrane may help finding the way to the trachea (see Further Reading).

If these intubation techniques are unsuccessful, an alternative awake technique is required (Table 32.1). Occasionally, unsuccessful awake intubation can be salvaged by using an FOB as a 'lighted stylet'. The tip of the FOB is advanced posteriorly past the epiglottis and down towards the estimated position of the glottic opening and then wedged against the anterior surface of the trachea. The light from the FOB can then be seen through the anterior neck, thus verifying the position of its tip in the trachea. Adoption of such specialised techniques requires practice in non-bleeding airways to optimise familiarity.

Airway Topicalisation and Sedation

Airway topicalisation (e.g. nebulised, atomised, or direct administration with gauze or pledglet) is largely ineffective in the presence of blood and alternative methods may be needed. Bilateral superior laryngeal nerve blocks, combined with transtracheal injection of local anaesthetic, may produce a superior result. It may be preferable to avoid tracheal topicalisation so the patient remains able to cough if blood enters the

trachea; the trade-off is that the patient may react when the tracheal tube enters the trachea. Of note, the presence of blood lubricates the airway, facilitating intubation without local anaesthetic and with only limited patient discomfort. In patients presenting with severe respiratory distress and a likely difficult direct laryngoscopy, an awake technique is indicated and is often well tolerated without topicalisation or sedation. If cautious sedation is required, ketamine may be particularly helpful due to the minimal respiratory depression.

Ventilation and Intubation via a Supraglottic Airway Device

An SGA can potentially partially and temporarily protect the trachea from blood soiling provided that the origin of the bleeding is above the glottis, and permit lifesaving ventilation. Insertion of an SGA and use of it as a conduit for intubation may be used in the awake patient, or as a rescue technique in the unconscious (or anaesthetised) patient after failed intubation or mask ventilation. An SGA (without subsequent intubation) should be considered only as a temporary solution as it offers limited protection from aspiration and prevents surgical access to the bleeding site.

Ideally, an SGA specifically designed to accommodate a tracheal tube should be used, and intubation should be guided by an FOB. If an SGA with a narrower stem is placed intubation can be facilitated by using an Aintree intubation catheter (Cook Medical Europe Ltd) (see Chapter 13). A second generation SGA with a large-bore drain tube may allow egress, or suctioning, of blood from the stomach, but may not provide effective protection against aspiration.

'Blind' intubation techniques (i.e. without guidance of an FOB) have an unacceptably low success rate, especially in children, whereas FOB-guided intubation achieves a higher success rate and should be used whenever possible. Finally, an SGA can be converted to a tracheal tube using a retrograde technique in which a guidewire or epidural catheter is passed via the CTM, directed cranially via the SGA, and then used to facilitate a railroaded intubation.

Cricothyroidotomy and Tracheostomy

Cricothyroidotomy or tracheostomy can be performed in the awake patient as a primary or pre-emptive airway, or after induction of anaesthesia, as a rescue technique for failed intubation. In adults, either technique should be performed using a technique that permits the placement of a cuffed tracheal tube of at least a 5 mm internal diameter. This will provide effective ventilation while protecting against further aspiration. A narrow-bore cannula ('needle') cricothyroidotomy is not suitable in the bleeding airway other than as a temporary oxygenation technique. In smaller children tracheostomy is the technique of choice.

Profuse Bleeding

If the bleeding is so profuse that use of an FOB or videolaryngoscope is likely to fail or has already done so, then a variety of options must be considered (Table 32.1). Awake, pre-emptive, tracheostomy or cricothyroidotomy should always be considered in such cases. However, in certain situations, other awake approaches may be preferable depending on clinical experience. Of these, the retrograde 'pulling' intubation technique is especially well suited in the management of an awake, sitting patient with a profusely bleeding airway (Figure 32.2). During

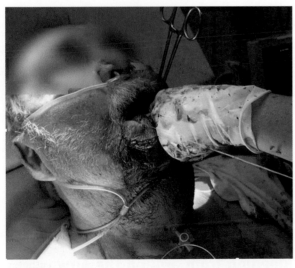

Figure 32.2 Awake and sitting patient with severe bleeding from pharyngeal site. The surgeon is compressing the bleeding site with a clamped swab in her gloved hand. A cannula has been placed through the cricothyroid membrane and an epidural catheter has been passed via the cannula. The distal end of the epidural catheter is still protruding from the cannula and the cranial end of the catheter is pulled out from the mouth in preparation for retrograde intubation with the 'pulling' method (Figure with permission from the Scandinavian Airway Management course, www.airwaymanagement.dk).

retrograde intubation, the tracheal tube is pulled into the trachea using an epidural catheter, inserted through the CTM, or through the crico-tracheal membrane, that is secured to the distal end of the tracheal tube (see Box 32.1). This technique has the following advantages: it is relatively simple, requiring readily available equipment (an epidural catheter), is independent of vision and thus works in bloody airways, allows intubation via the mouth or the nose as appropriate and even allows reintubation if necessary (by leaving the catheter *in situ* following extubation). The technique should preferably be used in the *awake* patient. One detailed approach is described at http://www.airwaymanagement.dk/retrograde.

There are other retrograde intubation techniques, including the use of a dedicated kit specifically designed for this purpose.

Finally, lightwand-guided intubation is another useful technique in this setting and can even be used in combination with retrograde intubation. This approach requires the availability of dedicated equipment, although a flexible endoscope may be used for this purpose, as briefly described above.

Bleeding from the Larynx

The same approach and various techniques discussed above can be applied in this situation with the exception of techniques that involve the use of an SGA, because in such cases the bleeding site is distal to the SGA and thus it cannot provide protection from the blood.

Bleeding from a Tracheostomy

A combination of direct external pressure and temporary overinflation of the tracheostomy cuff may lessen bleeding. Bleeding may be temporarily reduced or stopped by applying finger pressure to the root of the neck in the sternal notch. Alternatively, a narrow tracheal tube can be placed from above (or through the tracheostomy tube after removing any inner cannula) and the cuff inflated distal to the tracheal stoma. This will protect the lungs from aspiration of blood while giving access to the stoma for haemostasis.

Box 32.1 Retrograde intubation in the awake, bleeding and sitting patient: using readily available equipment, an epidural catheter. A link to a video of the procedure is available at: http://www.airwaymanagement.dk /retrograde

- The cricothyroid membrane, or the cricotracheal membrane, is identified with inspection and palpation and/or with ultrasonography.
- An 18G venous cannula or a Tuohy cannula is inserted, through the cricothyroid or cricotracheal membrane.
- An epidural catheter is inserted via the cannula and advanced in a cephalad direction until it exits the mouth or the patient spits it out or it can be pulled out with a gloved finger or a pair of Magill forceps.
- The epidural catheter is lubricated and threaded up a 5–6 mm ID tracheal tube that has had the proximal connector removed. The epidural catheter is passed in through the distal end of the tube, out through the Murphy's eye before being threaded again into the distal end of the tube and up and out of the proximal end of the tube. The proximal connection of the tube is reinserted so that the epidural catheter is fixed between the tube and the connector.
- The catheter is then pulled downwards from the end that protrudes from the cricothyroid or cricotracheal membrane, thus pulling down the tracheal tube through the mouth and into the larynx.
- When resistance is met, the tip of the tube is at the inside of the cricothyroid or cricotracheal membrane and can be pulled no further.
- The pulling on the distal part of the catheter is stopped and the tube is pushed distally until it is in the trachea. If the tube impinges on the arytenoid cartilages, it may be gently rotated or a FOB may be passed down the tube to visualise passage into the trachea.
- The cuff is inflated and the location of the tube in the airway is verified with capnography.
- The patient can be anaesthetised and haemostasis surgery performed.
- Extubation can be performed by pulling the tube (having released the catheter from the tube connector) while holding taught on the distal end of the catheter, thus letting the catheter unwind while withdrawing the tube. In this way, the catheter can be left in situ in recovery to potentially provide a guide for reintubation.

With permission from the Scandinavian Airway Management course, www.airwaymanagement.dk.

Bleeding from the Lungs: Haemoptysis

Management of the airway during haemoptysis is considered in a recent review by Ittrich (see Further Reading) and can be summarised as follows:

Mild haemoptysis is self-limiting in 90% of cases; in massive haemoptysis, positioning of the patient with the bleeding side down (if known) is advisable, and temporary intubation may be necessary. If the bleeding arises from a central, bronchoscopically accessible site, then haemostasis can be achieved by interventional flexible bronchoscopic local treatment. If the bleeding site is in the pulmonary periphery, then bronchial artery embolisation is the first line of treatment. Placement of an endobronchial blocker may create temporary haemostasis.

Initial placement of a single-lumen tube with a cuff in the unaffected main-stem bronchus may be lifesaving and even if the tube is in the affected main-

stem bronchus it may still be helpful as it can drive blood away from soiling the other lung.

Bleeding from the Gastrointestinal Tract

In cases of bleeding from the gastrointestinal tract that result in severe soiling of the upper airway and a need for securing the airway, the same approach may be used as when the bleeding originates from the airway itself.

Bleeding from around the Airway Compressing It?

This chapter deals with blood in the airway. If there is no bleeding in the airway, but only compression from around the airway, then visual techniques, including awake FOB-guided intubation, can be employed as usual in airway management.

The Unconscious Bleeding Patient

In the unconscious patient with a bleeding airway and an urgent need for a cuffed tracheal tube, typically a major trauma patient, the choices for airway management are still the same as those listed in Figure 32.1 and Table 32.1, but clearly without the 'awake' options. However, if the patient has sufficient spontaneous ventilation these techniques may still be attempted. The initial approach will most often be an attempt at intubation with direct laryngoscopy followed by FONA in case of failure. Alternatively, FONA may be chosen as the primary approach.

Post-operative Management

The managing team must formulate an airway rescue plan to deal with the possibility that bleeding may recur or that the airway becomes compromised at the time of extubation or soon afterwards.

Caveats

The options we list for the bleeding airway have various advantages and disadvantages, and the choice for any one technique relates to the clinical circumstances, available equipment and – most importantly – clinical experience and skills. It is crucial to gain familiarity with these techniques in the non-urgent situation, and we would strongly encourage healthcare providers who may handle this type of challenging patient to participate in workshops towards this end.

Further Reading

Abou-Madi MN, Trop D. (1989). Pulling versus guiding: a modification of retrograde guided intubation. *Canadian Journal of Anaesthesia*, **36**, 336–339.

Ittrich H, Bockhorn M, Klose H, Simon M. (2017). The diagnosis and treatment of hemoptysis. *Deutsches Arzteblatt International*, **114**, 371–381.

Kristensen MS, McGuire B. (2020). Managing and securing the bleeding upper airway: a narrative review. *Canadian Journal of Anaesthesia*, **67**, 128–140.

Kristensen MS, Fried E, Biro P. (2018). Infrared Red Intubation System (IRRIS) guided flexible videoscope assisted difficult airway management. *Acta Anaesthesiologica Scandinavica*, **62**, 19–25.

Windfuhr JP, Schloendorff G, Sesterhenn AM, Prescher A, Kremer B. (2009). A devastating outcome after adenoidectomy and tonsillectomy: ideas for improved prevention and management. *Otolaryngology–Head and Neck Surgery*, **140**, 191–196.

Yang SH, Wu CY, Tseng WH, et al. (2019). Nonintubated laryngomicrosurgery with transnasal humidified rapid-insufflation ventilatory exchange: a case series. *Journal of the Formosan Medical Association*, **118**, 1138–1143.

Chapter 33

The Airway in Anaesthesia for Transoral Robotic Surgery

Rasmus Winkel and Michael Seltz Kristensen

Introduction

Transoral robotic surgery (TORS) is becoming increasingly widespread. The use of a surgical robot allows access to surgical sites in the oropharynx, base of the tongue, laryngeal inlet and soft palate that would otherwise be inaccessible or require a mandibular split to obtain access. The surgery is performed through a rigid gag, and the arms of the surgical robot are controlled by the surgeon sitting at a remote console. The surgeon controls the robotic arms via hand controls and has a three-dimensional view of the surgical site, via optical lenses at the control station.

The robotic arms are manually guided to optimal positions and their relative positions are logged, the so-called docking procedure. Further movement of the robotic arms is done by the surgeon via the remote console. To remove the robotic arms from the oral cavity requires undocking of the robot and manually guided removal by the assistant. Renewed surgical access requires that the docking procedure is repeated. An assistant facilitates surgical access with retractors and camera positioning.

The surgeon can employ multiple surgical tools on the robotic arms, and the computer filters out involuntary motions of the surgeon's hands, thus providing a steady movement of the tools. There is, however, no tactile feedback, and the surgeon is thus limited to the inputs he or she can see. In order to raise team situation awareness, the camera view can be broadcast to one or more screens in the operating theatre.

This kind of surgery poses unique challenges as the multiple surgical instruments share the same space as the airway placed by the anaesthetic team.

Preparation

Airway management of the TORS patient poses some of the same challenges as other patients with airway pathology. A thorough preoperative assessment of the airway, including a preoperative nasendoscopy, should be standard, and will identify most difficult airways prior to anaesthesia. No patient should be anaesthetised for TORS without having their cricothyroid membrane assessed. In case of difficulty palpating it, ultrasound assessment should be used to mark it prior to induction of anaesthesia (see Chapter 7).

The choice of airway route (nasal, oral or front of neck) should be discussed with the surgeon, as their surgical access can be affected by the anaesthetist's choice of airway route.

Choice of Airway Equipment

Due to the nature of the surgery, only tracheal intubation or tracheostomy are valid airway solutions during the surgery.

Choosing the right tracheal tube for TORS is an act of balancing the requirements of the surgeon to the safety and comfort of the patient. The tube should be resistant to compression from the robotic arms, thus requiring a wire-reinforced tube. These tubes resist compression well, but if compressed above their resistance threshold they will buckle and then remain compressed.

If the surgeon uses laser during the procedure, the tube should also be laser resistant. Otherwise a plan for draping and protecting the tube should be formulated in close cooperation with the surgeon. Depending on the proximity of the surgical field to the tube, and the use of monopolar cautery equipment, there is also a risk of heat transfer to the tube, thus requiring the tube to be heat resistant.

If the patient is orally intubated, a floppy tube may require stitches to keep it out of the surgical field, introducing the risk of retained stitches at extubation.

A wire-reinforced, laser- and heat-resistant tube will often be able to stay out of the surgical field, but may cause bleeding and has an increased risk of submucosal placement, when introduced through the nose. Standard wire-reinforced tubes are gentler on the nasal cavity, but often lack the proper length to be placed nasally without risking pressure sores at the nares. Guide the nasal tube through the nose by threading it over a soft suction catheter to minimise the risk of submucosal placement.

If the surgery is near the laryngeal inlet, a double cuffed tube may be preferable, due to the risk of damage to the cuff (Figure 33.1).

At the authors' institution the heat-resistant wire-reinforced tubes are used orally and the extra length soft wire tubes are used nasally (Figure 33.2).

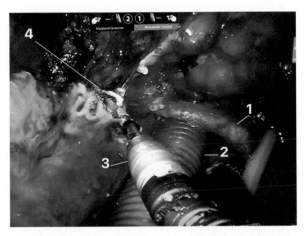

Figure 33.1 Illustration of the intimate relationship between the surgical field and the tracheal tube during transoral robotic surgery. 1 – epiglottis, 2 – tracheal tube, 3 – surgical instrument, 4 – surgical incision line.

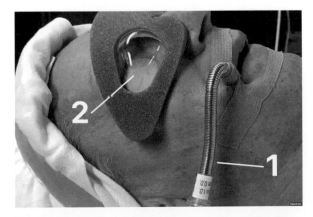

Figure 33.2 A patient for transoral robotic surgery, showing the need to lead the tracheal tube away from the surgical field. 1 – tracheal tube with reinforced wire, 2 – reinforced eye protection.

Intubation

The choice of intubation technique should be tailored to each patient individually.

Direct laryngoscopy remains a good way of placing the tracheal tube but in situations where the visibility is limited and a rigid wire-reinforced tube is placed, this may not be the optimal choice. The rigid wire-reinforced tube lacks external depth markings, and it is therefore difficult to assess the depth of placement unless there is a good view of the larynx. A videolaryngoscope improves laryngeal view and is therefore the tool of choice when placing rigid wire-reinforced tubes.

Awake intubation using either a videolaryngoscope or a flexible optical bronchoscope (FOB) should be the preferred method when anticipating difficult ventilation or intubation.

FOB-guided intubation in combination with rigid wire-reinforced tracheal tubes poses a risk of damaging the scope. A two-stage approach, placing a non-reinforced tube first and then exchanging this for the rigid wire-reinforced tube, via an airway exchange catheter, is a valid alternative. It should be noted that some clinicians dislike FOB-guided intubations for patients with airway malignancy. They fear that the blind nature of railroading the tube can cause bleeding and dislodgement of tumour tissue. This can be overcome by combining with a videolaryngoscope (see Chapter 19).

An elective tracheostomy prior to the robotic procedure is a good way of ensuring optimal access for the surgeon, as well as securing airway patency postoperatively. It should be considered in those patients that have difficult airway access prior to surgery, including those with poor access to the cricothyroid membrane due to pathology, obesity or other causes. About a third of patients undergoing supraglottic partial laryngectomy will require a tracheostomy prior to surgery. Post-operative airway access is almost invariably temporarily worse after TORS, even after tumorous masses have been removed.

Perioperative Complications and Safety Issues

Once the surgical robot is docked and ready, access to the tube and airway is extremely limited. Prior to the docking, it is therefore important to secure the airway sufficiently and make a plan with the surgical team should an airway issue arise during the surgery.

Undocking the robot and clearing the airway for emergency access should take no less than a minute, if performed smoothly in a timely fashion. It is important to identify which situations require this and to practise doing it, so every team member knows what to do. Accidental extubation, severe damage to the tube or cuff and occlusion of the tube by secretions or compression are all perioperative emergencies that require emergency undocking of the robot.

Perioperative and post-operative loss of airway control should always be considered a risk and can lead to the need for an emergency front of neck airway.

Post-operative Considerations, Extubation and Reintubation

The post-surgery airway plan involves the key decision of whether to extubate immediately or delay this. The decision is dependent on the patient, the surgical procedure and the expected ease of re-establishing a definitive airway, should this be required.

It is useful to discuss the likely effect of the performed surgery on airway management post-operatively with the surgeon prior to extubation. It should also be thoroughly documented in the patient's notes, to avoid surprises for the staff handling the post-operative phase.

Care should be exercised during extubation, especially when removing the rigid wire-reinforced tubes, as they can remove clots and cause bleeding with subsequent airway loss. Removal can also cause damage to flaps and suture lines. If the tube has been sutured in place, during the procedure, removing the stitches prior to extubation becomes as important as removing the throat pack in other procedures.

Placement of an airway exchange catheter or wire at extubation can facilitate reintubation if there is a loss of airway patency (see Chapter 21), but reintubation over such devices also risks causing bleeding and damage to flaps and suture lines.

Should an extubated TORS patient require reintubation, in the immediate post-operative phase, it is important to understand that the airway anatomy may have been substantially altered by the surgical procedure. Besides swelling, bleeding and haematomas, suture lines, resections of the epiglottis and surgical flaps can be present. Substantial areas of resected mucosa increase the adherence of clots in the airway, which limits the effect of suction and alters airway topology.

Rigid suction catheters may prove insufficient for clot removal; in such cases a tracheal tube attached directly to the suction tubing may function as a large-bore makeshift solution.

In some institutions, extubation is routinely delayed and the patient is transferred to the post-operative or critical care unit while intubated for 24–72 hours. At the authors' institution delayed awakening and extubation is only used rarely (less than 5%).

Post-operative risks to the airway consist of swelling due to manipulation, bleeding and haematomas.

Further Reading

Chi JJ, Mandel JE, Weinstein GS, O'Malley BW Jr. (2010). Anesthetic considerations for transoral robotic surgery. *Anesthesiology Clinics*, **28**, 411–422.

Jeyarajah J, Ahmad I, Jacovou E. (2018). Anaesthesia and perioperative care for transoral robotic surgery *Journal for Otorhinolaryngology and its Related Specialties*, **80**, 125–133.

Stubbs VC, Rajasekaran K, Gigliotti AR, et al. (2018). Management of the airway for transoral robotic supraglottic partial laryngectomy. *Frontiers in Oncology*, **8**, 312

34

Departmental and Hospital Organisation

Lauren Berkow and Alistair McNarry

Airway management does not happen in isolation. Although an individual secures the patient's airway, many upstream organisational events will influence how airway management is actually performed. Decisions concerning equipment purchases, staff training, post-operative care arrangements and even departmental staffing will all influence how an anaesthetic is administered.

Hospitals and departments should invest in an organised and standardised approach to airway management both inside and outside the operating theatres.

The 4th National Audit Report of the Royal College of Anaesthetists and the Difficult Airway Society (NAP4) is discussed elsewhere in this book. However, it is noteworthy that many of the 168 recommendations were directed towards institutions as much as to individuals.

The 'Organisation and equipment' chapter in NAP4 challenges anaesthetic departments to:

- Provide leadership for airway management throughout their entire organisation
- Standardise equipment across all sites in a hospital where an airway might be managed (e.g. critical care and emergency departments should have the same airway equipment as the operating theatres)

In order to have a full complement of airway devices available for use in any location and at any time, several upstream issues must be addressed:

1. The airway device is available within the institution
2. It is stocked in all locations where it may be needed
3. It is functional (batteries, leads, connectors and blades are available)
4. Documented procedures exist for its cleaning (if appropriate)
5. The clinician is *at least* proficient in its use
6. An institutional plan exists recognising that all airway devices can fail and that backup equipment

must be immediately available if the chosen device proves ineffective.

Role of the Organisation

The responsibility for acquiring training and experience with a particular device may lie with the individual clinician; however, ongoing training and the development of expertise will require departmental and institutional involvement. Adequate time should be allocated for clinicians to receive training.

NAP4 identified deficiencies in areas including preoperative airway assessment, and whilst conduct of the assessment remains an individual responsibility, institutions should provide space to conduct, scheduling to enable and resources to facilitate the necessary assessments and investigations required.

The organisation should allocate time for morbidity and mortality/quality improvement conferences that review challenging cases, address gaps and needs related to safe airway management, and discuss improvement plans and initiatives. As part of these, an environment should be created in which individuals are empowered to report mishaps and near misses. Institutions need to embed and support a 'no-blame' culture similar to that seen in the airline industry to avoid the reporting clinician becoming the 'second victim' in any adverse airway event. Such meetings must identify and address departmental and institutional factors (e.g. related to staffing, equipment availability or training) that may have contributed to the event, in order to reduce the likelihood of recurrence.

Airway Leads and Airway Teams

Airway Leads in the United Kingdom (UK)

NAP4 also called for an identified individual within an organisation to take responsibility for dealing with the organisational aspects of difficult airway management, a position endorsed by the Royal College of

Table 34.1 Major responsibilities of a UK airway lead (for complete list see http://www.nationalauditprojects.org.uk /NAPAirwayLeads)

Operations:
  Ensure airway equipment is appropriate and standardised as per airway guidelines
  Ensure local policies exist for airway management emergencies and facilitate their dissemination
  Liaise with other departments (ICU, ED) to ensure consistent standards and practices
  Assure consistency with airway assessment and planning

Safety:
  Overseeing airway audits and compliance with guidelines
  Assist with national surveys and audits

Education:
  Overseeing and expanding local airway training for all those involved in airway management

Anaesthetists in 2012. Airway leads were to be appointed in all hospitals and an outline of their duties is shown in Table 34.1. Currently, the airway lead system is essentially universal in UK hospitals. The project has been rolled out in Ireland and New Zealand and is progressing in Australia. Important roles of the airway lead include staff education, coordination between departments (e.g. anaesthesia, intensive care, emergency departments) and liaison with management and procurement to optimise patient safety and ensure availability of appropriate airway equipment. The presence of an airway lead does not remove the need for individual responsibility but does provide a central departmental point of contact for airway-related issues.

Airway Teams in the United States of America (USA)

Some hospitals in the USA have formed multidisciplinary airway teams to manage difficult airway patients and who focus on improving organisational preparedness. Team success relies on a multidisciplinary approach, education and training of team members on airway devices and algorithms, as well as simulation and team training. Table 34.2 describes several airway teams that have published data on outcomes.

Although the airway leads initiative and airway teams were developed separately, they share a common focus on the many system components required to enhance patient safety and ultimately reduce the chance of airway misadventure in an individual case. Teaching and training are fundamental to this approach, particularly as an organised team rather than relying on an educated individual.

There are three components of a successful airway team:

1. Operations: provision of necessary equipment and personnel

   Operations should focus on providing the necessary equipment and personnel required to deliver airway management when needed both inside and outside the operating theatre. Both NAP4 and the American Society of Anesthesiologists (ASA) recommend using standardised airway trolleys (referred to as airway carts in the USA) containing devices to perform laryngoscopy, rescue ventilation and surgical airways. Figure 34.1 shows examples of an airway trolley. A portable airway bag may also be useful.

   Personnel should be trained to be proficient with all the airway equipment on their trolley, and support personnel are required to maintain and stock the trolleys. A significant financial investment may be needed to create and maintain a comprehensive airway trolley, particularly when several are required throughout the organisation.

   Items recommended to be included in an airway trolley/cart:

   Supraglottic airway devices
   Videolaryngoscopes
   Flexible bronchoscopes
   Tracheal tubes of various sizes
   Tracheal tube introducers/stylets/bougies
   End-tidal capnography
   Equipment to perform an emergency front of neck airway

Precise airway team membership will depend on the needs of the individual institution. Anaesthetists, intensivists, otolaryngologists and other surgeons can provide valuable input, and other clinicians/staff who regularly manage airways should be included. This expands the skill sets of the team and enables multidisciplinary collaboration and creation of backup plans. Multidisciplinary teams reduce adverse events related to airway management (Table 34.2). Team members should share a similar mental model for problem solving, e.g. by sharing knowledge of and using the same guideline.

2. Safety and incident reporting

   To maintain safe practice and to enable the team to learn from events (errors, near misses and examples of excellent practice), airway

Table 34.2 Examples of multidisciplinary airway teams in the USA

Hospital/ Institution	Team Members	Equipment	Education/ Training	Outcomes measured
Johns Hopkins Difficult Airway Response Team (DART)	Anesthesiology Otolaryngology Trauma surgery Emergency medicine	Specialised cart (trolley) with flexible and rigid bronchoscopes, supraglottic airways and tracheostomy set	Airway course held quarterly Simulation and skills training *In situ* simulation Crisis management and team training	Airway-related adverse events and malpractice claims reduced to zero
Grant Medical Center Alpha Team	Anesthesiology Trauma surgery Respiratory therapy Pharmacist	Portable airway case	Simulation training Didactic seminars Equipment training	No deaths related to airway management in first year of programme
Boston Medical Center Emergency Airway Response Team (EART)	Anesthesiology Otolaryngology Trauma surgery Emergency medicine Nursing Respiratory therapy	Airway carts	Simulation training	None published to date

incident data should be recorded, analysed and the learning fed back. Event analysis can be used to continuously improve practice and increase the team's knowledge base. *In-situ* simulation identifies areas for improvement and allows for assessment of team performance in situation awareness and guideline/protocol compliance.

3. Education and training

Departments should provide education (distinct from training) for all anaesthesia providers at every stage of their career. External meetings and symposia/workshops supplement but cannot replace local education.

Education programmes should be repeated regularly, and all providers must be able to attend. Programmes should include airway assessment, airway algorithms and guidelines, review of departmental policies and procedures, and can usefully include a review of difficult airway cases.

Education should also include training on available airway devices and procedures, including videolaryngoscopy, flexible optical bronchoscopy, placement and advanced use of supraglottic airway devices and performance of an emergency front of neck airway.

Since teams may often not work together regularly, team training and multidisciplinary participation are crucial in ensuring that, in an airway crisis, all team members understand their role. Team training in crisis management improves communication and decision making, whilst addressing the complex area of human factors (see Chapter 36). The simulation environment provides an excellent opportunity for this as well as allowing for the rehearsal of rarely performed tasks or rarely occurring events.

Whether an organisation has an 'airway lead' or an 'airway team' this should offer a system that can support provision of reliable airway management, ensuring that the necessary personnel and equipment are always available. In addition, multidisciplinary team training promotes the formulation of coherent airway plans and the ability to effectively enact them, factors identified as important gaps by NAP4.

Standardisation of Policies and Equipment

Standardisation is a key component of institutional/ organisational preparedness for a difficult airway situation. It reduces medical errors and improves outcomes. In the context of airway management, standardisation should apply not only to equipment, but to personnel, use of guidelines and algorithms, and training.

Many published airway guidelines exist, and the hospital (or ideally hospital group, region, state or country) should choose which guidelines to endorse

(a)

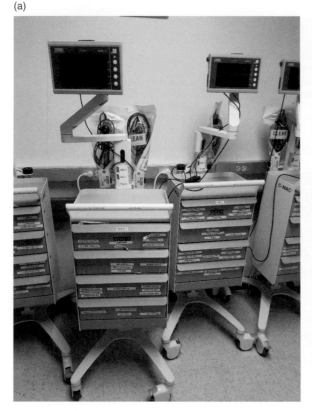

(b)

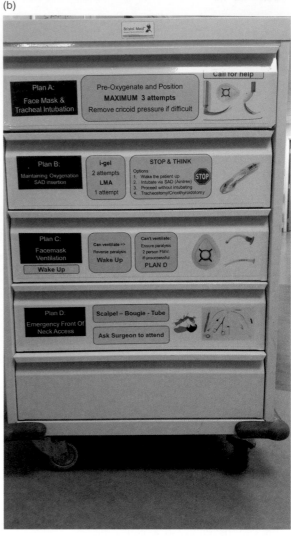

Figure 34.1 (a) Example of airway cart (trolley) for an airway team (USA). (b) Example of a DAS guideline-compliant airway trolley (UK).

and ensure that they are available. Cognitive aids such as the Vortex algorithm and PACE (Prompt, Alert, Challenge and Emergency) are useful; however, they must be adopted at an institutional level to ensure effective deployment.

Dissemination of Critical Patient Information

A particular challenge is how to share information about patients identified as having a difficult airway between different airway managers, institutions and even between countries. Often this information is not even documented in the medical record, prohibiting

any dissemination. As a minimum, institutions should have a method of identifying patients with a known difficult airway, ideally in the medical record. Ensuring the patient is aware of their airway difficulty and has a record of it is a key step. Difficult airway alerts and armbands are other methods that can be used. Each institution must ensure that they have an easy to follow pathway for both recording and forwarding the information – as this has been done poorly in the past.

Unfortunately, no single universal system for critical information reporting has yet been adopted throughout all nations. MedicAlert is a US-based organisation that facilitates the documentation of

Patient Name	
Date of birth	
Hospital number	
Home address	
Telephone	
GP address	
Tel	

To the patient: Please keep this letter safe and show it to your doctor if you are admitted to hospital.
Please show this letter to the anaesthetic doctor if you need an operation.
This letter explains the difficulties that were found during your recent anaesthetic and the information may be useful to doctors treating you in the future.

To the GP: Please copy this letter with any future referral.
READ CODE SP2y3 / ICD-10, T88.4 / SNOMED CT 718447001

Summary of Airway Management

Date of operation: Type of operation:

		Reasons/comments
Difficult mask ventilation?	**YES/NO**	
Difficult SGA insertion	**YES/NO**	
Difficult direct laryngoscopy?	**YES/NO**	Size of blade: DL grade: 1/2a/2b/3a/3b/4
Difficult videolaryngoscopy	**YES/NO**	Devices Blade sizes Best VL grade 1/2a/2b/3a/3b/4 Which device/blade
Difficult tracheal intubation?	**YES/NO**	
Extubation		.
Further investigation		.

Please provide further information regarding the difficulty encountered and technique used:

Recommended plan for future anaesthetics:

Is awake intubation necessary in the future?   Yes / No

Follow up care (tick when completed)

YES/NO One copy to patient   **YES/NO** Spoken to patient
YES/NO One copy to GP   **YES/NO** Anaesthetic chart complete
YES/NO One copy in case notes   **YES/NO** Information on front of case notes
YES/NO One copy in anaesthetic department   **YES/NO** Difficult Airway Society database
YES/NO One copy uploaded to electronic medical record.

Name of anaesthetist:
Grade: Date:

Please contact the anaesthetic department if you require further information:
Tel .... Email...

Figure 34.2 An airway alert form. (Adapted from forms developed by Difficult Airway Society and Royal United Hospital, Bath, UK.)

critical medical information and has a designated reporting form for difficult airway patients. Although it is a non-profit organisation, there is still a cost involved and other effective recording and dissemination methods may be available.

The Difficult Airway Society (DAS) has developed a UK database (https://das.uk.com/dad) where details of difficult airway cases can be held and accessed: initial uptake was slow but it is hoped this will increase.

Many medical coding systems include an entry for a difficult airway or difficult tracheal intubation: these include: Read Code (UK general practitioners), SP2y3, ICD-10 T88.4 and SNOMED CT 718447001. SNOMED CT (Systematized Nomenclature of Medicine – Clinical Terms) is a structured vocabulary for electronic health records; it is already used in 50 countries, but is not yet universally adopted. The clinician involved in documenting the presence of a difficult airway should use the coding system that is in most common use within their institution and region to ensure effective information transfer. No coding system should replace the patient discussion mentioned above.

An example of an airway alert form is shown in Figure 34.2.

Summary

Although individual practitioners provide airway management, their options will be dictated by decisions made at a departmental and institutional level. Departments should aim to standardise all available airway equipment in an institution to facilitate effective education and use. Multidisciplinary collaboration is a vital part of effective airway management. Effective airway management in a crisis requires adherence to the same mental model. Institutions should adopt standardised guidelines that are then embedded through education and training throughout the organisation.

Incident reporting of cases demonstrating excellence in airway management, as well as those where morbidity or mortality has occurred, should be reviewed regularly. Steps should be taken to ensure that anyone reporting a case does not inadvertently become a second victim. When available, a system/database for dissemination of difficult airway patient information should be used. As a minimum, individual institutions should document all difficult airway management details in the patient record. Airway leads/teams may facilitate each of the above goals for an organisation.

Further Reading

Long L, Vanderhoff B, Smyke N, et al. (2010). Management of difficult airways using a hospital-wide 'Alpha Team' approach. *American Journal of Medical Quality*, **25**, 297–304.

Mark LJ, Herzer KR, Cover R, et al. (2015). Difficult Airway Response Team: a novel quality improvement program for managing hospital-wide airway emergencies. *Anesthesia & Analgesia*, **121**, 127–139.

Martin T, Roy, R. (2012). Cause for pause after a perioperative catastrophe: one, two, or three victims? *Anesthesia & Analgesia*, **114**, 485–487.

Tsai AC, Krisciunas GP, Brook C, et al. (2016). Comprehensive Emergency Airway Response Team (EART) training and education: impact on team effectiveness, personnel confidence, and protocol knowledge. *Annals of Otology, Rhinology, and Laryngology*, **125**, 457–463.

Woodall N, Frerk C, Cook TM. (2011). Can we make airway management (even) safer? – lessons from national audit. *Anaesthesia*, **66**(Suppl 2), 27–33.

Website

https://www.rcoa.ac.uk/safety-standards-quality/support-anaesthetic-departments/airway-leads

35 Chapter

Training in Airway Management

Mark R.W. Stacey

Basic Principles

Control what you can

Learn it right

Practise it right

Perform it right

You are called to intensive care to assist with a patient who has been extubated prematurely. Before admission the patient was known to be a difficult intubation. You are faced with a severely hypoxic patient that your colleague (despite being intimately associated with the difficult airway guidelines) is unable to oxygenate. You wonder if you had approached your airway training differently 10 years before whether your management and skills in this case would have been different.

'In theory, there is no difference between theory and practice. In practice, there is.'

Airway skills at their simplest are designed to ensure delivery of oxygen from a source to the patient's lungs. The skills discussed below are theoretically easy to perform, but because of time constraints and the effect of stress caused by the significant effect of hypoxia on a patient, these skills may not be performed at their best, and a very high level of skill performance is required to optimally manage your patient during a crisis.

In order to learn any skill, it is useful to understand, to an extent, how our mind work, in terms of learning, teaching and performance. If we consider the limitations of working memory to be of the order of approximately four components or blocks of information then the learning, practice and performance of a skill needs to be focussed on not overloading the working memory.

The simplest model of the mind (from an idea by Willingham, see Figure 35.1) considers the working memory as a bottle neck between the skill you are trying to learn, teach or perform and your long-term memory. Long-term memory is huge but in order for it to be useful in any given attempt at performance of the skill, it is important that the skill that is being learnt is taught properly (i.e. learn it right), is practised properly (i.e. practise it right), so that ultimately it can be performed correctly (i.e. perform it right). In order to achieve this, it is important to focus on learning what has been called the inflexible content or inflexible knowledge of whatever one is trying to learn. The relevant inflexible content needs to be carefully considered, particularly in the arena of teaching airway skills, because of the significant negative effect of stress on the performance of that basic skill.

If we consider a systematic approach to solving the problem of which airway skills should be learnt and how to learn them, it is useful to consider five prescriptive principles as described by Merrill in 2002:

1. Learners are engaged in performing real-life tasks or solving real-world problems (the practice is context-specific training)
2. Existing knowledge is activated as a foundation for new knowledge (draw on what the learner already knows)
3. New knowledge is demonstrated to the learner (coaching)
4. New knowledge is applied by the learner (deliberate practice)
5. New knowledge is integrated into the learner's world (the learner moves from practice to performance)

In this fashion, the learner moves from learning to practice to practice under pressure to performance to performance under pressure. Making training real enhances the likelihood of the performance being successful. In view of the potential overload on the working memory it can be useful to divide the learning of a skill into learning a series of subskills.

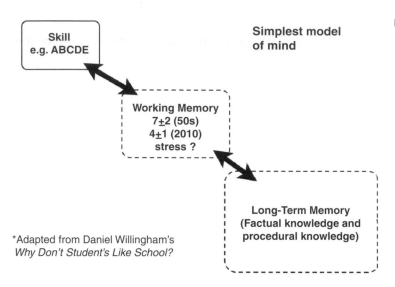

Figure 35.1 Simplest model of the mind.

Ergonomics (See Figure 35.2)

For each of the various airway skills discussed, the importance of considering ergonomics is part of successful outcome, e.g. position for laryngoscopy or face mask anaesthesia, performing an awake flexible optic intubation etc. Additionally, as Ericsson states (see Further Reading) the principles of deliberate practice will lead to improved performance.

Principles of Deliberate Practice

1. Establish a (reachable) **specific goal**. Vague overall performance targets like 'succeed' or 'get better' won't cut it.
2. **Focus** on improvement during practice. It must be intense, uninterrupted and repetitive ('drilling'). Not particularly pleasant, but highly rewarding.
3. You must receive **immediate feedback** on your performance. Without it, you cannot figure out what you need to modify or how close you are to achieving your specific goal.
4. You must get **out of your comfort zone**, constantly attempting things that are just out of reach.
5. It is **arduous** cognitively and physically (Figure 35.3).

Which Airway Skills Should Be Learnt?

Ideally one would like to focus on becoming competent moving to mastery with the aim of

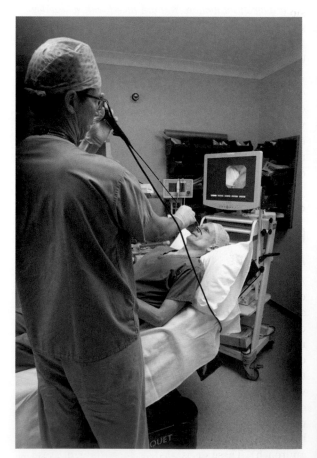

Figure 35.2 Ergonomics of awake flexible optical bronchoscope (FOB)-guided intubation.

becoming an expert over years of practice in the following skills. It is unrealistic to expect to become an expert in all airway skills, but certain skills have a higher priority.

- Assessment and planning airway management
- Maintenance of the airway and anaesthesia with bag valve mask
- Supraglottic airway insertion
- Laryngoscopy (both direct and video) and tracheal tube insertion
- Flexible optic intubation
- Extubation

With additional training for one rescue technique for the cannot intubate, cannot oxygenate situation (see current Difficult Airway Society (DAS) material for a worked example).

Specific more complex techniques (e.g. jet ventilation) should only be used by clinicians who are experienced in those techniques. Additionally, the introduction of an awareness of human factors (decision making, communication, stress management, situation awareness, fixation error) can be introduced as part of real-life task training and learning, once the basic skill is mastered.

If we look at learning these skills it becomes obvious that there are more than four components of information that need to be learned to fit into that working memory box. It is useful to divide the skills themselves into subskills and structure the learning material in such a way that you maximise the function of the working memory model.

Specific Inflexible Components for the Following Components of Airway Skills: Assessment

Assessment of the airway is important because it determines what specific airway skill is likely to be successful. There are a variety of assessment techniques: Mallampati, neck movement, Wilson, thyromental distance (see Chapter 5) – these are used in order to plan and decide which particular airway technique can or should be used, and what the relevant backup plans are (see Chapter 4). The complexity of this planning, appropriate decision making and performance is also important to address and should be simplified wherever possible (e.g. the Vortex approach). These decisions are important because if you start a procedure with the wrong decision leading to the wrong technique, it does not matter how skilful the individual is, the success of the airway procedure is likely to be compromised.

Maintenance of the Airway and Anaesthesia with Bag Valve Mask

Despite this being called a 'basic' airway skill, it is difficult to teach, learn and perform. Additionally, because it requires a certain degree of strength, fatigue will cause deterioration in performance over time. It is a difficult skill to teach because none of the current manikins enable the learner to develop the correct kinaesthetic ability to perform the skill and it is rarely practised on patients. When practice is failing, the instructor may have difficulty seeing or understanding what is wrong. In the author's department asking anaesthetists how many bag-valve-mask anaesthetics longer than 15 minutes they will do in a year, the answer is usually below 10. Even novices who start working independently on a rota have done fewer than 10. The introduction of supraglottic airways has meant that learning the skill of bag-valve-mask anaesthesia on patients has almost disappeared. Because bag-valve-mask anaesthesia is a pure kinaesthetic skill it needs to be practised in a physical manner. If it is not practised it is unlikely that one will be able to perform the skill successfully, when required, in a difficult airway setting. Understanding and practising difficult mask airway maintenance using a two-hand technique to optimise oxygenation may minimise the risk of the situation deteriorating to a cannot intubate, cannot oxygenate situation (also see Chapter 12). It is also arguable that a disproportionate focus on training for the rare cannot intubate, cannot oxygenate has diverted training from more important basic skills.

Laryngoscopy and Intubation (See Also Chapter 14)

Breaking the skill down into subskills enables rapid and accurate training and learning of the skill. If you ask a learner what they are thinking of when performing laryngoscopy their sole focus will be on inserting the tracheal tube to the exclusion of other aspects of the technique. A practical approach that minimises cognitive workload and maximises success is to divide the skill into subskills as follows. These subskills are initially practised and performed on a manikin before being used on a patient. The instructor's voice is in italics.

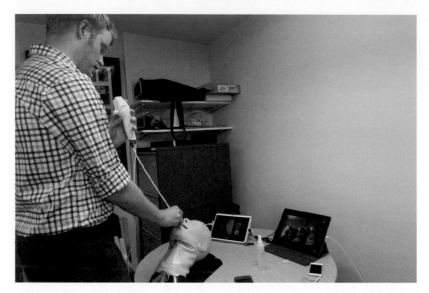

Figure 35.3 Demonstrating flexible optical bronchoscope (FOB) set-up using an iPad as a monitor. To enhance the stress on performance and evaluate situation awareness while focussed on an FOB-guided intubation. A similar technique can be used for other airway skills, but care should be taken if used for the cannot intubate, cannot oxygenate situation.

- **Skill 1:** '*Insert the laryngoscope.*' Put the laryngoscope in the mouth without touching the teeth or lips. This is performed regularly until the motor skill becomes smooth (develop automaticity). Precise feedback from the coach enables refinement of each subskill.
- **Skill 2:** '*Show me the larynx.*' This enables further practice of skill number 1 multiple times followed by skill number 2, which enables the learner to demonstrate the larynx. The learners can begin to appreciate the effect of fatigue degrading performance.
- **Skill 3:** '*Insert the bougie through the vocal cords.*' This diminishes the potential trauma of laryngoscopy, and teaches the learner the additional skill of how to place a tracheal tube over the bougie.
- The introduction of videolaryngoscopy can enable the learner and teacher to share the view thus enabling the teacher to make minor physical modifications of the technique to improve the view. It also enables the teacher to show the learner methods to optimise the insertion of the bougie/stylet ('*I can see what you're doing and what you're seeing*'). Practice such as this also can assist learners to overcome the difficulties they may have intubating with videolaryngoscopy despite a perfect laryngeal view.

Flexible Optical Bronchoscope (FOB)-Guided Intubation (See Also Chapter 16)

Flexible optical bronchoscope (FOB)-guided intubation is often considered to be a difficult skill to master and is a good example of how a structured training programme can optimise and enable a successful outcome, minimising the discomfort of anaesthetists (and patients) who may not consider the skill part of their armamentarium.

Successful FOB-guided intubation involves:

- Ensuring ergonomics is optimised (inflexible rule 1)
- Preparing the equipment and ensuring the FOB works (preparation inflexible)
- Remembering the four inflexible components (see Figure 35.4)
- Ensuring the assistant is briefed (and patient if awake)
- Managing yourself
- Managing the patient (if awake)

The process of learning starts on a manikin. The ergonomic set-up should be as real as the environment allows (Figure 35.3). As the skill improves and the trainer successfully negotiates the anatomical structures, time constraints are introduced ('*Move the scope from lips to carina, then nose to carina, without touching the sides of the airway in under 60 seconds*').

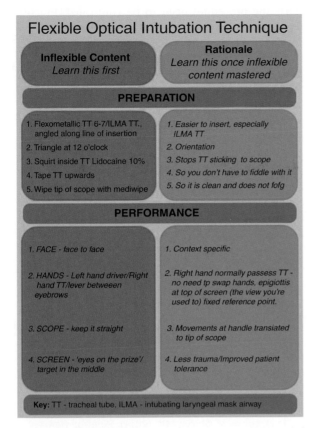

Flexible Optical Intubation Technique

Inflexible Content Learn this first	Rationale Learn this once inflexible content mastered
PREPARATION	
1. Flexometallic TT 6-7/ILMA TT., angled along line of insertion	1. Easier to insert, especially ILMA TT
2. Triangle at 12 o'clock	2. Orientation
3. Squirt inside TT Lidocaine 10%	3. Stops TT sticking to scope
4. Tape TT upwards	4. So you don't have to fiddle with it
5. Wipe tip of scope with mediwipe	5. So it is clean and does not fofg
PERFORMANCE	
1. FACE - face to face	1. Context specific
2. HANDS - Left hand driver/Right hand TT/lever betweeen eyebrows	2. Right hand normally passess TT - no need tp swap hands, epigiottis at top of screen (the view you're used to) fixed reference point.
3. SCOPE - keep it straight	3. Movements at handle transiated to tip of scope
4. SCREEN - 'eyes on the prize'/ target in the middle	4. Less trauma/Improved patient tolerance

Key: TT - tracheal tube. ILMA - intubating laryngeal mask airway

Figure 35.4 Inflexible flexible optical bronchoscope (FOB)-guided intubation training.

Once this is achieved an app such as SimMon (an app that turns an iPad into a monitor that can be controlled by an iPhone and mimics an anaesthetic monitor) can add simulated reality (and clinical pressure) (Figure 35.3). By decreasing oxygen saturation as the FOB-guided intubation is being performed the trainee can begin to understand the practicalities of situation awareness, communication and improved decision making on their perfor-mance. Once automaticity of the skill is developed and the detrimental effect of stress on performance is reduced, the learner can then move on to super-vised FOB-guided intubation on patients, and with appropriate scaffolding/systematic building on the learner's experiences gradually increasing the pres-sure on cognitive workload ('*I'll look after the patient, you just do the scope*' to '*you do everything as smoothly as possible*').

The author has found that given the paucity of FOB-guided intubations there is a need for the learner

to become accomplished and succeed quickly and that the most efficient method of teaching FOB-guided intubation is to teach it in a very didactic fashion. This may be challenging to both learners and teacher when some learners already have some knowledge or experience.

Historically the author would teach the skill as follows: '*you do this because of this, you do this because of this, you do this because of this*', and by the time the teacher had got to the third description the learner had forgotten the first instruction.

Now the author teaches by getting the learner to focus on learning four things. The script is as follows:

> '*I'm going to teach you four things and, until you can do those four things smoothly and in a nice controlled fashion, I'm not going to even teach you what those four things mean or why they are only four things.*'

The four inflexible components are listed under 'per-formance' in Figure 35.4.

Cannot Intubate, Cannot Oxygenate (CICO)

DAS has designed material for teaching the 'scalpel, finger, bougie technique' that maximises the use of the cognitive principles described above. Learning the management of a CICO situation in isolation has been compared to teaching pilots how to crash-land an aeroplane without emphasising the skills required to fly safely, particularly under adverse conditions. The use of cognitive rehearsal of potential airway disasters can potentially enhance the likelihood of a successful performance should a real CICO incident occur (so when inserting the scalpel into the cricothyroid mem-brane think '*blood!*' – this visualisation process is useful to aid real performance). Additionally, the teaching material can be used to highlight critical steps that are often performed poorly (such as the insertion tech-nique of the bougie). (See https://www.das.uk.com/content/fona_training.)

Practice and Stress Management (Stress Inoculation)

The difficulty is not the procedure – it is the cognitive hurdle.
You don't rise to the occasion – you sink to the level of your training.

It is important that the role of deliberate practice is understood. Many of the skills described above can be practised, and should be practised, on manikins. Ideally the motor skill is developed in a zero risk, low stress environment, without time constraints, supervised by a teacher, with the critical components of the skill being emphasised at appropriate moments.

Once the skill can be performed in a low stress environment in a smooth and straightforward fashion the trainer can increase the stress (e.g. using the SimMon app described above).

What is often seen is that because of the fixation error on the skill itself, which often occurs in an airway skill environment when one is stressed, the trainee may not even be aware that the monitor is present. When debriefing the trainer can then have a discussion around the human factor component of airway skills, in particular loss of situation awareness.

Having performed the skill in a low stress and high stress environment on manikins, it is then appropriate to move on to a very supervised environment on patients. Again, it is possible in a safe fashion to use structured, preferably objective, feedback by for example using video assessment to enable accurate feedback to the learner. As the learner gets more experienced the cognitive workload challenges can be changed. The simplest way to do this is to just say to the individual '*I am timing you*'. By them stressing themselves due to this artificial time pressure, they may fail or stutter in their performance. When they do fail, you can demonstrate to them the practical effect of that stressor on the performance (or lack of knowledge) of the inflexible components.

Summary

In order for an individual to learn the airway skills it is important for them to understand the following:

First of all, whatever elements that can be controlled, e.g. ergonomics, the patient, the nerves of the anaesthetist, the equipment, *before* the individual starts the procedure need to be controlled. Practise regularly. Additionally, a plan should be made to be employed if the initial technique is unsuccessful ('*what ifs/if then*' – what if I fail to intubate? If the *patient gets laryngospasm then . . .*). Furthermore, if help is required it is important to know where the help is located.

Then, in order to approach the airway skills in a safe fashion, the skill needs to be learned right, performed right and practised right. Practice will require appropriate feedback and the teaching session needs to be designed around a strategy of managing cognitive workload so that as the learner gets more confident the stress on the learner is increased to demonstrate the potential complications of failure. This training process is more likely to lead to a successful outcome.

Further Reading

Ericsson A, Pool R. (2016). *Peak: How All of Us Can Achieve Extraordinary Things*. London: Vintage.

Hess E. (2014). *Learn or Die*. New York: Columbia University Press.

Kaufman J. (2013). *The First 20 Hours: How to Learn Anything Fast*. London: Portfolio Penguin.

Leslie D, Oliver M, Stacey MR. (2014). Point-of-view high-definition video assessment: the future of technical skills training. *British Journal of Anaesthesia*, **112**, 761–763.

Merrill MD. (2002). First principles of instructional design. *Educational Technology Research and Development*, **50**, 43–59.

Stacey M. (2017). Practice under pressure: what neurology can learn from anaesthesia. *Practical Neurology*, **17**, 439–443.

van Merrienboer JJG, Kirschner PA. (2013). *Ten Steps to Complex Learning*. New York: Routledge.

Willingham D. (2009). *Why Don't Students Like School?* San Francisco: Jossey Bass.

Chapter 36

Human Factors in Airway Management

Mikael Rewers and Nicholas Chrimes

What Is Meant by 'Human Factors'?

Human factors (ergonomics) is the scientific discipline concerned with the understanding and optimising of interactions between humans and other elements of a system. It involves considering the individual, team, environmental and organisational factors that influence overall system performance (Table 36.1). It is as concerned with augmenting the human contribution to success as it is with protecting against the potential to contribute to error.

This chapter provides an overview of the principles of human factors in relation to airway management.

Table 36.1 Common human factors in airway management

CATEGORY	FACTORS	THREATS	SAFEGUARDS
Individual			
Situation awareness (also at team level)	Attention/vigilance, perception, problem detection, memory, recognition, comprehension, anticipation	Distraction, lack of gathering all cues, distorted time perception, memory lapse, inadequate knowledge, inability to apply knowledge into context, poor communication, lack of 'shared mental model', assumption, fixation	Continuous systematic scanning, cross-checking information, establishing/maintaining a 'shared mental model', declaring a situation, 'thinking ahead'
Decision making (also at team level)	Identify available options, judgement to select and implement, re-evaluation	Poor situation awareness, poor judgement, failure to re-evaluate	Cognitive aids, considering advantages/disadvantages, re-evaluating after each airway attempt
Personality	Confidence, insight, willingness to act	Overconfidence, denial, pride, guilt, diffidence	Humility, willingness to ask for help, recognition of own limitations, reflection
Technical	Competence, manual dexterity	Inadequate skills, inadequate airway assessment	Expertise, experience, supervision, training
Performance-shaping factors	Stimulation, mood, satiety, alertness, health, motivation, interest	Stress, hunger, fatigue, illness/injury, apathy/improper motivation	Calm, refreshed, sleep hygiene, alert, engaged
Team			
Behavioural	Coordination/leadership, role allocation, teamwork, communication	Ineffective coordination/teamwork, role ambiguity, unclear communication, multiple ambiguous/conflicting terminologies	Effective coordination/leadership, clear roles, cooperative teamwork, consultation, calling for help, team brief, names, closed loop communication, prompting, common goal, 'speaking up', 'mini team time-out'

Table 36.1 (cont.)

CATEGORY	FACTORS	THREATS	SAFEGUARDS
Social	Interactions, familiarity	Conflict, awkwardness, intimidation	Harmonious relationship, understanding each other's ideas or concerns
Work preparation	Planning, preparing	Limitation in strategies/plans, lack of available time to plan	Strategy with contingency plans, checklists, taking only a few seconds to plan can be beneficial for decision-making and teamwork
Environmental			
Equipment	Design, availability, access, maintenance, function	Inconsistent storage locations, clutter, poor user interface, design defects, equipment faults, inappropriate alarm settings or alert signals	Suitability, proximity, visibility, readiness, well-designed equipment/alarms
Workspace	Size, layout	Crowding, obstructed views, poor equipment position	Adequate space, optimal layout
Ambience	Lighting, sound, temperature	Inadequate lighting, noise	'Sterile cockpit', 'Focus'
Organisational			
Job factors	Task complexity, staffing, workload	Task difficulty, inadequate staffing, excessive workload, time/production pressure, night shift	Assistance/backup
Policies/Procedures	Guidelines, protocols, reporting, standards	Lack of incident reporting or multi-professional morbidity/mortality meetings	Learning through multi-professional morbidity/mortality meetings
Training/Supervision	Programmes	Lack of training, inadequate supervision	Education, feedback, supervision, case discussion
Culture	Management, norms, patient safety	Judgemental culture, skewed norms, 'waiting for errors to occur'	Non-judgemental culture, praise colleagues for good work, resilience

How Much Do Human Factors Impact on Airway Management Outcome?

Human error is implicated in up to 80% of anaesthetic incidents. The 4th National Audit Project (NAP4) in the United Kingdom concluded that human factor-related issues such as poor judgement, communication and teamwork contributed to 40% of major complications in airway management and were deemed to be major factors in 25% of these cases. In a follow-up study, Flin et al. identified an average of four contributing human factors per NAP4 case; the most frequent were failures to anticipate, wrong decision, task difficulty, inappropriate staffing, time pressure, tiredness, hunger, stress, poor communication and limitations in competence. The study also revealed protective factors such as good teamwork and effective communication. Overall, the contribution of human factors related issues to patient harm during airway management is at least as important as that resulting from technical issues.

Stop and think: is there any data on airway management outcomes in your department? What does the data show?

Why Do Human Factor-Related Adverse Events Occur in Airway Management?

Error Triggers

Human errors are inevitable, no matter how well trained and motivated an individual is.

'Threats' refer to aspects of the individual, team, work environment or organisation that can influence work performance by increasing the *chance* of an error (Tables 36.1 and 36.2). Threats will not inevitably lead to errors, nor will errors always result in adverse consequences. For the most part, additional contributing elements are necessary for an error to evolve into an adverse event. Small errors can trigger significant adverse outcomes and vice versa.

> Stop and think: what threats can you identify in your clinical practice? How will you address these?

Table 36.2 Selected 'threats' from Table 36.1 with examples

CATEGORY	THREATS	EXAMPLES OF RESULTING ERRORS IN AIRWAY MANAGEMENT
Individual		
Situation awareness	Distorted time perception	• Distorted time perception leads to team failing to recognise how long patient has been hypoxic
	Assumption	• Assumption that lack of $etCO_2$ trace or low SpO_2 are errors
	Fixation	• Repeated attempts at intubation, prolonged hypoxia, airway trauma and potential precipitation of CICO
Personality	Denial, pride, guilt	• Refusal to acknowledge oxygenation is not occurring
		• Trying to prove you can intubate the patient
		• Clinician belief that they should have predicted or have precipitated the difficult airway
Technical	Inadequate skills	• Reluctance to perform front of neck airway rescue or awake flexible optical intubation
		• High failure rate of front of neck airway rescue techniques
	Inadequate airway assessment	• Impaired situation awareness of airway risk
		• Diminished ability to deal with airway challenges
Performance-shaping factors	Stress, hunger, fatigue, illness/injury, apathy/improper motivation	• May act as a distraction which impairs situation awareness
		• May promote taking shortcuts e.g. inadequate airway assessment, planning, positioning or preoxygenation
Team		
Behavioural	Ineffective coordination/teamwork, role ambiguity, unclear communication	• Duplication of tasks combined with failure to allocate other tasks: multiple people focused on getting emergency airway trolley, no one watching monitors
	Multiple ambiguous/conflicting terminologies	• E.g. surgical airway, eFONA, CICO rescue, infraglottic rescue; these terms may not be mutually understood by all team members leading to confusion and delays in execution
Social	Conflict, awkwardness, intimidation	• Failure to mention important information: e.g. 'There's no $etCO_2$ trace', 'The patient is cyanotic', or 'The SpO_2 has been <80% for 2 mins'
Environmental		
Equipment	Inconsistent storage locations, clutter	• Difficulty locating airway rescue or CICO equipment
	Poor user interface, design defects, equipment faults, inappropriate alarm settings or alert signals	• Difficulty obtaining/interpreting information: misinterpreting airway pressure waveform or etO_2 waveform as $etCO_2$ trace
		• Alarms set too broadly fail to alert team to hypoxia (trigger too late)
		• If alarm settings are too sensitive clinicians develop 'alarm fatigue' and ignore them delaying recognition of a crisis
		• Inconsistent tone modulation with SpO_2 change between different types of monitors
		• Tone modulation on SpO_2 monitor switched off

Table 36.2 (cont.)

CATEGORY	THREATS	EXAMPLES OF RESULTING ERRORS IN AIRWAY MANAGEMENT
Workspace	Crowding, obstructed views, poor equipment position	• Lack of visibility of monitors: failure to recognise falling SpO_2, lack of $etCO_2$ trace or other clinical abnormalities
Ambience	Noise	• Impaired communication, difficulty hearing SpO_2 tone modulation or alarms
Organisational		
Job factors	Excessive workload, time/ production pressure	• Failure to develop an airway strategy, avoidance of awake flexible optical intubation, inadequate preoxygenation
Training/ Supervision	Lack of training, inadequate supervision	• Inexperienced staff (airway operators & assistants) with poor decision making, inadequate airway skills
Culture	Skewed norms	• Acceptance of high risk behaviours, failure to assess airway, failure to plan
	'Waiting for errors to occur'	• Only allows safety improvements to be implemented retrospectively (underestimation of risk)

CICO: cannot intubate, cannot oxygenate, **FONA:** front of neck airway

Table 36.3 Common human factor-related errors seen in airway crises

ACTIONS	RESULTS
Inadequate attempts at upper airway rescue: omission of optimisations or entire techniques	Unnecessary front of neck airway rescue
Fixation on intubation: to the exclusion of upper airway techniques, airway trauma	Precipitating CICO, delayed CICO rescue
Poor decision-making when oxygenation is present, ignoring options to wake or convert, repeated instrumentation	Precipitating CICO
Fixation on upper airway techniques: failure to declare CICO and move to front of neck airway techniques	Delayed CICO rescue

CICO: cannot intubate, cannot oxygenate

Stress

An airway crisis can be a high-stakes, time-critical situation. Excessive stress compromises the cognitive, communication and technical skills of clinicians, which may diminish their ability to resolve the crisis. Although the susceptibility of different individuals to performance impairment due to stress will vary, all clinicians will suffer from this phenomenon, if the pressure exceeds their limits.

Stress-related cognitive impairment may lead to fixation, distorted time perception, impaired knowledge recall and impaired judgement. These issues may combine to lead even experienced clinicians to make fundamental errors, considered inconceivable in the non-stressed state.

Failure to 'do the basics' under pressure is a recognised problem in real-life airway emergencies.

No preceding attempt was made to place a supraglottic airway device (SGA) in over half of the cases of emergency front of neck airway in NAP4. Some common human factor-related errors seen in airway crises are listed in Table 36.3.

Fixation Error

Fixation is the cognitive error that occurs when a clinician focusses on a limited aspect of care, to the exclusion of other more relevant considerations. In airway management, fixation on intubation, ignoring the option to supply oxygen to the patient using a face mask or SGA, is a common error. Not only does this prolong hypoxia, the airway trauma from repeated instrumentation can diminish the chance of success at these alternatives and increase the chance of a 'cannot intubate, cannot oxygenate' (CICO) event

Table 36.4 Selected 'safeguards' from Table 36.1 with examples

CATEGORY	SAFEGUARDS	EXAMPLES OF REDUCING HARM IN AIRWAY MANAGEMENT
Individual		
Situation awareness	Continuous systematic scanning	Using a systematic pattern to collect cues from: • Patient (e.g. airway, chest movement) • Monitors (e.g. SpO_2, $etCO_2$) • Equipment (e.g. displays, tactile feedback) • Time (e.g. from induction to expected critical desaturation) • Team members (e.g. medication administered, previous airway attempts)
	Cross-checking information	• E.g. checking pulse oximetry probe position and blood pressure if SpO_2 is falling
	Establishing/maintaining a 'shared mental model'	• 'Could this be a … situation? Or could it be something else?' • 'Has anyone experienced such a situation before?' • 'Is this an emergency requiring immediate action?'
	Declaring a situation	• 'We now have a CICO situation, prepare for front-of-neck-airway rescue'
	'Thinking ahead'	• 'Will there be any difficulties with oxygenation or airway techniques?' • 'What access is available to the airway (mouth, nose or cricoid membrane)?' • 'What could happen next to the patient?' • Get required resources ahead to the OR: 'Who or what is available? Where to find it? How to call? How long does it take for them to arrive?'
Decision making	Cognitive aids	• Reminder to optimise upper airway rescue techniques, prompt for CICO rescue or opportunities when oxygen delivery achieved
	Identifying available options	• 'Which techniques are possible? Has the clinical situation changed? What are the alternatives?'
	Considering advantages/disadvantages	• 'What are the benefits, possible success, risks and potential complications of the chosen technique?' • 'Has the airway operator maintained regular training in this technique?' • 'Is time, equipment or assistance available?'
	Re-evaluating after each airway attempt	• 'Is oxygenation/ventilation possible now? Or is it worsening?' • 'Have any complications occurred after previous attempts? Or are there new/other problems?'
Personality	Humility, willingness to ask for help, recognition of own limitations, reflection	• Improved decision making leading to effective actions
Technical	Expertise, experience, supervision, training	• Preparedness to effectively manage challenges • Extending the safe apnoea time may create less time pressure and stress and therefore improved decision making
Performance shaping factors	Calm, refreshed, sleep hygiene, alert, engaged	• Improved situation awareness and decision making
Team		
Behavioural	Clear roles, prompting	• Allocating someone to observe monitor or declare time since desaturation improves situation awareness
	'Mini team time-out'	• E.g. flags anticipated difficulties
	'Shared mental model' and a common goal	• Enhance teamwork efficiency
	Effective leadership	• Coordinated team activity
Social	Harmonious relationship, understanding each other's ideas or concerns	• Team members are more likely to speak up to flag potential errors or make suggestions, e.g. suggesting alternative airway techniques if airway operator has difficulties in intubating

Table 36.4 (cont.)

CATEGORY	SAFEGUARDS	EXAMPLES OF REDUCING HARM IN AIRWAY MANAGEMENT
Work preparation	Strategy with contingency plans	• Clear plan to optimise each of FMV, SGA & TT with defined triggers for moving between these and to CICO rescue • Have all equipment (checked in advance) & drugs ready by the patient
	Checklists	• Ensure airway equipment is available
Environmental		
Equipment	Suitability, proximity, visibility, readiness, well-designed equipment/alarms	• Standardised location & layout of airway equipment • Clear labelling: use of icons rather than text to improve identification under stress • Minimise equipment options: less clutter, simpler decisions, easier to maintain proficiency
Workspace	Adequate space, optimal layout	• Monitors that are easily visible to the airway team may help improving situation awareness
Ambience	Focus	• Minimising extraneous noise during induction, emergence or a crisis
Organisational		
Job factors	Assistance/backup	• Practical & reliable systems to specifically declare an airway emergency and source advice/assistance
Policies/Procedures	Learning through multi-professional morbidity/mortality meetings	• Regular processes for collaboration, exchange of ideas
Training/ Supervision	Education, case discussion	• Multi-professional simulation-based training • Case review and evaluation in a safe learning environment
Culture	Non-judgemental culture, praising colleagues	• 'I think you developed an excellent airway strategy for the patient'
	Resilience	• Examine why things regularly go right, and try to integrate these behaviours into standard clinical practice

CICO: cannot intubate, cannot oxygenate, **SGA:** supraglottic airway device, **FMV:** facemask ventilation, **TT:** tracheal tube

(also see Chapter 3). Fixation error is a major contributing factor in many airway-related deaths.

Stop and think: have you ever suffered a fixation error?

How Human Factors Play a Role in Avoiding Adverse Events in Airway Management

Just as threats increase the chance of error, the term 'safeguards' can be used to refer to aspects of the individual, team, work environment or organisation that contribute to enhanced work performance by decreasing the chance of an error (Tables 36.1 and 36.4).

Resilience

Humans are often wrongly regarded as the 'weakest link' in a system. Clinicians perform well most of the time, because they are flexible and can rapidly adjust their work so that it matches varying conditions. Human adaptability is therefore a safeguard, responsible for reducing the risk of patient harm, both via neutralising threats before they trigger an error and from intercepting errors before they result in patient harm ('resilient' behaviours).

One of the challenges to improving patient safety, therefore, is that waiting for errors to occur results in an underestimation of risk and only allows safety improvements to be implemented retrospectively, often after patient harm has occurred. A resilience-based approach instead examines why things regularly go right by observing daily work and the successful management of potentially harmful situations, and then tries to integrate these behaviours into standard clinical practice.

Stop and think: have you neutralised threats or prevented errors from causing patient harm? Could these strategies be shared and implemented more widely?

Non-technical Skills

Non-technical skills can be defined as the cognitive (e.g. situation awareness and decision-making) and behavioural skills (e.g. teamwork, leadership and communication) that are integrated with technical skills to contribute to safe and efficient task performance. Just as technical skills require regular practice to ensure competence when they are required, non-technical skills practices must be embedded in routine clinical work so that they become second nature and are more likely to be effectively implemented when a critical situation arises.

Situation Awareness

Airway management takes place in an environment of high cognitive load, so that maintaining a dynamic awareness of the patient's condition is paramount. On an individual level, this can be achieved by continuous systematic scanning of the environment and gathering cues (e.g. laryngoscopy view, monitors, time) to 'get the whole picture' of the situation. Cross-checking can increase the reliability of information, e.g. ensuring a decreasing SpO_2 or absent capnography trace is not dismissed as artefactual. On the team or organisational level, situation awareness can be supported by task delegation and communication. Establishing and maintaining a mutual situational understanding ('shared mental model') in the team ensures that all are 'on the same page'. In a crisis situation, this can be done by 'thinking out loud', inviting inputs and discussing patterns of cues. Sharing knowledge and prior experience can help identifying problems, making decisions and setting a common goal for the patient. Declaring a situation is vital, e.g. 'We now have a cannot intubate, cannot oxygenate event, prepare for ...'. 'Thinking ahead' about potential outcomes by asking 'What could happen next to the patient?' may facilitate anticipating complications and possible progress paths, and thereby planning (Table 36.4).

Planning and Preparation

Proper planning and preparation can both help prevent the occurrence of an airway crisis and decrease the cognitive load involved in managing a crisis by simplifying decision-making and improving situation awareness. NAP4 stressed the importance of having a strategy for airway management – a coordinated sequence of plans accounting for foreseeable contingencies (i.e. backup plans in case the preceding plan fails). The strategy should include identification of the triggers for abandoning a failed plan and implementing the next one. The goals for such strategy should be avoiding hypoxia, minimising failures and complications of airway techniques and preventing progression to an unnecessary CICO situation.

Stop and think: do you develop and communicate an airway management strategy for every patient?

Decision-Making

Decisions are based on situation awareness, which, in turn, can be affected by factors such as communication or available resources. Cognitive aids can facilitate decision-making by prompting consideration of the available options. The merits of these options in a given context can be assessed by asking 'What are the benefits and risks of the chosen airway technique? Has the airway operator maintained regular training in this technique? Is time, equipment or assistance available?' It is vital to assess the efficacy of each implemented airway attempt (re-evaluation) by asking 'Is oxygenation/ventilation possible now?' This will lead to a new situation, thus affecting situation awareness and again decision making etc.

Coordination: Leadership and Role Allocation

Coordination represents a particular challenge during complex airway management as the airway operator may be both the most experienced clinician and the only person in a position to make decisions about what equipment/interventions are required, but it can be difficult to maintain situation awareness while 'head down' during airway attempts.

To address this, it can be useful to separate the leadership role into three components and assign these to separate individuals as the 'coordinating team':

- Information gatherer (afferent limb): systematically screens the patient, monitors and environment, prompts time/options etc. to maintain situation awareness
- Decision maker: may also be the airway operator
- Resource allocator (efferent limb): calls for help, assigns roles, sources equipment etc.

The clinicians assuming each of these roles must be explicitly declared to the team to provide role clarity. Between each airway attempt, a 'shared mental model' should be established/maintained, and decisions are based on this.

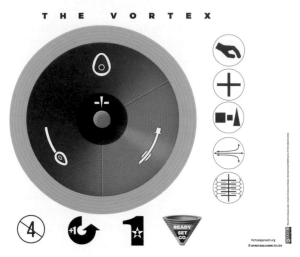

Figure 36.1 Vortex Approach. (Reproduced with permission from Nicholas Chrimes.)

Stop and think: how often have you seen someone explicitly declared the leader during a crisis? What do you think are the barriers to this occurring? How could such barriers be overcome?

Calling for Help

There are many potential barriers to clinicians calling for help including cultural resistance, pride, inadequate escalation processes and simply being so distracted by an evolving crisis that seeking assistance is overlooked. A cognitive aid that prompts to call for help in response to specific events during an airway emergency can facilitate overcoming some of these issues. Figure 36.1 shows an example of this.

Stop and think: what events during airway management do you think should mandate a call for help?

Teamwork and Communication

Training together and working in teams enables appropriate flattening of hierarchies, which is essential to break down barriers to effective communication in both everyday and crisis situations.

Effective communication should be practised all the time, not only in critical situations. The airway strategy for each patient should be explicitly communicated to all involved in airway management before the case starts (pre-brief).

Communication should be clear, unambiguous, mutually understood and ideally include 'closed loops' (i.e. a team member repeats instructions from a colleague, and reports back once tasks have been executed).

Challenging erroneous decisions ('speaking up') is essential to preventing harm. If a nurse or junior doctor knows what is required, they should make their concerns heard and challenge a senior anaesthetist persisting with inappropriate airway management. Advocacy-inquiry is one method to be used in sharing what is observed, what your views are about this and why you are concerned, and inquiring about the underlying reasoning behind the observed decision or action. For example, 'I can see that you persist with several intubation attempts', 'I think we should move on to SGA now, as we cannot face mask ventilate or intubate despite having made our best effort, and I am concerned about airway trauma and precipitating CICO', 'What are your reasons for continuing intubation attempts?'

Graded assertiveness is another tool to be used to flatten hierarchies and to enable more junior staff to challenge inappropriate behaviour of seniors. An example is shown in Box 36.1.

Simple interventions can help establish clear role allocation and improve communication. Senior staff can break down established barriers by seeking input from others. Explicitly making a simple statement like 'If I seem like I'm doing something that doesn't make sense, please query it' can be a powerful tool to provide team members with permission to speak up. A team brief is a formal process where team members introduce themselves, are assigned clear responsibilities and are made aware of the strategy. It can be carried out at the start of a shift as well as immediately before airway management. Even during an airway crisis, if the opportunity arises, a 'stop and think' moment can also help ensure team members understand the situation, goals and strategy for achieving them ('shared mental model'), and invite for inputs.

Writing team members' names up in a prominent position in the room is another easy way to facilitate communication and role allocation but remains vulnerable to the issue of new staff subsequently entering the room, especially once a crisis is declared. A recent initiative, the 'theatre cap challenge', encourages

Box 36.1 The PACE tool as an example of graded assertiveness in the situation of multiple attempts at intubation

Probe – "Are you going to try to intubate again?"

Alert – "This is your third attempt at intubation"

Challenge – "I don't think you should have a fourth intubation attempt"

Emergency – "I'm going to call one of your colleagues to help as you've had too many goes"

operating theatre staff to put their name and role on the front of their theatre cap, to overcome this.

Stop and think: what strategies could you implement to improve role allocation and communication?

In addition to non-technical skills, many other human factors help influence human performance.

Cognitive Aids

Cognitive aids are structured tools presenting key information in an easy-to-use form and are designed to be referred to in 'real time' during managment to improve cognition and adherence to best practice. These 'prompts' can be used to facilitate situation awareness, prompt decision making and guide key actions. However, integrating them into clinical work requires training and practice. Algorithms in difficult airway guidelines are typically too detailed and context-specific to be used during a high-stakes, time-critical emergency. Conversely the Vortex Approach (Figure 36.1) and the DAS ICU Intubation Checklist (Figure 36.2) are examples of cognitive aids that both facilitate planning and present information in a simplified

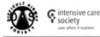 **Intubation Checklist : critically ill adults – to be done with whole team present.** The Faculty of Intensive Care Medicine RCOA

Prepare the patient

- ☐ **Reliable IV / IO access**

- ☐ **Optimise position**
  - ☐ Sit-up?
  - ☐ Mattress hard

- ☐ **Airway assessment**
  - ☐ Identify cricothyroid membrane
  - ☐ Awake intubation option?

- ☐ **Optimal preoxygenation**
  - ☐ 3 mins or $ETO_2 > 85\%$
  - ☐ Consider CPAP / NIV
  - ☐ Nasal O_2

- ☐ **Optimise patient state**
  - ☐ Fluid / pressor/ inotrope
  - ☐ Aspirate NG tube
  - ☐ Delayed sequence induction

- ☐ **Allergies?**
  - ☐ ↑ Potassium risk?
    - avoid suxamethonium

Prepare the equipment

- ☐ **Apply monitors**
  - ☐ SpO_2 / waveform $ETCO_2$ / ECG / BP

- ☐ **Check equipment**
  - ☐ Tracheal tubes x 2
    - cuffs checked
  - ☐ Direct laryngoscopes x 2
  - ☐ Videolaryngoscope
  - ☐ Bougie / stylet
  - ☐ Working suction
  - ☐ Supraglottic airways
  - ☐ Guedel / nasal airways
  - ☐ Flexible scope / Aintree
  - ☐ FONA set

- ☐ **Check drugs**
  - ☐ Consider ketamine
  - ☐ Relaxant
  - ☐ Pressor / inotrope
  - ☐ Maintenance sedation

Prepare the team

- ☐ **Allocate roles**
  One person may have more than one role.
  - ☐ Team Leader
  - ☐ 1st Intubator
  - ☐ 2nd Intubator
  - ☐ Cricoid force
  - ☐ Intubator's assistant
  - ☐ Drugs
  - ☐ Monitoring patient
  - ☐ Runner
  - ☐ MILS (if indicated)
  - ☐ Who will perform FONA?

- ☐ **Who do we call for help?**

- ☐ **Who is noting the time?**

Prepare for difficulty

- ☐ **Can we wake the patient if intubation fails?**

- ☐ **Verbalise "Airway Plan is:"**

- ☐ Plan A:
  Drugs & laryngoscopy
- ☐ Plan B/C:
  Supraglottic airway
  Face-mask
  Fibreoptic intubation via supraglottic airway
- ☐ Plan D:
  FONA
  Scalpel-bougie-tube

- ☐ **Does anyone have questions or concerns?**

Figure 36.2 DAS ICU Intubation Checklist. ((Reprinted with permission of the Difficult Airway Society. Copyright © 2017 Difficult Airway Society. Higgs et al. (2018) British Journal of Anaesthesia, 120, 323–352).

way in order to make it accessible to highly stressed clinicians.

Modifying the Clinical Environment

There are many disturbances in a typical operating room, impeding clinicians' ability to work. 'Below 10 thousand' is an initiative derived from the 'sterile cockpit' concept in aviation: when an aircraft is below 10 thousand feet, only essential conversation is allowed. Translating this to airway management, the declaration of 'Focus' can be used to highlight that a critical intervention is occurring and direct those in the room to minimise extraneous noise and other interruptions.

Proper equipment position and workspace layout are other environmental factors important for optimal work performance (Table 36.4).

Stop and think: what modifications could you make in your clinical environment?

Competence and Training

Improved competence with technical skills may influence clinical judgement by improving confidence in performing procedures such as awake tracheal intubation or making the decision to move to an emergency front of neck airway in a CICO situation. Reluctance to perform both of these procedures was documented as a cause of patient harm in NAP4.

Common sense dictates that use of techniques to extend the safe apnoea time can minimise the chance of desaturation during a difficult airway situation, reducing team stress and potentially improving situation awareness and decision making.

Gjeraa et al. suggest that non-technical skills and technical skills have an intertwined relationship, so it is important to train and assess both – not only technical skills.

NAP4 recommends having a nominated airway lead in each department to e.g. organise local airway management training (in knowledge, skills, attitudes and resources) to maintain standards of performance (see Chapter 34).

Recurrent multidisciplinary simulation-based training is encouraged, accompanied by regular discussions of the best use of non-technical skills in clinical practice (see Chapter 35).

Summary

While management of an airway crisis is inherently stressful, human factor-based interventions can be used to address this by reducing stress (e.g. increasing safe apnoea time, proper planning and preparation, calling for help) and optimising performance when stressed (e.g. cognitive aids, non-technical skills).

The combination of resilient human behaviours, combined with environmental and organisational human factor strategies, act as safeguards against threats, errors and patient harm.

Conclusions

Human actions can contribute to adverse events, but humans also correct many errors and optimise working conditions systematically. Non-technical skills and their interplay with technical skills should be practised daily, not just in emergency situations. Establishing and maintaining a 'shared mental model' and a common goal enhance situation awareness. Prompting cognitive aids enhance situation awareness and decision making. Re-evaluate after each airway management attempt: 'Is oxygenation/ventilation possible now?' Share your experience and cases with your colleagues – reflect and learn from them together.

Acknowledgements

The authors would like to thank Peter Dieckmann and Stuart Marshall for constructive feedback on this chapter and sharing ideas.

Further Reading

Flin R, Fioratou E, Frerk C, Trotter C, Cook TM. (2013). Human factors in the development of complications of airway management: preliminary evaluation of an interview tool. *Anaesthesia*, **68**, 817–825.

Gjeraa K, Jepsen RM, Rewers M, Østergaard D, Dieckmann P. (2016). Exploring the relationship between anaesthesiologists' non-technical and technical skills. *Acta Anaesthesiologica Scandinavica*, **60**(1), 36–47.

Gleeson S, Groom P, Mercer S. (2016). Human factors in complex airway management, *BJA Education*, **16**, 191–197.

Rall M, Gaba DM, Howard SK, Dieckmann P. (2015). Human performance and patient safety. In: Miller RD (Ed.), *Miller's Anesthesia*. 8th ed. Philadelphia: Elsevier, Saunders. pp. 106–166.

Schnittker R, Marshall S, Horberry T, Young KL. (2018). Human factors enablers and barriers for successful airway management – an in-depth interview study. *Anaesthesia*, **73**, 980–989.

Weller JM, Long JA. (2019). Creating a climate for speaking up. *British Journal of Anaesthesia*, **122**(6), 710–713.

Websites

https://resilienthealthcare.net/reads/

https://www.abdn.ac.uk/iprc/ants/

http://vortexapproach.org/

Chapter 37

Decontamination of Airway Equipment

Subrahmanyan Radhakrishna

Anaesthetic equipment and machines can be potential sources of cross-contamination of microbiological pathogens and hence causes of healthcare-associated infections (HAIs), which are an important concern across the world. Anaesthetists must take an active role in reducing cross-contamination. This chapter gives a brief insight into the processes involved and ways of preventing cross-contamination.

Healthcare-Associated Infection (HAI)

HAI has a negative impact on the health industry, with an estimated 300,000 cases per annum in the National Health Service (NHS) in England with respiratory tract infection the commonest. Scrupulous hand hygiene has been emphasised for reducing HAI. In the USA an estimated 1 million HAIs are reported annually, which is approximately 1 in 20 patient admissions with an annual cost of 30 billion dollars. Australia does not have a national surveillance for HAIs and therefore reports low figures of 165,000 per year which may not reflect the true scale of the problem. New Zealand has started a national trial to assess the extent of HAIs to help introduce corrective measures.

Bacteria top the list of causes of HIAs but they may also be caused by viruses, prions and fungi. Hepatitis A, B, C and the human immunodeficiency virus (HIV) are all potentially important viruses that may be transmitted between patients. Coronavirus-19 and its implications for anaesthetic practice is discussed in detail in the next chapter.

Prions are transmissible disease-causing proteinaceous particles. As they lack nucleic acid, they are resistant to almost all standard decontamination and sterilisation methods. Despite their resistance to sterilisation, cleaning with detergents is an important aspect of prion decontamination as it will wash away the hydrophobic prions reducing their numbers to low safe levels. Prions are the cause of variant Creutzfeldt–Jakob disease (vCJD), which was a disease of great concern in the UK in the 1980s to 1990s. It is a rare disease but necessitates the use of single-use equipment for surgical and anaesthetic procedures to minimise risk of transmission. Local policies based on national guidance must be followed diligently.

Decontamination Methods

The definitions of decontamination and the various components of decontamination used here are taken from the Medicines Healthcare products Regulatory Agency's (MHRA) Microbiology advisory committee glossary of terms.

Decontamination

Decontamination is a broad term that includes cleaning, disinfection and sterilisation. It effectively removes contaminants or infectious agents that may potentially cause harm.

Cleaning

Cleaning, using detergents and water, is an important step that removes organic debris from equipment and is the only method of removing prions. Disinfection and sterilisation are only effective after cleaning has reduced the bioburden (i.e. amount of organic debris on the contaminated equipment).

Disinfection

Disinfection is a process used to reduce the number of viable infectious agents, but which may not necessarily inactivate some microbial agents, such as certain viruses and bacterial spores. Disinfection does not achieve the same reduction in microbial contamination levels as sterilisation. Effect of different decontamination methods on various vectors of infection is shown in Figure 37.1.

Method	Spores	Mycobacteria	Bacteria	Viruses
Steam	###	###	###	###
Gas plasma/act H_2O_2	###	###	###	###
Chlorine Di-oxide	###	###	###	###
Para-acetic acid	###	###	###	###
SuperOxidised Saline	###	###	###	###
Dry Heat**	###	###	###	###
Orthophthaldehyde	#	###	###	###
Aldehydes - other	#	###	###	###
Thermal Washer Disinfector	X	###	###	##
Low Temperature Steam	X	###	###	##
Alcohol	X	##	###	##
NaDCC	X	X	###	###
Cleaning*				

Figure 37.1 Effectiveness of various agents against four important infectious agents. Prions cannot be destroyed by any of the agents, they can only be removed by washing and cleaning with water and detergents. X, not effective; #, mildly effective; ##, fairly effective; ###, strongly effective. Act H_2O_2, activated hydrogen peroxide, NaDCC = Sodium dichloroisocyanurate.
*Cleaning is an essential process to remove all debris. Without this decontamination will not be effective. Cleaning with detergents is currently the only way of reducing prion proteins from the surface of equipment.

A high-level disinfectant is a chemical agent that can kill bacteria, viruses and spores. It is only sporicidal under certain conditions.

Sterilisation

Sterilisation indicates the elimination of *all* pathogens including spores. For a medical device to be labelled sterile, the theoretical probability of there being a viable microorganism present on the device should be equal to or less than 1×10^{-6}.

Steam sterilisation is performed at temperatures above 120 °C and most anaesthetic equipment including videolaryngoscopes and flexible optical bronchoscopes (FOBs) cannot withstand such temperatures.

Reusable FOBs can be sterilised using low temperature sterilisers such as gas plasma or hydrogen peroxide sterilisers that are as effective as steam sterilisers against spores and mycobacterium (Figure 37.1). A select few videolaryngoscopes can also be similarly sterilised.

Ethylene oxide sterilisation is a slow process, but it is often used at an industrial level for equipment (including single-use devices) that are delivered sterile.

Single-Use versus Reusable Equipment

The arguments about single versus reusable equipment (e.g. cost, quality, environmental impact and infection risk) are often more complex than they initially appear.

A single-use device is a device that should be discarded after a single use. Some devices such as laryngoscopes and suction may be retained for a single patient episode (duration of an anaesthetic procedure) but used a few times on the same patient. A single-use device should not be reprocessed or reused. Reusable equipment may be used multiple times and on multiple patients and therefore requires reprocessing between uses.

Sterile single-use equipment prevents cross-contamination and reduces the costs related to reprocessing, but raises concerns about quality, cost and the environmental impact of supply chain and disposal. On the other hand, reusable equipment has the potential to cross-infect even after decontamination. Decontamination and sterilisation services can be costly and balance of economic and environmental costs are further complicated when this service is offered at a site distant from the point of clinical use.

If single-use equipment is chosen it is important that it performs to the same levels as reusable equipment it replaces. However, for many devices single-use alternatives are simply not available so that cleaning reprocessing of some equipment will remain necessary for some time.

Airway Equipment: Problems and Solutions

Pathogens may be grown from anaesthetic equipment after use and this has the potential to cause transmission of disease-causing agents between patients. Cultures taken from laryngoscope handles have yielded both commensal and pathogenic organisms, including after cleaning and disinfection. Failure to clean and decontaminate laryngoscopes and their handles has been reported to have caused fatalities in adults and neonates through transmission of organisms including Group A streptococcus and *Serratia* species.

Reusable FOBs require special care as their working channels are long, narrow, difficult to clean and can lodge debris and organisms. In respiratory medicine, 48 outbreaks of infection (including *Pseudomonas aeruginosa* and mycobacteria) related to bronchoscopy have been reported between 1970 and 2012 and in the USA this led the Food and Drugs Administration (FDA) to issue a notice highlighting the issue.

Single-use FOBs may be a solution to this problem and are increasingly available and used in anaesthetic practice. Limiting factors have included image quality, handling and cost, but a number of acceptable devices now exist, and cost comparisons suggest single-use scopes may be an effective and affordable solution for many departments. Single-use FOBs may also become contaminated after use and it is recommended that they should only be used during an anaesthetic episode lasting less than 3 hours.

Many of the currently available supraglottic devices including the i-gel and many laryngeal masks are single use. Conversely, the ProSeal LMA is reusable and needs to be cleaned and sterilised before use.

Anaesthetic masks, catheter mounts and bougies are mostly single use. Single-use anaesthetic circuits which are marketed as single use are often used for up to 7 days provided a pleated heat and moisture exchange (HME) filter is placed between the patient and the anaesthetic circuit as shown in Figure 37.2. The filter should be changed after each patient use. A second HME filter is inserted by some to protect the machine. This filter is useful only as a backup to protect the machine, if the user forgets to put an HME between the patient and the

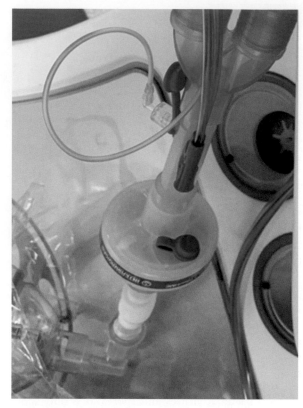

Figure 37.2 A heat moisture exchanger (HME) filter between the patient end and the circle system. The filter must be changed after each patient. The filter protects the circle from contamination.

circuit. It is also important that the anaesthetic circuit when not in use should have its patient end capped or closed to prevent contamination (Figure 37.3).

Preventing Cross-Contamination in Airway Management

Prevention of cross-contamination of airway equipment may require some important changes to current practice.

Good hand hygiene practices by the anaesthetic team are easy to implement and should be mandatory. Hand-washing in water and soap between procedures or change of gloves between procedures is an important step to prevent contamination of anaesthetic surfaces and equipment with blood, saliva and body fluids.

Single-use equipment is often practical and feasible. This includes oropharyngeal and nasopharyngeal airways, tracheal tubes, catheter mounts, bougies, angle pieces and nosocomial filters. Standard direct laryngoscopes were traditionally reusable and processed in the

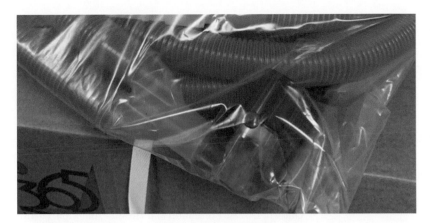

Figure 37.3 Manufacturers supply a protective cap (red) that is fitted to the patient end of the circle system inside their sterile package. A circle system is single use but can be retained for 7 days provided an HME filter is used for each patient and the patient end of the circle is kept closed between each use. The red cap may be used for the purpose or the end may be closed by inserting over an appendage on the anaesthetic machine specifically provided for that purpose by some manufacturers.

hospital sterile services department (SSD). However, steam sterilisation of direct laryngoscopes can damage the light components. With the outbreak of vCJD single-use laryngoscopes became increasingly popular. Current single-use direct laryngoscopes are of good quality and very affordable.

The advent of videolaryngoscopy has introduced a new complexity as some are reusable, and some are single use with reusable parts. The problems of processing reusable parts of videolaryngoscopes are similar to those of direct laryngoscopes. Cleaning and disinfection should be undertaken according to instructions from the device manufacturer. Automated washer disinfectors are generally more reliable than manual cleaning and disinfection, but many hospitals rely on manual chemical cleaning for quick processing and reuse. Chlorine dioxide wipes are popular, but the quality of disinfection and cleaning can vary between individuals, introducing an element of uncertainty into the system. Chemical disinfectants may also be used but can cause skin irritation and emit irritant fumes. Staff undertaking manual processing should be trained and should wear personal protection equipment (PPE) and undertake the processing in a dedicated area. The cleaning process should include a device-tracking process. Cables and monitors should also be cleaned after use.

Reusable FOBs should be transported in a sterile tray to the point of use. Anaesthetists should place FOBs on dedicated, cleaned and disinfected surfaces and their hands should be gloved or cleaned and disinfected. Single-use FOBs should be treated with the same level of care to avoid contamination of the device before introduction to the patient's airway. Once used the reusable FOB should be cleaned, paying particular attention to irrigation of the working channel with sterile saline, and returned to the SSD for high level

decontamination. Failure to do this promptly will encourage contamination and blockages from drying debris especially in the working channel. A sterile FOB is assumed to retain its sterility for 4 hours except when it is stored in special dedicated cabinets: this recommendation of 4 hours is one of convenience and not based on any evidence. Research shows that endoscopes can be stored for 7 days if they have been effectively reprocessed and appropriately stored.

In a life-threatening situation, when it is in the best interest of the patient, the medical team may use a device that is not decontaminated to the usual level. Such events should be documented, and after appropriate multidisciplinary consultation efforts should be made to mitigate the consequences of any potential infection.

Tracking Equipment Use

Reusable equipment should be tracked through the decontamination processes.

- Each device should have a unique identifier.
- As part of the reprocessing cycle, processed equipment should be labelled
  - indicating that it has been appropriately cleaned
  - identifying details of reprocessing (machine, cycle, date).
- A record of this is kept at the decontamination location.
- When the device is used, this information is entered into the patient record.

Should there be problems with a sterilising process or device, or a patient is identified as having a transmissible infection, it is then possible to track the device's decontamination history and to identify any other patients exposed to risk.

Further Reading

Association of Anaesthetists. (2020). *Guidelines. Infection prevention and control 2020*. Available at: https://anaesthe tists.org/Home/Resources-publications/Guidelines/Infectio n-prevention-and-control-2020.

Department of Health and Social Care. (2013). *Management and decontamination of flexible endoscopes (HTM 01–06)*. Available at: https://www.gov.uk/government/publications/ management-and-decontamination-of-flexible-endoscopes.

Department of Health and Social Care. (2016). *Decontamination of surgical instruments (HTM 01–01)*. Available at: https://www.gov.uk/government/publications/ management-and-decontamination-of-surgical-instruments-used-in-acute-care.

McCahon RA, Whynes DK. (2015). Cost comparison of re-usable and single-use fibrescopes in a large English teaching hospital. *Anaesthesia*, **70**, 699–706.

McGrath BA, Ruane S, McKenna J, Thomas S. (2017). Contamination of single-use bronchoscopes in critically ill patients. *Anaesthesia*, **72**, 36–41.

Medicines and Healthcare products Regulatory Agency. (2010). *Sterilization, disinfection and cleaning of medical equipment: guidance on decontamination from the Microbiology Advisory Committee (the MAC manual)*. London. p. 14.

Medicines and Healthcare products Regulatory Agency. (2011). *Medical Device Alert*. MDA/2011/096. Crown Copyright. https://mhra-gov.filecamp.com/s/ywDEZLgX0 nEPtNCx/fo/3gd4DFg85VgXQoG9/fi/f22KmJZol3Qswky0

Office of Disease Prevention and Health Promotion. (2013). *National Action Plan to Prevent Health Care Associated Infections: Road Map to Elimination*. Available at: http://th econversation.com/heres-how-many-people-get-infections -in-australian-hospitals-every-year-82309.

Airway Management in a Respiratory Epidemic or Pandemic

Tim Cook and Massimiliano Sorbello

Epidemic and Pandemic Infection

This chapter is written during the 2019–20 coronavirus pandemic. It is a period of dramatic change and learning. We have attempted to write a chapter that is accurate but the fast-moving evidence means that there may be changes between our writing and publication. While the chapter focuses on coronavirus disease 2019 (COVID-19) the principles can be broadly applied to any contagious respiratory pathogen.

On the last day of 2019, the World Health Organization (WHO) was informed by the Chinese authorities of an unexplained cluster of pneumonias in Wuhan in the Hubei province. Over the coming months this cluster grew to an epidemic in China – affecting more than 80,000 patients, and then to a pandemic (declared by WHO on 11 March 2020) affecting all countries and at the time of writing (early April 2020) affecting more than 1.9 million patients and more than 100,000 deaths. It is likely that the worst is yet to come and that numbers may increase many-fold before we see beyond the pandemic.

The illness, due to a coronavirus (of the common cold variety) called SARS-CoV-2, causes a predominantly respiratory illness: COVID-19. In the vast majority of patients, it is a mild, or even unnoticed illness. Indeed, it is so mild that its epidemiology is hard to study because it is impossible to determine how many people have had the illness simply by symptoms. Population studies exploring antibody presence will in due course determine that but at present there is uncertainty.

The virus is very infectious and for each patient with the disease the infectivity rate (i.e. the number of patients each individual will infect without counter measures, termed R_0) is 2.5–3. For comparison, the R_0 of influenza is around 1.3 and of Ebola 2.0. Because of its geometric progression, after 10 cycles of infection, perhaps in one month, a single patient with influenza would have infected 14 others, while COVID-19 would have spread to 59,000 patients. It is this potential for spread and the high fatality rate that accounts for its devastation.

Controlling the illness is about containment – to reduce R_0. If this can be reduced to below 1 the epidemic will eventually peter out. Outside hospitals this relies on restricting physical contact and many countries have been placed in lockdown for several months. Within hospitals, containment is intended to prevent cross-infection from infected patients to staff (or vice versa) or other patients.

Current best estimates are that 30–80% of the population will contract the virus – there is no preexisting immunity. The fatality rate depends on which denominator is used – the number of infections, or the number of detected cases. Overall, it is likely that the overall infection fatality rate is approximately 1%. By comparison for influenza it is between 0.1% and 0.01%. The disease severity is summarised in Figure 38.1.

COVID-19 causes a severe viral pneumonia in a significant number of patients. In the early stages this may be associated with pulmonary microthrombotic disease. Typically, 7–10 days into the illness this can progress to severe acute respiratory syndrome typically with hypoxaemia without hypercapnia. While some patients can be managed with continuous positive airway pressure (or high flow nasal oxygen (HFNO)) the failure rates are high and tracheal intubation for controlled ventilation in intensive care is often required. Myocardial and renal failure and thrombotic complications may also occur but the predominant illness is respiratory. Treatment is currently supportive, although multiple therapeutic interventions are being explored. Mortality in those requiring ventilation is approximately 50%.

Mortality will vary by country, affected by overall healthcare structure and by the dynamic preparation that was possible before the epidemic surge hit, to both slow down spread within that country and to expand hospital and critical care services. Risk factors for mortality include increasing age (rising from the mid-50s), non-white ethnicity and those with cardio-vascular or respiratory disease, hypertension, diabetes, immunosuppression or cancer. Obesity is also prominent in some series.

Airway management is primarily required for the initiation of ventilation. However, during and after the peak of the epidemic patients with mild disease, but with unrelated conditions, may present for surgical care and it may be impossible to determine who does or does not have the infection.

Viral Transmission, Infection Control and Personal Protective Equipment

Viral Transmission

Airway management during a respiratory epidemic requires clear understanding of infection control measures. This understanding is fundamental to preventing cross-infection but also impacts on the planning, ease and speed of airway management and so affects patient and staff safety.

Spread of a respiratory illness may occur by three routes: contact, droplet or airborne (Figure 38.2). During a respiratory illness coughing and sneezing cause forceful expulsion of particles from the respiratory tract. In general terms particles of > 5 μm (but as large as 2000 μm) are subject to gravitational forces and fall near to the patient – mostly within 1 m, but perhaps up to 2 m away. If another person is close by these droplets may enter their respiratory tract via their mucosa. The particles settle on whatever surface they first meet and can remain there and be viable for many hours or even several days, becoming fomites. Anyone touching those surfaces may become contaminated with the virus. Droplets may account for well above 99% of the particulate volume of a cough or sneeze. Coughing and sneezing also produce an aerosol of smaller particles (< 5 μm) which may spread much further – up to 6 or 7 m – and may also remain in the air for a longer period of time. These small particles, if inhaled, may reach the alveoli. Certain medical procedures – including almost all aspects of

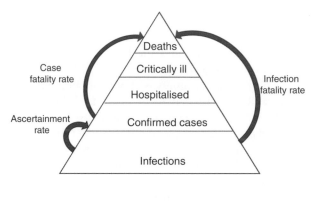

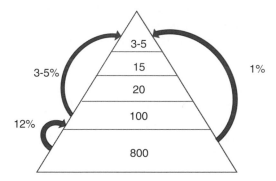

Figure 38.1 The epidemiology of coronavirus disease 2019. The upper figure explains the terms used in describing infections, cases, deaths etc. and the ascertainment, case fatality and infection fatality rates. The lower figure gives an estimate of the likely numbers when 100 cases are identified in a community.

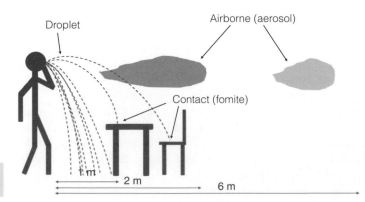

Figure 38.2 Modes of viral transmission for respiratory pathogens.

Table 38.1 Aerosol generating (medical) procedures. The numbers in brackets indicate the rank order of decreasing risk for the top four procedures as reported by Tran et al. (2012)

Respiratory aerosols

Tracheal intubation, extubation (1)
Non-invasive ventilation (2)
Tracheostomy and front of neck airway (3)
Face mask ventilation (4)
Positive pressure ventilation of the airway (irrespective of mode) if the airway is not sealed
Open tracheal suctioning
Bronchoscopy and bronchoalveolar lavage
Induction of sputum
High flow nasal oxygen
Dental drilling procedures
Chest compressions and/or cardiopulmonary resuscitation*
Supraglottic airway insertion and removal**

Blood or tissue fluid aerosols

Surgical procedures using high-speed devices (e.g. drilling, pulse lavage, sternotomy)

---

* Chest compression is not considered by all organisations to be an aerosol generating procedure but the international consensus is that it is.
** Supraglottic airway insertion and removal is assumed but not proven to be an aerosol generating procedure.

---

airway management may also create respiratory aerosols – especially when the airway is at positive pressure and gas leaks from it. Aerosol generation and infectivity is complicated – aerosols may or may not contain viable virus and whether they do will depend on the stage of the illness, the location in the respiratory tract they were generated from and other factors including the type of mucus secreted and the extent to which that particular patient secretes the virus, which is not readily predictable from the severity of symptoms.

For SARS-CoV-2 spread is thought to be predominantly via droplet and contact transmission.

If another individual or healthcare worker is > 2 m away from a patient the risk of droplet transmission of infection is very low. Aerosol generating procedures (AGPs) are listed in Table 38.1 'The list is pragmatic and better evidence is needed to understand AGPs and risk better.'

Infection Prevention, Control and Personal Protective Equipment

There is a natural focus amongst staff on the equipment component of PPE but other aspects of infection control are equally important. PPE is only one part of a system to prevent contamination of those working near patients with COVID-19. The illness represents a risk to those staff, other staff and patients.

Other elements of a system to reduce cross-infection include:

- Preventing patients, visitors or staff who have or have been exposed to COVID-19 entering hospitals without reason
- Meticulous hand-washing and personal hygiene
- Managing patients with known or suspected COVID-19 separately from those without it, through a cohort or isolation
- Definition of clear personnel/patient pathways
- Restricting staff and visitors in the location of patients with COVID-19 to only those needed
- Wearing of a surgical face mask by suspected or infected patients
- At least twice daily cleaning and decontamination of surfaces and equipment
- Minimising unnecessary patient and surface contact during patient care
- Best practice in donning, doffing and disposal of PPE
- Prompt disposal of single-use equipment after use
- Decontamination of reusable equipment according to manufacturer's instructions
- Appropriate waste management

Numerous non-governmental organisations have made recommendations about PPE and all are generally in agreement with each other. It is logical to match the PPE used to the mode and risk of viral transmission. This approach is summarised in Table 38.2.

Wearing a fluid resistant face mask may protect both the wearer and those around from viral particle dispersal and so may be added to contact precautions. Where there is increased risk of aerosol exposure – e.g. if viral spread is considered airborne or during AGPs – a fitted face piece mask should be worn – variously designated as FFP2/N95/FFP3 depending on their ability to filter 0.3 μm particles (respectively >94%/95%/99%). These need to be checked for seal ('fit tested') before the user is signed off to use a specific design and then fit checked (i.e. confirming a good seal), before each use.

When a viral aerosol has been created, sufficient time should be left for viral clearance before the room is cleared. This *aerosol clearance time* is dependent

323

Table 38.2 Personal protective equipment: matching use to the mode of viral transmission and relevant locations. Levels of protection are incremental: droplet precautions are also designed to prevent contact transmission; airborne precautions also to prevent droplet and contact transmission. A fluid resistant surgical face mask may be added in non-clinical and contact zones if prevalence of disease is high

Precaution	When to use in a patient being treated as COVID-19 positive	What is it?
Non-clinical areas	No additional risk	Standard infection control precautions
Contact precautions	> 2 m away from patient	Gloves Apron
Droplet precautions	Within 2 m of patient	Gloves Apron Fluid resistant surgical mask +/− Eye protection* (risk assess) Patient to wear fluid resistant surgical mask
Airborne precaution**	Aerosol generating procedure	Gloves Fluid repellent long sleeved gown Eye protection* FFP3 mask A powered air purifying respirator suit is an alternative

* Eye protection may be goggles or a visor. Personal spectacles are insufficient.

** In areas where aerosol generating procedures are undertaken regularly airborne precautions may be worn on a sessional basis: a plastic apron is added over the gown and this and the gloves are changed between patients.

Adapted from Cook TM, *Anaesthesia* 2020, with permission.

In some healthcare settings and during epidemic surge, surgical face masks may be worn throughout the facility.

more on room ventilation than whether a room is positively or negatively pressured, which simply affects where the virus goes. Approximately two thirds of all virus is cleared by one 'air exchange' so after two air exchanges approximately 15% of the viral aerosol remains and after five <1%. In a typical hospital there may be 6 air exchanges per hour on a ward and >20 in an operating theatre.

Airway Management

Intubation for Initiating Critical Care

The commonest cause for airway management in a respiratory epidemic is for establishing ventilation of the lungs at the start of intensive care management. The patients are not intrinsically anatomically difficult (though some may be) but there is physiological difficulty (as with any critically ill patient) and extreme logistical difficulty, due to the need to perform procedures wearing PPE and the importance of avoiding self-contamination.

The basic principles of airway management are the same as for any critically ill patient (see Chapter 28) and only important differences are described here. Throughout the procedure the aim should be to be:

safe for the patient and staff

accurate in terms of using techniques which are proven to work in easy and difficult settings and which are familiar. Aim to succeed at the first attempt because multiple attempts increase risk to sick patients and staff. Do not rush but make each attempt the best it can be.

swift by achieving first-attempt success and managing the airway promptly

- Tracheal intubation of the critically ill COVID-19 patient is a high-risk procedure for the patient (desaturation, rapid deterioration, haemodynamic collapse) and the team (contamination risk, psychological pressure and human factors) so intubation of any COVID-19 patient should be performed in as close to elective conditions as possible, including anticipation of the decision to intubate.

- Safe airway management in this setting is reliant on institutional preparation (i.e. provision of sufficient numbers of appropriately trained staff; equipment for routine and difficult airway management; availability of tracheal intubation checklists; PPE etc.). This must be in place well before airway management occurs.
- Personal preparation is equally important – being appropriately trained and aware of the specifics of local practices and standard operating procedures.
- Airborne precaution PPE should be used for intubation. Everyone involved should be trained and practised in its use before being involved. Double gloving is recommended to reduce fomite contamination. Note that goggles and visors may be prone to fogging and anti-fogging treatment may be needed.
- Airway management should take place in a well-ventilated room, ideally a negatively pressurised side room with > 12 air changes per hour where possible.
- A dedicated tracheal intubation trolley or pack is needed that can be taken to the intubation location, which may be ICU, the emergency department or the ward.
- The number of staff involved should be limited. Some guidelines recommend only two (the intubator and an assistant), others three and some four. The roles of airway management, administering drugs, monitoring the patient, managing difficulty and complications all need to be achieved by the intubating team and two may be too few to do this. Some recommend a backup clinician in airborne precaution PPE stays outside the room ready to enter if needed. The number of staff in the intubating team may vary according to local arrangements and staff availability during the peak of an epidemic.
- The best-skilled airway manager present should manage the airway to maximise first-pass success.
- Full preparations of equipment (first line and backup) should be undertaken outside the room. Single-use equipment is favoured except where it is considered that reusable equipment would be more suited to the principles of safe, accurate and swift airway care.
- The team should undertake a full briefing, defining all individuals' roles and primary and backup plans before entering the room. Use a checklist for this – examples are shown in Figure 38.3 and 38.4.
- Communication when wearing airborne precaution PPE is very difficult. This needs planning before entering the room.
- Cognitive aids such as an airway kit dump, a checklist, an algorithm for use in the event of difficulty are recommended to avoid cognitive overload and improve communication. These should be understood before starting and present in the intubation room for use.
- Take the algorithm or cognitive aid you plan to use into the room or display it there.
- Touch as little as possible in the room to avoid fomites.
- The procedure should be fully explained to the patient.
- Full monitoring, including continuous waveform capnography, should be used before, during and after tracheal intubation.
- Airway assessment is likely to be limited but may include a MACOCHA score (see Chapter 28) and identification of the cricothyroid membrane.
- All airway devices should have a viral filter or a heat and moisture exchanger (HME) filter placed close to the patient before use.
- Pre-oxygenation should be thorough. Techniques that increase positive pressure in the airway (mask continuous positive airway pressure (CPAP), non-invasive ventilation) or aerosol generation (starting HFNO) should be avoided. Simple mask pre-oxygenation with a Mapleson C ('Waters') circuit is likely ideal.
- Low flow nasal oxygen is not considered an AGP and may provide useful apnoeic oxygenation.
- Induction should include a hypnotic (ketamine 1–2 mg kg^{-1} or etomidate 0.2–0.3 mg kg^{-1} are favoured in different countries, especially in cases with haemodynamic instability) and a rapidly acting muscle relaxant (rocuronium 1.2–1.5 mg kg^{-1} is favoured by many, suxamethonium 1–2 mg kg^{-1} is acceptable but has the disadvantage that it may wear off too soon). Vasopressors should be immediately available for managing hypotension. In order to prevent

Emergency tracheal intubation checklist
COVID-19

Personal Protective Equipment	Prepare Equipment	Prepare for Difficulty	In the Room	Post-procedure and Safety

OUTSIDE ROOM

PPE – be thorough, don't rush
- Wash hands
- Buddy with checklist
- Put on PPE
  - Long sleeved gown
  - FFP3 (or equivalent) mask
  - Gloves
  - Eyewear
  - Headwear and wipeable shoes as per local protocol
- Final buddy check
- Names on visors

Allocate roles:
A: Team leader and intubator
B: Cricoid force and intubator's assistant
C: Drugs, monitor, timer
D: Runner (outside)
Decide who will do eFONA

How does runner contact further help if required?

Check kit (kit dump)
- Mapleson C with HMEF attached (preferred to BVM)
- Catheter mount
- Guedel airways
- Working suction
- Videolaryngoscope
- Bougie/stylet
- Tracheal tubes x2
- Ties and syringe
- In-line suction ready
- Tube clamp
- 2nd generation SGA
- eFONA set available

Do you have all the drugs required?
- Ketamine (or other)
- Muscle relaxant
- Vasopressor/inotrope
- Maintenance sedation

Weight?

Allergies?

If the airway is difficult, could we wake the patient up?

VERBALISE the plan for a difficult intubation?
Plan A: RSI
Plan B/C: 2-person mask ventilation & 2nd generation SGA

2nd generation supraglottic airway

Facemask
- 2-person
- Adjuncts
- Low flow
- Low pressure

Plan D: Front of neck airway: scalpel bougie tube

Confirm agreed plan

Does anyone have any concerns?

INSIDE ROOM

- Airway assessment
  - MACOCHA
  - Identify cricothyroid membrane
- Apply monitors
  - Waveform capnography
  - SpO_2
  - ECG
  - Blood pressure
- Checked i.v. access (x2)
- Optimise position
  - Consider ramping or reverse Trendelenburg
  - Firm mattress
- Optimal pre-oxygenation
  - ≥ 3 min or $ETO_2 > 85\%$ (No NIV, no HFNO)
- Optimise patient condition before tracheal intubation
  - Fluid/vasopressor/ inotrope
  - Aspirate nasogastric tube
  - Delayed sequence induction?
- Now proceed

AFTER AND LEAVING

- Airway management
  - Inflate cuff before any ventilating
  - Check waveform capnography
  - Push/twist connections
  - Clamp tracheal tube before any disconnection
  - Avoid unnecessary disconnections
- Other
  - Insert nasogastric tube
  - Consider deep tracheal viral sample
- Careful equipment disposal
- Decontamination of reusable equipment
- Complete and display intubation form
- Remove PPE
  - Observed by buddy
  - Use checklist
  - Meticulous disposal
  - Wash hands
- Clean room after 20 minutes

Figure 38.3 Emergency tracheal intubation checklist for COVID-19. (Adapted from Cook TM et al., *Anaesthesia* 2020, with permission.)

AIRWAY MANAGEMENT
Rev. 1.1

One of the most critical issues regarding 2019 nCoV patients is the transitory phase between initial symptoms and potentially severe evolution requiring critical care, while taking into account the comorbidities. The choice of supplementary oxygen delivery interface and the decision to provide invasive ventilatory support is crucial.

These decisions have the potential of impacting outcome and may lead to consequences on saturation of critical care beds. Non-invasive support methods (CPAP, BiPAP, NIV, HFNO) might correct hypoxemia and counterbalance respiratory failure though univocal data are missing and may either delay or avoid endotracheal intubation (with potential complications and effects on outcome). Nevertheless, data from the SARS epidemic provide evidence showing that these ventilatory techniques might favor the risk of airborne viral spreading. Given the nature of nCoV 19 in terms of contagiousness, should the patient require, or be expected to necessitate invasive ventilator support, an elective endotracheal intubation should be preferred, or even anticipated, rather than waiting for an emergency procedure (in the precipitating patient) as to minimize complications of intubation itself and also to reduce both the risks of procedural errors and the contamination of healthcare providers.

Adoption of early warning scores (EWS), shared and predefined strategies, multidisciplinary team training and simulation of possible scenarios are highly recommended, taking also into account the available levels of care and feasibility of critical care settings and of assistance in a non-ICU environment. The decisional elements for airway management, oxygenation and invasive ventilator support thus include competencies and organization and available human and environmental resources.

Vigilance in prevention, strict adhesion of donning/doffing of PPE, preparedness for the care of infected patients remain priority and of utmost importance.

HIGHLIGHTS
▸ INTEGRATED COMPETENCIES FOR EVERY PHASE/STEP
▸ AIRBORNE PROTECTION FOR EVERY EVERY PHASE/STEP IN CRITICAL CARE SETTINGS (IF POSSIBLE)
▸ ANTICIPATE NEEDS, MAXIMIZE FIRST-PASS SUCCESS

DOUBLE-CHECK INDICATIONS FOR ENDOTRACHEAL INTUBATION
▸ Adopt Early Warning Scores for intubation/quoad vitam prognosis (consider DNR cases)
▸ Identify Isolated room/(negative pressure environment if possible)
▸ Balance benefit of CPAP/BiPAP/NIV/HFNO versus risks of airborne diffusion
▸ IF INTUBATION s required, prefer ELECTIVE procedure (in emergency >> patient risk)

TEAM PREPARATION
▸ Minimize the number of team members:
1. The most expert team member should perform the intubation and advanced airway control/ventilation (with donned PPE) [INSIDE the chamber]
2. EXPERT assistant on protocols and devices (doctor/nurse with donned PPE) [INSIDE the chamber]
3. Second doctor with donned PPE if complex maneuver/difficult airway is expected/planned [INSIDE the chamber]
4. PPE available with donned PPE [OUTSIDE the chamber]
5. Donning/doffing Observer [OUTSIDE]

CARRY OUT PRELIMINARY BRIEFING FOR ROLE DEFINITION, STRATEGY DEFINITION, IDENTIFICATION OF DONNING/DOFFING OBSERVER

PPE DONNING
▸ Second level PPE (recommended for airway management including aerosol-generating procedures i.e. bronchoscopy, awake endotracheal intubation) hair cover s/hoods, FFP2/N95 mask, goggles or face shield, long sleeve fluid-resistant gown, double gloves, overshoes
▸ Third level PPE (suggested for selected cases of aerosol-generating procedures) Helmet, FFP3 mask, face shield, goggles, long sleeve fluid-resistant gown, double gloves, overshoes

DONNING/DOFFING OBSERVER EXTERNALLY CHECKING, INDIVIDUAL DONNING

CLINICAL CHECKLIST (wearing PPE)
▸ COMPLETE EVALUATION OF AIRWAYS AND OXYGENATION (accept difficult airway management risk overestimation)
▸ HEMODYNAMIC EVALUATION ▸ PRE-EMPTIVE HEMODYNAMIC OPTIMIZATION

AIRWAY INSTRUMENTATION
▸ HEPA FILTER on EVERY OXYGENATION INTERFACE (face mask, circuit, endotracheal tube, supraglottic airway devices, introducer, airway exchange catheters, respiratory circuit)
▸ AIRWAY CART READY (DISPOSABLE devices preferable)
▸ SUCTION: CLOSED SYSTEM
▸ ANTIFOGGING
▸ MEDICATIONS: PREPARED AND DOUBLE-CHECKED
▸ EMERGENCY CART READY (DISPOSABLE devices preferable)

AWAKE INTUBATION NOT INDICATED:
▸ PREOXYGENATION (according to respiratory and hemodynamic status)
• 3min' at TV FIO_2=100%
or 1min' at FVC 8 breaths FIO_2=100%
or CPAP/PSV 10 cmH_2O + PEEP 5 cmH_2O FIO_2=100%
▸ RSI in all patients (limit BMV unless unavoidable and apply Cricoid Pressure only in case of ongoing regurgitation)
▸ NASAL PRONGS 1-3 l/min FIO_2=100% FOR APNOIC PHASE (NODESAT)
▸ FULL DOSE NEUROMUSCULAR BLOCK RESPECT onset time for laryngoscopy
▸ 1° LARYNGOSCOPY: prefer VIDEOLARYNGOSCOPE with separate screen + endotracheal tube pre-loaded on introducer
Re-oxygenate with low TV/pressure between attempts -Early switch (after failed second attempt) to supraglottic airway devices (prefer second generation - intubable SADs)
> INTUBATION THROUGH SUPRAGLOTTIC AIRWAY DEVICES: flexible endoscope with separate screen (prefer DISPOSABLE)
▸ EARLY CRICOTHYROTOMY IF CI-CO

AWAKE INTUBATION INDICATED (only if really mandatory):
▸ AIRWAY TOPICALIZATION: no aerosol/vaporization
▸ TITRATED SEDATION (INFUSION PUMP) - sedation depth monitoring
▸ FLEXIBLE ENDOSCOPE WITH SEPARATE SCREEN (PREFER DISPOSABLE)
▸ RESCUE: INTUBATION THROUGH SUPRAGLOTTIC AIRWAY DEVICES (see above)
▸ EARLY CRICOTHYROTOMY if CI-CO

TUBE POSITION CONTROL - PROTECTIVE VENTILATION
▸ CAPNOGRAFIC CURVES repeated and with standard morphology (if in doubt take it out)
▸ AVOID unuseful circuit disconnections (if needed: ventilator on stand-by/clamp endotracheal tube)
▸ CONSIDER indications for advanced techniques: ECMO - experts advise

PPE DOFFING
▸ During and after PPE doffing, hands hygiene mandatory
▸ Donning/doffing observer externally checking, individual doffing
▸ Waste disposal

TRANSPORT
▸ Follow bio-containment regulations

S - Secure airway: anticipated intubation
T - Team briefing
O - Organize (competencies - team - pathways)
P - Prepare (devices)
C - Checklist - controls- crisis management
O - Optimize (hemodynamics - oxygenation)
V - Vigilated donning/doffing
I - Invasive airways - evaluation and integrated airway management
D - Debriefing

SIAARTI — PRO VITA CONTRA DOLOREM SEMPER

M. Sorbello, I. Di Giacinto, F. Bressan, R. Cataldo, G. Cortese, C. Esposito, S. Falcetta, G. Merli, F. Petrini on behalf of SIAARTI Airway Management Research Group

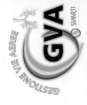

COVID-19

GESTIONE VIE AEREE — GVA — SIAARTI

Reference

Figure 38.4 Airway management checklist. (Sorbello M et al. SIAARTI Airway Management Research Group, with permission from SIAARTI http://www.siaarti.it/SiteAssets/News/COVID19%20-%20documenti%20SIAARTI/SIAARTI%20-%20Covid-19%20-%20Airway%20Management%20rev.1.2.pdf)

coughing and increased risk to medical staff aim to give the muscle relaxant early and in full dose. It may be prudent to warn the patient that they may feel weak before they are unconscious. Wait for full neuromuscular blockade before attempting tracheal intubation – likely 60–90 seconds.

- After induction of anaesthesia, avoid face mask ventilation unless needed. If it is needed use a low flow, low pressure technique as described below.

- Intubate as normal and pass the cuff 1–2 cm below the cords to avoid bronchial placement. As auscultation may be difficult when wearing PPE and stethoscopes are a fomite source, they are best avoided. If there is doubt lung ultrasound or chest X-ray may be needed later.

- Seal the airway by inflating the tracheal tube cuff and then attach to the ventilator. Avoid circuit disconnection and push twist all connections.

- Confirm tracheal intubation with continuous waveform capnography, noting that this is present even during cardiac arrest.

- During intubation aim to communicate with simple instructions and closed-loop communication (e.g. repeating instructions back).

- After intubation it may be timely to place a nasogastric tube and if COVID-19 status has not already been confirmed to use closed tracheal suction to take a deep tracheal aspirate for virology.

- If there is difficulty during tracheal intubation, use a standard failed tracheal intubation algorithm with a cognitive aid. Simple reliable techniques and avoiding pressurising the airway are both strongly favoured. Early insertion of a second generation supraglottic airway (SGA) may be favoured over mask ventilation. Intubation though an SGA may not be considered a suitable technique. The threshold for transitioning to emergency front of neck airway may be lower and when this is performed the scalpel-bougie technique is likely to be favoured over cannula techniques and high-pressure source ventilation.

- Cleaning the room and decontaminating equipment is essential. Discard disposable equipment and decontaminate reusable equipment according to manufacturer's instructions. Doffing of PPE after leaving should be meticulous and evidence suggests that having a 'buddy' verbalise instructions reduces errors. After a suitable aerosol clearance time the room should be cleaned – usually about 20 minutes after the last AGP was performed.

- Place a prominently visible 'intubation record' in the patient's room so it can be referred to if an airway emergency arises. Where there was airway difficulty this intubation record should be supported by a patient-specific airway plan which is displayed in the room and communicated between shifts.

Airway techniques

In choosing techniques that are likely to be reliable, several national bodies have recommended:

- Rapid sequence induction with cricoid force where a trained assistant can apply it. Take it off if it causes difficulty.

- Videolaryngoscopy for tracheal intubation

- Two-person, two-handed mask ventilation with a VE-grip to improve seal (see Chapter 12)

- A second generation SGA for airway rescue, also to improve seal

Simulation of techniques before use is likely to be of benefit. This applies to donning and doffing of PPE and to intubation while wearing it. Staff who are at increased risk of COVID-19 or of developing more severe disease should be allowed to refrain from airway management where practical. Some have also recommended shielding of staff with cancer, who are immunosuppressed or pregnant.

Managing the known or predicted difficult airway is challenging. Awake techniques are likely to be associated with significant coughing and aerosol generation. Patient reassurance may be difficult. Awake techniques can be used but require skill, patience and meticulous attention to detail to minimise aerosol generation. Prudent sedation should be considered. There may also be a lowered threshold to undertaking techniques after general anaesthesia – supported by skilled operators and a very clear strategy regarding what steps will be taken if initial plans fail.

Airway management after intubation is focussed on avoiding accidental breathing circuit disconnections, accidental extubations and minimising AGPs. This impacts on choices for circuit humidification, use of closed suctioning, modes of ventilation and sedation, careful planning of sedation pauses, physiotherapy and patient movement (including proning).

Extubation after Critical Illness

Extubation is particularly challenging. In most ICUs, extubation is followed by a period of time on HFNO or CPAP and despite this approximately 10% of patients may require reintubation within 24 hours.

Extubation itself may be challenging and is a relatively high-risk AGP. It is unknown whether use of anaesthetic drugs to reduce coughing at extubation such as opioids, lidocaine or dexmedetomidine have a role here. Staff should don airborne PPE in preparation for extubation. Extubation should be carefully planned, preceded by physiotherapy, closed tracheal suction and pre-oxygenation. The HME filter should remain on the tracheal tube throughout extubation. During or immediately after extubation a surgical face mask should be applied to the patient's face. A technique for 'droplet-free extubation' has been described at www.airwaymanagement.dk/extubation. As HFNO may not be considered suitable after extubation provision should be made to facilitate prompt reintubation at any time.

The timing of extubation in the course of recovery from COVID-19 remains controversial. This is also true for the role of tracheostomy. As more severe cases of COVID-19 are associated with more prolonged secretion of virus and higher titres, both extubation and tracheostomy may be delayed. If tracheostomy is performed the same meticulous planning, focussed on expert airway management and safety for the patient and staff, is required. Anaesthetic and operator communication must be clear, particularly regarding the point at which the anaesthetist hands over responsibility for the airway to the operator. Standard techniques may be modified to reduce aerosol generation when the trachea is opened: there is emphasis on full muscle relaxation and passing the tracheal tube further down the trachea until the point of exchange to the tracheostomy at which time lung ventilation may be paused until the tracheostomy is in place.

Novel Techniques

In a pandemic situation there is considerable innovation. For example, in the COVID-19 epidemic there have been numerous suggestions for intubating boxes or intubating and extubating under plastic sheets. Innovation is often tempting, but safety often rests in performing well-established and well-practised techniques simply, accurately and swiftly. Innovation may add complexity, unintended consequences and unexpected risk. Innovative techniques, even in a pandemic, require evaluation to ensure safety, efficacy and avoidance of complications for both the patient and the intubating team.

There may also be a temptation to use techniques which the operator is not practised in. The above principles apply. A high-risk situation is rarely, if ever, a time to try untested and unfamiliar techniques for the first time.

Do not use techniques you have not used before or are not trained in. Again, for the reasons stated above, this is not a time to test new techniques.

Airway Management during Cardiac Arrest

Whenever a critically ill patient is anaesthetised and intubated there is a risk of cardiac arrest. The same patients may also experience cardiac arrest due to their illness. Although controversial, there is general international consensus that chest compression is an AGP. Some also consider defibrillation to be an AGP, but this is less certain.

The UK Resuscitation Council recommends that defibrillation may be undertaken prior to donning PPE. Airborne precaution PPE should be donned before starting chest compression-only CPR. Mouth-to-mouth ventilation should not be undertaken. Airway management, two-person mask ventilation, SGA insertion or tracheal intubation should be undertaken only by those trained and skilled in the procedure. Resuscitation efforts should be followed by careful disposal of single-use equipment, decontamination of reusable equipment and careful doffing and disposal of PPE.

Airway Management for Anaesthesia

During an epidemic some patients with or without the illness will present for incidental surgery or for surgery related to complications of the disease. Elective procedures should be minimised and carefully isolated. As the epidemic proceeds, it may become increasingly difficult to determine who may or may not have the infection and at some point, all patients will be treated as if they do. The principles described above apply equally in this setting. Safe airway management requires preparation, communication, correct use of PPE, skilled use of reliable techniques and decontamination, doffing and disposal after the procedure.

The airway management techniques employed likely differ little from normal settings. Use of face mask ventilation is avoided whenever possible. The threshold for use of an SGA over face mask ventilation may be lowered but also for tracheal intubation. Insertion and removal of an SGA may be considered an AGP but use during anaesthesia is not an AGP unless there is significant airway leak. Preventing a leak during use of an SGA may be minimised by appropriate consideration of the operation, patient, patient position, device, insertion technique, skill and experience of the airway manager and ventilation mode. Low pressure, controlled ventilation or spontaneous modes of ventilation will minimise airway leak. Tracheal extubation is associated with coughing at extubation and this may be mitigated by use of an SGA instead of tracheal intubation, exchange for an SGA at the end of surgery or use of medications as described above.

Protection of the anaesthetic machine and other equipment with dedicated covers should be considered, and waste disposal and room disinfection performed carefully after the procedure.

Summary

The fundamental principles of airway management in the setting of a respiratory epidemic are not changed from normal. However, it is essential to maximise safety of both the patient and all staff involved in caring for them. The airway manager should fully understand and apply principles of infection prevention and control, including matching PPE to the prevailing mode of viral transmission. Airway management should be meticulously planned, safe for the patient and staff, be undertaken by skilled operators using reliable, well-practised techniques and should aim to achieve high first-attempt success rates so that securing the airway is timely and swift.

Further Reading

Brewster DJ, Chrimes NC, Do TBT, et al. (2020). Consensus statement: Safe Airway Society principles of airway management and tracheal intubation specific to the COVID-19 adult patient group. *Medical Journal of Australia* (in press).

Cook TM. (2020). Personal protective equipment during the COVID-19 pandemic – a narrative review. *Anaesthesia*. doi:10.1111/anae.15071.

Cook TM, El-Boghdadly K, McGuire B, et al. (2020). Consensus guidelines for managing the airway in patients with COVID-19: Guidelines from the Difficult Airway Society, the Association of Anaesthetists, the Intensive Care Society, the Faculty of Intensive Care Medicine and the Royal College of Anaesthetists. *Anaesthesia*. doi:10.1111/anae.15054.

Gralton J, Tovey E, McLaws ML, Rawlinson WD. (2011). The role of particle size in aerosolised pathogen transmission: a review. *Journal of Infection*, **62**, 1–13.

Lockhart SL, Duggan LV, Wax RS, Saad S, Grocott HP. (2020). Personal protective equipment (PPE) for anesthesiologists and other airway managers: principles and practice during the COVID-19 pandemic. *Canadian Journal of Anaesthesia* (in press).

Meng L, Qiu H, Wan L, et al. (2020). Intubation and ventilation amid the COVID-19 outbreak: Wuhan's experience. *Anesthesiology*. doi:10.1097/ALN.0000000000003296. [Epub ahead of print]

Nicolle L (2003). SARS safety and science. *Canadian Journal of Anaesthesia*, **50**, 983–988.

Sorbello M, El-Boghdadly K, Di Giacinto I, et al. (2020). The Italian coronavirus disease 2019 outbreak: recommendations from clinical practice. *Anaesthesia*. doi:10.1111/anae.15049. [Epub ahead of print]

Tran K, Cimon K, Severn M, Pessoa-Silva CL, Conly J. (2012). Aerosol generating procedures and risk of transmission of acute respiratory infections to healthcare workers: a systematic review. *PLoS One*, 7, e35797.

van Doremalen N, Bushmaker T, Morris DH, et al. (2020). Aerosol and surface stability of SARS-CoV-2 as compared with SARS-CoV-1. *New England Journal of Medicine*, **382**, 1564–1567. doi:10.1056NEJMc2004973.

Yao W, Wang T, Jiang B, et al. (2020). Emergency tracheal intubation in 202 patients with COVID-19 in Wuhan, China: lessons learnt and international expert recommendations. *British Journal of Anaesthesia* (in press). doi:https://doi.org/10.1016/j.bja.2020.03.026.

Index